NURSING HOMES AND ASSISTED LIVING

NURSING HOMES
—— AND ——
ASSISTED LIVING

The Family's Guide to Making Decisions and Getting Good Care

—— SECOND EDITION ——

Peter S. Silin

The Johns Hopkins University Press
Baltimore

First edition published in 2001 as *Nursing Homes: The Family's Journey*

The Johns Hopkins University Press
2715 North Charles Street
Baltimore, Maryland 21218-4363
www.press.jhu.edu

Library of Congress Cataloging-in-Publication Data
Silin, Peter S., 1954–
Nursing homes and assisted living : the family's guide to making
decisions and getting good care / Peter S. Silin. — 2nd ed.
p.   cm.
Rev. ed. of: Nursing homes. 2001.
Includes bibliographical references and index.
ISBN-13: 978-0-8018-9351-3 (hardcover : alk. paper)
ISBN-10: 0-8018-9351-8 (hardcover : alk. paper)
ISBN-13: 978-0-8018-9352-0 (pbk. : alk. paper)
ISBN-10: 0-8018-9352-6 (pbk. : alk. paper)
1. Older people—Nursing home care. 2. Nursing home patients—
Family relationships. 3. Older people—Nursing home care—
Psychological aspects. 4. Older people—Nursing home care—Social
aspects. I. Silin, Peter S., 1954– Nursing homes. II. Title.
RC954.3.S556 2009
362.16—dc22   2008056008

A catalog record for this book is available from the British Library.

Special discounts are available for bulk purchases of this book.
For more information, please contact Special Sales at 410-516-6936 or
specialsales@press.jhu.edu.

The Johns Hopkins University Press uses environmentally friendly
book materials, including recycled text paper that is composed of at
least 30 percent post-consumer waste, whenever possible. All of our
book papers are acid-free, and our jackets and covers are printed on
paper with recycled content.

To my parents, Ann and Melvin Silin. I love you.
To Bobby G. Thanks for being my friend.

Decision

Do I go or do I stay?
Should I wait another day?
The house is so comfy, I love it quite clearly.
My things and my treasures I'm devoted to dearly.
My books and my paintings, my living room chairs,
My oversized bed and my tables in pairs.
So many memories over the years,
So many laughs, a sprinkling of tears.
It takes courage to leave all that good stuff behind me,
"But the fence needs replacing," my daughter reminds me.

While the leaves have been falling,
The gardener's been calling.
"No cleanup," he says. "There's an excess of rain."
I see in the window a storm-loosened pane.
The railing outside is shaky and loose.
Some shingles have fallen from off of the roof.
The basement's a mess, I'm developing stress
And I still can't decide: Is it no? Is it yes?

Is there room in the Village for a packrat like me?
I will make the decision responsibly.
I will visit Goodwill and make countless donations
Of what's gathering dust in forgotten old spaces.
I will sort, I will pack, and then do it some more.
I'll decide what I need and the rest I will store.

So do I go or do I stay?
I will not wait another day.

The decision's been made: Lasell it will be.
An exciting new home that will set me free.

Ruth Margolin-Silin

Contents

Preface   xiii

Acknowledgments   xv

PART I

CARING DECISIONS

CHAPTER 1

When Someone You Love Goes into Care   3

Becoming a Caregiver 3 • Becoming "the Family Member" of
Someone in Care 4 • Learning the Role of "the Family Member" 6
• Types and Levels of Care 7 • Other Considerations 14

Alastair   16

CHAPTER 2

Deciding about Care   19

How to Talk about Care 19 • Choosing the Right Time 26 • Stress
and Burnout 28 • When a Parent Chooses to Live at Risk 30
• Making the Decision 32 • Your Legal Right to Make Decisions for
Your Relative: A Warning 33 • Advance Directives and
Medical Decisions 35

Lydia Jean   40

CONTENTS

CHAPTER 3

Family Decision Making   42

Family Relationships and Care Decisions 42 • How to Make
Family Decisions 44 • Family Meetings 46 • Keep Your
Relative Involved 51

Mary   53

CHAPTER 4

Guilt, Loss, and Grief   58

What Is Guilt? 58 • Conflicts That Give Rise to Guilt 60
• Families and Guilt 61 • Adult Children 62 • Guilt, Culture,
and Society Today 64 • When Guilt Has Other Purposes in
Your Life 65 • Not All Relationships Were Ideal 66 • Guilt and
Dementia 68 • Dealing with Guilt 69 • Letting Go 74
• Grief and Loss 77 • Handling Grief 79

Marjorie   82

PART II

THE RESIDENCE

CHAPTER 5

About Nursing Homes and Assisted Living Facilities   87

Keeping Your Relative at Home 88 • Where to Start Finding a
Nursing Home or Assisted Living Facility 91 • Applying for Seniors
Housing 95 • About Good Care and Good Caring 96 • Models of
Care 98 • On Abuse 100 • Specialized Dementia Care Units 110
• Costs 111 • Nursing Homes and Legal Responsibility 119

Mildred   121

CHAPTER 6

Viewing the Residence   124

Staffing 126 • Programming 127 • Policies 129
• Dining 130 • Physical Plant 131
• Surveys and Accreditation 132

John and Joyce   133

CHAPTER 7

Staff Roles: Who Does What?   139

Receptionist 139 • Administrator 140 • Personal Care: Nurse's
Aides 141 • Nurses 143 • Dietitian and Food Services Staff
144 • Social Worker 145 • Recreation Therapists 145
• Rehabilitation Staff 147 • Housekeepers/Building Maintenance
Staff 148 • Pharmacist 149 • Physicians 149
• Other Staff Members 150

Mabel   152

CHAPTER 8

Nursing Home and Assisted Living Systems   155

How the System Works 157 • A Typical Day 158

Cyrus   161

PART III

MOVING IN AND SETTLING IN

CHAPTER 9

Preparations for Moving Day   167

How to Prepare Your Relative 167 • Get to Know the Home
in Advance 170 • Equipment 172 • Valuables 173 • Clothing
and Laundry 174 • Plan Ahead for Moving Day 176 • Plan to
Take Care of Yourself 178

Betty   180

CONTENTS

CHAPTER 10

Moving Day   182

Stay Calm 182 • If Your Relative Refuses to Go 183 • Walking through the Door 184 • When You First Arrive 185

Joan   188

CHAPTER 11

Settling In   192

Resident Adjustment 192 • Changes and Differences in Behavior 193 • Dementia and Behavior 200 • Sex and Relationships in Nursing Homes and Assisted Living 203 • On Staying Healthy 205 • Your Emotional Adjustment 207 • The Gap in Your Life 208 • Phases of Adjustment 210 • Acceptance 212 • New Relationships 213

Bill   215

PART IV

BEING THE FAMILY MEMBER OF SOMEONE IN CARE

CHAPTER 12

Care and Care Planning   221

Basic Standards of Care 221 • How Care Is Organized 222 • Care Conferences 224 • Charts 227 • Medication and Care Planning 228 • Medication and Pain Control 230 • Restraints 232 • Toileting and Incontinence 234 • Falls 236 • Pressure Sores 237 • Depression 238 • Alcohol, Drugs, and Other Addictions 238 • Roommates 241

Louise   244

CONTENTS

CHAPTER 13

Communication and Problem Solving   247

Working the System 247 • Communication 248 • Gaps in the System 251 • When Things Go Missing 251 • Your Role 252 • Making Complaints 254 • Throwing Bouquets 261

Alvin (part 1)   *263*

CHAPTER 14

Visiting   267

How Often to Visit 268 • Visiting Someone Who Has Dementia 270 • Going Out and Going Home 271 • Ending a Visit 273 • Companions 274 • A Few More Words about Sex 276

Jane   *277*

CHAPTER 15

Out-of-Town Caregivers   280

Professional Geriatric Care Managers 285

Lloyd   *286*

CHAPTER 16

Making a Home Better   289

Include the Resident in the Change 290 • Individual Actions 290 • Working with Other Families 292 • Working with the System 294 • Working with Government 300

Ann   *302*

CONTENTS

CHAPTER 17

Difficult Decisions at the End of Life   306

Living and Dying 306 • Talking about Death 307 • Facing
Feelings about Dying and Death 309 • Decisions about Dying and
Death 310 • Hospice and Palliative Care 313 • Younger People and
Death 314 • What Occurs during the Dying Process 315 • After
Death 316 • Saying Good-bye to the Home 317

Donald   319

Alvin (part 2)   325

APPENDIX 1

Accessing Care in Canada   327

APPENDIX 2

Questionnaires   333

APPENDIX 3

Some Common Medical Abbreviations   345

Resources   347

Index   357

Preface

This book began as a small project for a nursing home where I provided social work services from 1996 to 1999. I asked the family members in a support group I was facilitating to write stories about what they went through during the time their relatives were admitted to the home and how they coped afterward. I thought those stories would be helpful to family members of people who were just being admitted. Reading those stories, I thought, would be like having a hand to hold or a friend to talk to as they went through a difficult process.

As I began to gather the stories, I was also giving tours of the home for prospective residents and their families, and I worked with the husbands, wives, sons, daughters, and friends of current residents. I saw that each of those people had to learn how this is done. So I decided to write a short introduction to the booklet of stories the families were writing, which could give some practical information. The more carefully I listened to families, the more I realized how much information they needed. I also saw how complicated a task it is to be the family member of someone in care. The project grew from there.

This book was written by listening to family members like you. The stories are by caregivers who have been through what you are going through. For some, their relatives had been in care for only a short time when they wrote about their experiences; for others, it had been several years. Their voices (some disguised in part) are interspersed among the chapters.

In the sections I wrote, I have alternated pronouns, rather than always writing "your mother" or "father" or "wife" or "husband," "your relative," etc. All the information is meant for all of you, whether you are a spouse, partner, child, or sibling of someone going into care. If you are someone who is thinking about nursing homes or assisted living or seniors residences, this is also written for you.

The first edition focused primarily on nursing homes. In the years since I wrote that edition, the number of assisted living and other alternative residences for older people has exploded. The landscape may be more complicated, but no matter where they are going, people have to face the same issues: leaving their home, a future that can be scary, and declining health or capabilities. The change, grief, and loss apply, no matter what kind of housing option they choose. In this edition, I may talk about nursing homes, assisted living, or seniors residences when I am talking generally. To understand the differences, please read the section entitled "Types and Levels of Care" in chapter 1.

Acknowledgments

This book is the story of the hundreds of residents of seniors residences and their families with whom I have worked since 1980. Thank you.

Special thanks, too, to the family members who had the courage to share their stories with those who need them. You have given a wonderful and special gift.

I want to acknowledge the staff in the nursing homes and assisted living residences where I have worked, especially all those compassionate nurses and nurse's aides who have shown me what good care and caring look like.

Thanks also to Professor Lillian Wells, at the University of Toronto, who encouraged and supported me along the way.

Thanks to Peter Belson for his ongoing support and gracious gift of time and experience. Also to my many colleagues in the National Association of Professional Geriatric Care Managers. Among those especially were Martha L. Henderson, general nurse practitioner and faculty (retired), University of North Carolina at Chapel Hill; Rhoda Goldberg, of We Care Elder Services, Inc., in Sarasota, Florida; Elizabeth Bodie Gross, of Quality Health Unlimited in Barrington, Illinois; Dale Tushman, a counselor and geriatric care manager in Brunswick, Georgia; and Barbara Payne, of Elder Care Strategies in Ashburn, Virginia.

Thanks also to Wendy Harris, medical editor at the Johns Hopkins University Press, who encouraged me and took a chance on me.

PART I

CARING DECISIONS

CHAPTER 1

When Someone You Love Goes into Care

Becoming a Caregiver

If you are a caregiver reading this book, you may be preparing for a relative to enter a seniors residence. If you are looking down that road, you may be imagining the day when the person you are caring for finally walks through the door of the home. You may be anticipating (or already having) some fear, anxiety, or guilt. You may be hoping the day will never come. Or you may be feeling so exhausted from caregiving that you think the day can't come fast enough. Perhaps you are feeling a combination of all of these emotions.

You are in the middle of a process. It may have started only a few weeks ago when your husband had a stroke. Or you might look back over several years and remember when your wife began to forget things and do things out of character. Now you know this is due to Alzheimer disease, but back then these incidents gave you only a vague sense of discomfort. You may look even further back and remember the time you were walking down the street with your mother and noticed that she couldn't walk as fast as she used to. That was the first time you thought to yourself, "My mother is getting old," and you felt a little sad and protective.

During this process, which we could call "becoming a caregiver," you learned the ins and outs of having to take care of someone who is disabled. Even if the caregiver role came overnight, learning how to do it took some time. The longer you did it, the better at it you became. You learned whom to talk to, where to go for help, who was available. You learned how "the system" functioned. You also learned what to watch out for, what to do if certain events occurred, and how to plan for potential problems so they didn't occur, or so they didn't occur a second time. You developed some expertise in being a caregiver.

Becoming "the Family Member" of Someone in Care

A caregiver's process often leads to and entails another process—that of being and becoming "the family member" of someone in a nursing home or other seniors residence. It begins when you first realize that you have become a caregiver and wonder what will happen over time. It continues when you start telling yourself, "No, not yet, it isn't time." Then later, when it becomes more necessary, you visit several different residences. You talk with the doctor or your siblings or your friends about what to do. As the time draws closer and the name moves up a waiting list, you label clothes and read admission agreements. Finally, the telephone rings and a voice tells you that there is a room available—tomorrow.

If you are beginning this process, you need to know that learning your role as "the family member" will continue after you have turned around and gone home on that first day when your husband has moved. For some people it is easy, for some it is harder, but for all it is an adjustment. It doesn't happen in one day or one week or even one month. If you already have a relative in care, you know that this process can take months.

Your new role will bring about many changes in your life. Your relationship with your relative will change. You won't be doing the same things for him, nor will you be relating in the same way or having the same responsibilities. This means that how you live your day and plan your time will change.

You will also have a whole new set of relationships. You may come to know the receptionist, the marketing person, nurses, nurse's aides, recreation therapists, housekeepers, and dietary people in the home. You will have a relationship with the laundry personnel, the social worker, and the administrator. You may come to know the other residents of the home and their families.

You will develop a relationship with "the system." You will come to learn how the residence functions. Or, as it will sometimes seem to you, how it does not. You will learn how to find lost laundry, how to solve a problem, whom to talk to about why your husband is not eating or how he is sleeping. You will learn to sign him out when you take him for a drive or appointment and to sign him back in when you return.

Along with these new relationships will come three sets of expectations. Even before admission, your expectations have probably been developing. We can call this your "mental care map." It includes your expectations of the staff: how they carry out their jobs, how they relate to your relative, and how they relate to you. It includes your expectations of what care looks like, what your role will be. These are formulated on many things: your experience, your fears, what you have read in a newspaper and seen on television. In some ways, you will find your care map is accurate; in some ways it will not be and will require you to shift.

You will also find that the staff has expectations of you: when good times to talk to them are, what your role is, how they can help you, how independent your husband is expected to be. They have expectations of how they carry out their jobs, and these may be different from yours. In some places the staff have good experiences with families, in others there can be a climate of defensiveness. It will not be about you, but you may sense it, somehow, a feeling that you can't quite put your finger on.

Most important, your wife may have expectations. She will have her own care map. She will have her own fears and other feelings. She may have expectations of how often you should visit, whether she can go home, what kind of help the staff will provide.

Becoming the family member also clearly entails an emotional process. It will unfold for both you and your husband during the transition to care and in the months afterward. Although your experiences will be different—being the resident is obviously different from being the family member—you go through the adjustment simultaneously. It is a family journey.

So, when the day comes and you walk through the door of a nursing home or assisted living residence with your wife or father or sister, you will be in the middle of a process, not at the end. You are changing from one phase to another and, as in the earlier parts of the process, you will learn new skills and face new challenges. The hard part of the process is not doing the practical tasks, it is dealing with the emotions that arise while you do them. This book is written to help you as you go through that process and experience those emotions throughout the time your husband is in care, and after.

As you read and as you go through the process of becoming "the family member," please keep this is mind: whatever else changes, and no matter where you or your relative go, you will always take with you the caring part of your relationship. It is the part you will always do best and the part that will matter most. Other people can give medications, provide recreation, or dress, wash, and feed the person you love, but they can't give the same love and attention that you can. They do not have the history that you do. No matter where your mother, husband, father, sister, or brother is, you are still a son, wife, daughter, or brother.

Learning the Role of "the Family Member"

Encountering nursing homes or other services for older people is a new experience for most people. This "becoming" process is one in which you may feel out of control, or like the tail is wagging the dog. These are feelings that increase exhaustion and lead to anxiety. In some ways, learning a new role in this sphere is like in any other; the better at it you become, the more in control you will feel and the more confidence you will have. Eventually, you become an expert. When you become an expert, it will take less emotional and physical energy for you to accomplish what you need to accomplish.

Developing expertise will also help to level the playing field. You are coming into contact with people who already have experience in the system because they work in it—they *are* the system. The staff have confidence, knowledge, and skills in an area where you do not. Yes, you are the expert in your family member, but the expertise you develop will help you to talk to them and participate fully in the care and services they provide. It will also help you to advocate for your father if you need to. Once you can talk their language and know their system, you will be able to obtain the care and services for your mother that she deserves.

Types and Levels of Care

Many different types of seniors residences are available to meet a variety of needs. Different states and provinces have different names for the options and have different regulations. It can be confusing. You may find names like "independent living for seniors," "congregate care," "assisted living," "retirement communities," "nursing homes," "board-and-care homes," or "skilled nursing facilities."

To make a rational decision about what type of housing is appropriate, you should understand what your father needs now and what he will need in the future. Obtain from the doctor a clear picture of his diagnosis and what it means. What is the expected progression and time frame? If he has an illness, contact an organization that deals with that illness, such as the Alzheimer's Association or the National Parkinson Foundation. They will give you a full picture of what to expect. Remember, you are not just choosing for now or the next few months, you are planning, potentially, for years.

When you start looking for housing (see chapter 5, "About Nursing Homes and Assisted Living Facilities"), think about what services your family member needs, rather than about whether you want a nursing home or assisted living facility. Then find out who is allowed to provide what in your area. When you have a picture of present and future needs and pair it with whether those needs would be met by assisted living, a nursing home, or another type of care in your area, you can look for housing. When you ask specific places about services, you will want them to be clear about what they can and cannot provide and when you will be able to move your father. To find out about the local regulations for the provision of housing in the United States, you can contact the local chapter of the Assisted Living Federation of America (www.alfa.org), the state long-term care ombudsperson, or your local area agency on aging. (The latter two are found through www.eldercare.gov, or you can find your state ombudsperson at www.nursinghomeaction.org/static_pages/ ombudsmen.cfm.) In Canada you can talk to your local Health Authority. In either country, you can also obtain information from the local Alzheimer's Association (www.alzheimers.ca or www.alz.org).

Below is an explanation of the types of housing about which you will hear.

INDEPENDENT LIVING

The basic level of care is usually called congregate care or seniors independent living. (The "ors" can go on and on.) There is a dining room, and one, two, or all meals may be served there. Usually they provide some housekeeping, some laundry services, some recreation, and transportation for outings. There will be an emergency call system in the living unit so that if a resident falls or has an injury, he or she can call a staff person for help. There may be a nurse on the staff. There tends not to be any personal care.

Independent living residences are set up to be able to offer this basic level of housing, but they are not licensed and do not have facilities for higher levels of care or service. In independent living, residents are generally expected to be fairly independent. They are supposed to be able to make their own decisions, get themselves to meals and appointments, and choose on their own whether to participate in the recreational opportunities available. The residences do not officially have the staff or mandate to call your father when there is an outing or bingo, they do not monitor whether he is drinking, they will not help him sort his mail and write checks. Unofficially, they may do so.

A place may be independent living only but allow you to engage private help when your father needs personal care and reminders. Or the facility may provide basic independent living, but have packages of personal care services available (for up to many hundreds of dollars a month). These personal care services are what constitute assisted living, so the residence must be careful about what they offer if they do not wish to fall under the stricter state regulations that accompany a higher level of care. Nonetheless, many independent living residences have helpful staff members, working beyond their job descriptions or the policy/mandate of the residence, who will work with residents and families to allow them be able to continue to live in the residence if their abilities begin to fail. If they do this, remember that it is temporary.

ASSISTED LIVING

The meaning of assisted living and the services that are provided in assisted living residences vary enormously from state to state and between provinces. In some areas, assisted living services can be almost identical to nursing homes. They have nurses, provide some direct nursing care, provide care for people with dementia, and have specific dementia care units. Sometimes there are regulations on what the nurse, if there is one, can do. In other states or provinces, assisted living facilities are allowed to provide only a certain number of personal care services and a certain amount of help. They may not provide direct nursing care, or they may limit the admission of people with dementia, depending on how far it has progressed. Often, however, even in these places, residents stay beyond the point at which the regulations say they should be allowed to stay. Some areas define the limits to assisted living as being when a resident is no longer able to make decisions regarding his or her care or lifestyle.

One way to distinguish nursing homes from assisted living is the model on which they are based. Assisted living is a social model; nursing homes are based on a medical model. They former tend to be more homelike and characterized by emphasis on non-nursing/non-medical services. Historically, nursing homes derived from hospital types of care. Assisted living is the child of what used to be called a retirement home, often a house where older people would go to live if they had no family.

In assisted living, residents generally, but not always, have their own apartments or rooms. Often there are cooking facilities in the unit, or at least a fridge and countertops, but all meals are provided. There should be a call system in the apartment/room/suite living area and one in a bathroom area for emergencies. Even if there is no direct nursing care, an assisted living residence may be all that even a fragile older person needs for a long time.

The difference between assisted living and independent living is that assisted living offers, in addition to the basic independent living services, at least help with

- personal care needs such as dressing bathing, toileting, grooming
- medication dispensing or reminding
- getting to and from a dining room
- personal laundry.

Both independent living and assisted living usually have accommodations suitable for couples. If Mum does not need help, but Dad does, the residence may still take them both (if they fit with the available levels of care), but the rates will most likely be different. It allows Mum to be free of some of her caregiving tasks and know that there are people around who can help and monitor. Assisted living is one of the ways in which housing is changing so that couples do not have to be separated as they age.

The assisted living services provided may differ enormously between facilities, and you must be careful about what you are paying for as a basic rate and what additional costs there will be. There may be a structure. For example, a residence may provide two services per day at a basic rate and charge for more than that. Or your basic rate may include, for instance, thirty minutes a day of care services, and if you need more you have to pay an additional fee. Fees may jump if Dad needs some nursing care (if they provide it at all). Make sure you get these things in writing. Remember, too, that the costs can increase enormously as someone becomes frailer. This might mean that you could afford the basic rate, but cannot afford the "All-Inclusive Platinum Deluxe All-You-Can-Eat" rate that Dad now needs, and he will have to move.

There is significant variation in how assisted living facilities are regulated in both Canada and the United States, and standards also differ widely. In the United States, more and more states have been increasing regulations and monitoring of assisted living residences. But do not be fooled into thinking that you do not have to monitor your father or the facility. If he is going into assisted living, he may be capable of telling you what is going on. But you will still have to know if he is taking his medications, how he is eating, and if he is engaging in a supportive and healthy social life. You will still have to figure out if he is changing his clothes and washing, or if those services (for which you may be paying extra) are being provided the way the facility says they will be. In short, you will have to make sure that the needs for which he entered the facility are in fact being met.

The longer your father is in an assisted living residence, the more his mental faculties may decline. As he becomes frailer, he still may not need nursing care, but he will increasingly need some kind of monitoring. Remember, there may be fewer staff members here than there would be in a nursing home, so fewer people to monitor areas of potential problem. If there is a problem with the facility, the regulatory agencies with which you can register a complaint may have less ability to become involved with the problem than they would with a nursing home. The state ombudspeople now have responsibility for complaints about assisted living. The industry association, Assisted Living Federation of America (see the resources section at the back of this book), has voluntary standards.

Some assisted living is subsidized by most Canadian provinces. There are also private, unfunded assisted living residences. Sometimes provincial governments have contracted for units in private facilities. In the United States, Medicaid in some states will cover assisted living, but the facilities may not wish to become part of the Medicaid funding because of the limitations on what they will be paid. For the moment, because of the limitations on funding, an assisted living facility may not be an option for you unless you have private means for payment.

The limits of service for many assisted living residences may be at the point where a resident needs skilled nursing care. This kind of care requires a huge investment in staff, equipment, and even building design. It is often not cost effective for the residence to provide.

SKILLED NURSING CARE FACILITIES

Skilled nursing care facilities are what we think of as nursing homes. These homes provide full-time nursing coverage. Nurses perform treatments, dispense medications, and so on. They are responsible for monitoring the health of the residents. Nurse's aides help with bathing, dressing, walking, toileting, grooming, and eating. There are other supplementary professionals, such as social workers or physical therapists. Nursing homes are highly regulated by the provinces and health authorities and, in the United States, by the states and the federal government. The basis of regulations in the United States was the 1987 Nursing Home Reform Law. To be able to receive Medicare funding, a U.S. home must be licensed as a skilled nursing care facility.

In some areas, nursing homes are hospital-like settings for people who are bedridden or who need a great deal of medical and/or nursing care. They have a much higher staff-to-resident ratio than assisted living or other kinds of homes, and residents in them are much more disabled. Even in these facilities, however, acute medical services such as X-ray or emergency services may not be available, nor a physician present.

REHABILITATION CENTERS

Hospitals will often discharge someone who still needs care to a rehabilitation center. Theoretically, rehabilitation centers provide residents the physical, occupational, or speech therapy they need to regain maximum possible function. Under Medicare, people going to an inpatient rehabilitation center must be able to tolerate three hours of intense rehabilitation daily. To receive Medicare funding, you have to be admitted from a hospital; you cannot be admitted directly from home. So even if you need some rehabilitation services that would prevent hospitalization, if you are currently living at home, you are out of luck as far as Medicare funding. After rehabilitation, the idea and the ideal are that you will return to your own home. Many people are not able to do so and will then have to move to either assisted living or a nursing home. Many nursing homes have rehabilitation programs, sections, or beds. Many say they do, but the amount and quality of their rehabilitation leave, shall we say, something to be desired. The advantage for the nursing home is that it receives a higher funding rate for an individual in the rehabilitation phase of a medical condition than when the condition becomes chronic. If your father is in a rehabilitation bed in a nursing home, his bed may be converted to a regularly funded nursing home bed later, when he no longer is receiving actual rehabilitation. It becomes tricky for nursing homes that want to balance their funding sources.

GROUP HOMES

In some areas there are adult group homes, board-and-care homes, or residential apartments. This is another instance when a name can mean different things in different provinces or states. They usually have to be licensed to provide care. Depending on the type of residence, regulations governing them are often minimal. Some offer only limited assistance in a family setting. Some have full nursing care. They may be "homey" or they may be depressingly spartan. One of the trade-offs for the familylike atmosphere of a small facility can be limited recreation and activities because there are fewer staff members. Some of these homes are excellent, but some may be decidedly less so. Several provinces and states have been actively developing different forms of group homes and residential care that are supported and monitored by professionals and are publicly funded to some extent.

CAMPUS-OF-CARE / CONTINUING-CARE RETIREMENT COMMUNITIES

The past few years have seen the growth of a model of seniors housing called "campus of care." This means that in one building, or on the same grounds, there are multiple levels of housing—supportive housing, assisted living, and nursing homes. Sometimes they are provided to a resident in the same unit, or sometimes you may need to change floors or even move to another building on the same grounds as your health or care needs increase. Your father could start off in supportive living, then move to an assisted living area (or start receiving assisted living services), and then, as his needs increase, move to the nursing home. Here your father would not have to make one big move after another. He and your mother could move to one unit in the campus-of-care complex together, and if one needed more care later, at least they would be in the same complex. Or they could move to the same complex, but one might be in independent living and the other in the nursing home on site.

The campuses of care are often called continuing-care retirement communities (CCRCs). In order to gain entrance, you may be required to be in good health and even have to have a physical. You may also have to pay a sizeable entrance fee in addition to monthly fees.

Other Considerations

BUYING AND RENTING UNITS

In some residences and CCRCs there are options to buy a unit as well as rent. Or you may end up purchasing a contract with the right to live in the residence (or on the campus) but not actually be purchasing the unit. The choices can be confusing, especially with CCRCs. For instance, they may offer you a contract guaranteeing lifetime access to health care with no extra monthly fees should you need that additional care. (This is sometimes called a "lifecare" community or contract.) Or you may be able to access increased health and personal care if you need it but have to pay an additional fee for it. As mentioned, you may have a sizeable entrance fee. Your estate might receive money back after your death.

If you are considering buying a unit or a contract, be extremely cautious. Make sure it is the right place for you by spending some time there and getting to know the complex and the community as well as you can. Find out about selling or getting out of your contract if you are not happy or your financial circumstances change and you are no longer able to pay the monthly services fee, or if you cannot pay the additional care fees. It is a good idea to have the contract reviewed by an attorney, preferably an elderlaw attorney. (To find an elderlaw attorney, see the National Academy of Elder Law Attorneys website at www.naela.org.)

WHEN THEY ASK YOU TO LEAVE

I once had a client with dementia who had just moved to an assisted living residence. Her behavior was disturbing to some of the other residents, most of whom also had dementia. But more significantly (from what I could tell), her behavior was disturbing to the *families* of other residents. The residence's manager informed me that my client had to move in three days.

A seniors residence can ask your mother to leave if they feel she is no longer suitable to their situation. There are many reasons they may give. It might be because of the amount of help she needs, because she is making a disturbance in a dining room, because of funding limitations, because they cannot provide a safe situation, or because of other issues. Whereas in nursing homes federal or provincial regulations make it hard to discharge someone, in assisted living it may be much easier. In some states and provinces, assisted living is covered under landlord-tenant legislation; in others, it is not. In the United States, discharges from nursing homes are regulated by the Nursing Home Reform Law. Other legislation, such as the Fair Housing Act and the Americans with Disabilities Act, is sometimes used to fight unfair evictions and policies. If a residence does try to evict your mother, make sure you know your rights. At the same time, think about whether the situation might not be the best place for her anymore. Even if you don't like the *way* it is initiated, leaving the residence may be the best thing for your mother.

Alastair

His suitcase was packed and the car was at the front door. We went down the front steps together. Our son, Donald, looking sad and stressed, put the bag into the trunk. My husband got into the car without saying a word. We drove the kilometer to St. Mary's Home. He had no doubt visited parishioners there many times during his active ministry. He read the sign aloud, then said nothing more. Donald and I fought back the tears.

We were met by the receptionist, who called the head nurse. All residents who had dementia were housed on the secure second floor, which meant that a key was needed to activate the elevator. Upstairs we were shown to his room. Again he said nothing. We told him that he would be staying here until he was feeling better and that I would be coming to see him twice each day. When it came time to go home, we headed for the elevator. The image of his face as the elevator doors closed is burned into my brain. That day, July 18, 1996, was a major turning point in, and the saddest day of, my life.

Alastair had retired fourteen years earlier, and for the first ten of those years we had a wonderful retirement, with several trips of great interest. In January 1992 we visited Trinidad, where we had met and been married. Several times during that visit, I was uneasy about his behavior. He had always had a way with words and was never visibly upset when asked to speak extemporaneously, but when he was invited to speak at a school graduation ceremony in Trinidad, he lost his train of thought several times. As the months went by, he began to have frequent fainting spells, and after each episode his memory failed him more and more often. He was asked to perform a marriage ceremony, something that he had done hundreds of times, but this time he had the couple take the vows twice.

We consulted our doctor, who ran innumerable tests both in and out of the hospital. Finally, imaging of Alastair's brain showed that he had had many little strokes and each one had done damage. I learned that these little strokes were called TIAs [transient ischemic attacks] and that they caused a dementia called multi-infarct dementia.

The doctor encouraged me to have Alastair attend adult day care. He enjoyed this for more than two years, but his memory continued to deteriorate. He became more and more confused, and we went from crisis to crisis.

I had visited homes for the aged many times during our marriage and, like most people, I felt sorry for the poor old souls who were ending their days there in what I thought must be misery. If I thought about it at all, I was sure that we would never be living as those people were. Now it was our turn and our day had arrived. Days and weeks of adjustment followed. The staff advised me not to take him for a walk outside for the first couple of weeks. They also said it wouldn't be a good idea to take him home until he had settled into his new quarters. There was a lot of pain and a lot I had to learn in those first few months.

Gradually the visits became less painful. Alastair and I began to develop a routine of a daily walk around the beautiful little park across from the home. He started coming for a trip home every Sunday for dinner. Even though speech was becoming more and more difficult, he always had a big smile for family members as they arrived.

Soon I began to make friends with the relatives of other residents, especially with two of the other wives. A bright light at St. Mary's was the chaplain. He preached a great sermon, had a keen sense of humor, obviously loved the elderly residents—especially the ones who had dementia—and had a fine singing voice. When he walked into the room, the energy level rose immediately.

I also got to know the other residents. Some of them were unable to communicate, but others were very interesting. Ninety-one-year-old Gladys, a rotund English lady with a booming voice, was one of the most colorful. One day I visited St. Mary's wearing an outfit that she liked. While Alastair and I were waiting for the elevator, Gladys came up to us and told me in a voice that could be heard across the room, "You're a pretty lady." Two of the other old ladies were seated side by side in the nearby sitting area. One leaned over to the other and said, "She's all right, but she isn't that pretty!" The chaplain had enjoyed the whole episode and with a chuckle added, "That's what I like about these people: they're so honest." When he realized that his remark hadn't been particularly gallant, he tripped all over himself trying to make amends.

Every Thursday evening a student from Sri Lanka comes as a volunteer to entertain at the piano. The residents enjoy his music and have a great time when members of the staff get up and dance with them. One of the ladies is unable to say anything that makes sense, but her face is radiant when she dances. Hands, arms, and feet make joyous rhythm with the music.

By now we have settled into a routine. I know that Alastair is being well cared for and I have started to get on with remaking my life and developing new interests. I am again taking the art classes I began after our retirement. I am registered for exercise classes and life writing at the community center. All three activities are great tonics and most enjoyable. The support of our family and friends has also been with me throughout this time of separation from my husband.

Life is not the disaster I thought it was in July 1996. In fact, I can almost say what my mother said to me one day from her nursing home bed when she was almost ninety-five, "Well, it's not such a bad old life after all!"

CHAPTER 2

Deciding about Care

Ideally, the process of going into a seniors residence will be one in which your husband participates. If it is your husband's choice, it is easier on him as well as on you. He will adjust better, because having a choice means he still has some control over his life. To make it his choice, he will need time to get used to the idea and emotionally prepare himself to accept it. If he refuses or is unable, then you will have to make the decision. Sometimes there are options in between full participation and none.

How to Talk about Care

Most people find they don't know how to start having this conversation. Once you have started, it will become easier. Throughout your relationship there have probably been times when you had to make decisions together and times when you or he have changed and it meant that your relationship had to change. This decision is new, but you probably have had experience with this kind of process. Think about this conversation as one you need to have in order to make a difficult decision together. If your husband participates, it is a shared decision. It will not be something you are doing alone or something you are doing to him. You share the burden and you share your sadness, too. As you talk, it can become a decision made in the context of your relationship that can bring you closer and lighten your emotional burden.

Be clear in your own mind what it is you are talking about. Are you talking about a nursing home, about assisted living, or about having a professional caregiver live at home with your husband and you? You will want to look on your own at what is available so that you know what to tell him. You need to be clear on what the problem is and what potential solutions are. This can be part of the discussion, and it will make things easier.

Talking about moving or a nursing home is talking about a solution. It can make more sense to talk about the problem, and then make some tentative decisions. So, in starting a conversation with your husband about care, talk generally. Frame it as planning for the future for both of you. You can say, "I am noticing that doing the lawn and garden is getting much more difficult for you, and sometimes you have forgotten to take your pills." Or you can say, "I have been thinking about what we would do if something happened to either one of us." You can tell him what you would want and how you would want him to handle things. This can lead naturally to a discussion about his condition and what he wants.

For many months I worked with a delightful ninety-five-year-old woman who had lived in her apartment for thirty-five years. We talked about how hard it was for her to go to the store to buy groceries and how tired she was of cooking every day. That was how she eventually decided to move. The move was the solution.

You can also focus on the condition or disability rather than on the solution. Ask your husband how he sees his health. I often ask people about their memory. Many memory-impaired people do not know they are failing or will not acknowledge it, but some will. Often they tell me that they have "slipped somewhat" or use a similar expression. I ask them what will happen if they slip more. If they are physically impaired, I ask them what kind of help they need and who is giving them that help. We look together at their needs and what we think will happen. Then sometimes I can say to them, "It sounds like you are getting a lot of help from your wife. I wonder how she is handling it?" This can lead us to a discussion that will bring up the alternatives. When we talk about alternatives, we can talk about a nursing home as one of them.

Even persons with dementia can participate in making decisions about care, depending on how the choices are presented and the extent of the dementia. They can still talk about what they want and feel even if they will not remember the conversation. The conversation can also be valuable for you: it can help you gauge how your husband will react to the transition and to care.

Talking with your husband about the need for care may be frightening for you: it makes you acknowledge what you are facing. You also may be anxious because you don't know how he will react to the subject of a nursing home. When I have asked people what their worst fear is, they say they are afraid their husband will become angry and lose his temper.

Ask yourself what your worst fear is, and then ask yourself what will happen if that situation occurs. Follow it through, maybe talking it out with someone: "Okay, and what will happen if he does become angry? What will happen then?" "Okay, and then what will happen?" Follow it till the end. Fear can be like a wall or "Do Not Enter" sign: it stops us from moving forward. Most of the time, when we ask ourselves the questions such as "Then what would happen?" we find that the fear is greater than the event, and this helps us move through it.

Your husband may react with anger because at some level he knows his memory is failing or he can no longer manage on his own. Acknowledging his need to be cared for can be a message about many things—his health, age, and mortality—that he wants to hide both from others and from himself. When you talk to him about care, you make him face all these issues. Think about times you have been angry in your life. Often, if is because you have been afraid or anxious. Your husband's anger also helps keep you away—if he gets angry, then you will stop talking about it. This kind of behavior is especially true if your family tends not to face and deal with anger directly.

When you do finally talk about housing, the first step is to ask your husband what he hears you saying—does he think that you will abandon him or that you don't love him anymore? Acknowledge his feelings and fears. When he sees that you understand his feelings, it will be easier for him to move to the next step of being able to discuss the issue. Be ready to discuss your own feelings. What will it be like for you if he goes into care?

When you bring up the subject of a seniors residence, especially with a parent, your mother's first reaction may be a fear of being abandoned—that she won't see you anymore and will be cut off from the family. She may also have a sense of rejection and a feeling of being old and useless. In our society, there is some truth in that fear— there often *is* no "place" of usefulness for older people, especially those who are impaired. Watch for that reaction, and ask if she is feeling it. If she says no, address these issues anyway. She needs to hear about her value, both as a person and as a member of the family.

Think about other tough decisions you have made, especially ones you have made with someone else. Were they made in one conversation? Whatever your husband's reaction is at first, you may have to return to the subject several times before there can be a discussion. The first time, he may be angry; the fifth time, he may be more willing to listen. It may take a few conversations to talk about the feelings before you are able to make some decisions on the issues. This is normal. A housing decision is a decision about change, and it is a process. Acceptance is the end of the process of emotions that unfold and are passed through. Give the process time. You don't have to resolve it in one sitting.

You may want to tell a friend or family member that you will be having these conversations, and then talk to him or her after they have occurred. This can help you talk through or "debrief" yourself on what happened and what it was like for you. You don't have to give the details. Just have someone who can support you while you face this task. You may find several friends have already had the same conversations or are having them.

Once you start talking, you may find that your husband acknowledges his need for care. Many people know when they are ill, and know that their spouses cannot care for them much longer. Residents have told me that they chose a nursing home because they knew they needed help and did not want to burden their children with their care. They knew that their children needed or wanted their own lives. They wanted to maintain their own independence. Some have told me that they were lonely or not eating or afraid of falling when they lived at home. Despite their fears about going into care, they were willing to acknowledge their needs and make the decision that followed.

Younger people with disabilities or a progressive disease also usually know at some level when they need some kind of care. They see how they are managing, and they see the strain on their caregivers and families. This may make it easier for them to "work through" the process. On the other hand, younger people may have more resistance, anger, and grief, because they see going into care as the loss of so much of their lives. They feel cheated, and in a sense they have been (and so have you). Acceptance may take longer. Anger with the caregiver can be greater as these persons deal with their loss and sense of abandonment. As the recipient of that anger, you, the stressed caregiver who is perhaps also working and parenting young children, may become angry in return. If you can, instead of reacting, try to say something like, "I know you are angry. I am angry and sad about this, too." Try to remember that, although the anger is directed *at* you, it is not *about* you. If you are having trouble, bring in a professional who can help you both. Younger people especially should be given every opportunity to explore for themselves all possible alternatives. Going through this exploration process is part of the path to acceptance.

You can introduce the idea of a residence as insurance—"in case." This is why it is a good idea to start planning as far as possible in advance of when you will need a home. You might say, "I know you don't need it now, but we should take a look." You can use the same approach to put his name on a waiting list. Talking about the issue of care as a possible future gives your husband time to become accustomed to the idea without being frightened by its immediacy. You can also say that you want to look at alternatives, maybe senior housing complexes, maybe board-and-care homes. However you broach the subject, try to do it in a way that allows him to have choice and a feeling of control.

If there is a possibility of rehabilitation, make sure you discuss this. Many people who enter nursing homes, assisted living, or board-and-care homes do go home later or do manage at a different level of care. Younger people sometimes move to group homes. In your discussion, talk about use of the nursing home as helping to increase the possibility that he can move or return home and function better.

It may be easier if a physician, home health nurse, or social worker in the hospital tells your husband that he needs more care than he can receive at home. He may listen to a professional in a position of authority more than to someone in his own family. He will not experience it as rejection or criticism from you when it is coming from a professional. If he is going to become angry, it will be with the doctor. When someone else has initiated the conversation, it also allows you to deal with his reaction as a sympathetic person and someone who is on his side. It allows you to say, "What are we going to do now?"

When people think about nursing homes and care, they often have in mind pictures of what facilities were like years ago. They don't know how care alternatives have changed. For example, they are not aware of, or have not seen, assisted living residences. So when your husband becomes angry or refuses to consider care, he may be refusing the picture he has in mind. If he will agree to take a look at some of the options, his reaction may change. I walked into one assisted living home a few months ago and thought, "Nice place. Meals are cooked, cleaning done—I could live here."

If you are one of several adult children who are concerned about one or both parents, it may be that one of you would be better at bringing up the subject than another. Often, a mother will listen to a son, or father to a daughter, or sometimes there is one child who is closer to a parent than another. You all might want to sit down with one parent who is the caregiver and discuss your concerns (see chapter 3, "Family Decision Making"). Or you may want to sit down with both of them at the same time. Talking with them both can take the burden off the parent who is the caregiver; you can be the one to speak to the parent who needs care. Sometimes a parent will listen to an adult child more than to a spouse.

When meeting with both parents, define the issue as a family problem as opposed to there being something wrong with your father. List some of the issues and describe how they affect everybody. When your father hears from you a description of your mother's situation as she tries to take care of him, he may be more willing to accept his condition and the need for some kind of care. The idea is not to have him feel guilty but to help him develop a realistic view of his condition and its repercussions in the family.

Often the resistance will come from the person who is not going into care. Your mother may say it is because of your father, but in the end, it may be because she is afraid of being alone, feeling guilty, or having nothing to do. Your father may be able to face the concern; it may be your mother who cannot face her grief.

However you bring up the subject, in the end you may have to just do it. You may have to set a deadline for yourself and just start talking. The fear of doing so will probably be worse than the actual event; afterward you may have a sense of relief. You may also have a sense of sadness, knowing that this process has begun and it will happen.

Contrary to what you may think, many people who have long resisted moving to a seniors residence, or even a nursing home, end up being content once they are there. Although they never would have admitted it, life at home was a struggle. They were not eating well, small personal care tasks were painful and slow, they were lonely, they were afraid of falling. They find that it is a relief to have someone helping them dress, that it is enjoyable to have well-cooked meals and to have people around them. They feel safe. Some of the shame is gone.

Despite themselves, some people in care in a good facility have thrived. Their struggle was with the idea of giving up their independence and pride in being on their own. Once they got through those feelings, they would not go back to what they had. They realize they are the same people they were at home. What is important for people in a residence is to maintain a sense of dignity about themselves despite the fact that they need help.

Unfortunately, no matter how you bring up the subject of care, your husband may not be able to accurately look at his condition and will not be able to participate in the decision. His memory may be so bad that he will not remember what you have talked about. He may be so scared or angry or "in denial" that he will refuse to talk about it, and you will not make any progress. He may be so overwhelmed that he can't hear or react to the stress you are having.

The process should not stop and you should not give up because your husband will not participate in the decision. This is often the point at which people surrender, feeling defeated, guilty, or overwhelmed by having to do it on their own. Do not give up. Instead, this may be the time when you, as a caregiver, need to go out and develop a support network of friends, professionals, or support groups so that you can continue.

As you know, your caregiving process will continue even if you give up discussing care options. Most likely, your husband's need for care will increase, as will the burden on you. If he is not participating in the decision, you may have to begin the process without him. That means you will look for the home, ask the questions, and put his name on a waiting list. Your job will then be to help him—and yourself—prepare as the time comes closer. This is discussed further in chapter 4 and chapter 9.

Choosing the Right Time

I used to say there is no "right time" for someone to move to a care facility or assisted living. I now think, however, that there is one—it is when everyone agrees that the time has come. That is the point at which you have made a decision together. Another answer might be, "When your wife recognizes the need and is ready to act on it."

For the person receiving care, one way to look at the decision is to figure out what she will receive in care, as opposed to what she will receive at home. One of the biggest differences is in socialization. This is especially true of people who are able to go to assisted living. Over and over I hear people tell me how they appreciate having other people around and things to do. They no longer feel isolated, they feel safe. Almost everything else can be bought at home—products, foods, care. What you cannot buy at home is a community.

As far as the caregiver and the caregiving process go, the only "right time" for your wife to move is when you can no longer provide her care, for whatever reason. Caregivers' abilities to handle a burden vary enormously, depending on their circumstances and their emotional makeup. However, for all caregivers there are both warning signs and alarm signs. When you don't pay attention to the warnings, they will become alarms. Those are the times when you get into a crisis.

One of the reasons people find themselves in a crisis is that they close their eyes to the fact that their situation is progressive. For whatever reason, they do not want to hear it. If you find yourself avoiding asking the doctor what is going to happen, or refusing to consider the word *Alzheimer,* or becoming angry when people try to talk to you, this is a signal that you have shut down.

The problem with waiting for the alarm to sound is that when you finally hear it, your options may be limited. The waiting list for the residence of your choice could be one, two, or three years long. If you and your wife are in crisis, it can mean that there is greater physical and emotional risk to both of you than if she had moved earlier. It can mean that your emotional and financial reserves are strained to a breaking point. Waiting for the alarm may not do anyone a favor, and you may end up causing some damage to yourself and your wife.

Please, have the courage to be good to both of you: "plan, don't panic." Here are some of the warning signs that the caregiving burden is becoming overwhelming:

1. *Is your physical health beginning to suffer?* Don't wait until you are exhausted. Don't wait until you are never getting a good night's sleep or you are getting colds. By that time, you may not be able to provide care the way you should.
2. *Is your emotional balance beginning to be affected?* You find that you are crying or are feeling hopeless or even are feeling nothing. You find that your sex drive is gone, you are not eating, or your sleep is disturbed. These are signs of depression.
3. *Is your wife's health beginning to suffer?* There may come a time when, despite your best efforts, your wife's health will suffer and she will be at risk. This may be because she is not eating, taking her pills, or allowing herself to have the physical care she needs. Is she developing pressure sores or other rashes?
4. *Is your wife's safety becoming an issue?* She may be opening the door to strangers, wandering out of your home and getting lost, leaving the oven on, or leaving lit cigarettes around.
5. *Are you physically unable to provide care?* You cannot lift or do the tasks required.
6. *Are you feeling resentful, short-tempered, or angry?* These are signs of stress and can lead to you becoming abusive.
7. *Are people, including your doctor, beginning to tell you that it is time?* Usually, people on the outside notice the changes in you and in her; because they don't carry the guilt or other feelings, they can be more objective.

8. *Is the community unable to meet your wife's needs or your needs through the services it can provide?* Despite their help, are you having the physical or emotional symptoms listed above?

9. *Are you hiding the extent of your wife's disability and your physical or mental state from your family or friends?* Hiding something from family or friends means that you are closing off your support network. It also means that you are trying to deny what you know to be true but don't wish to see—that your wife needs help. You may be holding back feelings of shame or guilt. All of these factors increase the risk to yourself and your wife.

If you answer yes to one of these questions, it is a warning. If you answer yes to three or more, alarm bells should be going off. If you answer yes to six or more, then I hope your wife is on a waiting list for care. If not, my guess is that you are either unwilling or unable to make a decision. You need to talk to someone, most likely a professional. You are at risk.

Stress and Burnout

Have you ever put something on a shelf and then added more and more things to that shelf? The first items are fine, but as you add more, the shelf may begin to bend. You may not notice it at first, and so you keep piling on more things. If you kept adding things after that, the shelf would break. Caregiving is the same. You can take on some burden, but after a while you may begin to bend. You may not notice it at first, but this is the beginning of stress.

If you are not already overburdened from being a caregiver, it is possible that you will become so at some point during the process. It is essential that you learn to recognize your stress and be alert to how you are dealing with it. Stress will affect your health. It will have an impact on your heart and your immune system. It will affect your ability to be an effective caregiver as you deal with nursing homes and other systems. Behaviors resulting from stress can include increase in the use of alcohol and drugs, compulsive eating, and emotionally or physically abusing the person for whom you are caring. These behaviors can spin out of control: they can increase your isolation, further affect your health or caregiving ability, and even kill you.

If the last sentence wasn't enough for you, read this—it is important: at a physiological level, stress is the condition our bodies are in when we are primed to fight or flight. For instance, under stress

- skeletal muscle strength increases
- blood clotting time decreases
- heart rate increases
- sugar and fat levels increase
- intestinal movement is reduced
- digestive system work is decreased
- the bladder relaxes
- mental alertness increases
- blood vessels to some internal organs, such as intestines and kidneys, constrict
- blood vessels to skeletal muscles, such as those that move the arms and legs, dilate.

At the same time, we have increased blood pressure and decreased lymphocytes, the cells that fight disease. This is why the stress is dangerous—it gives you high blood pressure, it lowers your immune system responses so you become sick more easily, and it puts pressure on all of your body systems.

The stress response is what enabled us to escape from the wooly mammoth a million years ago. But then, when the mammoth was gone, our body system would return to a state of relaxation. With ongoing stress, such as in caregiving, there is no time out. Your body is exhausted. Its functioning is impaired, and there is no time for repair. This is burnout. The bottom line is that stress and burnout cause physical damage to your body.

Once you have burned out, it is difficult to restart. You will be unable to be an effective caregiver. So if you burn out, you have defeated yourself and will cause the very event that you are working so hard to prevent.

Some of the signs of burnout are similar to the signs that you are becoming overburdened:

- depression
- irritability, anger, poor emotional control
- lack of motivation, concentration, and energy
- feelings of hopelessness, helplessness, and despair
- sleeplessness
- stomach problems and headaches
- decreased sexual desire
- anxiety attacks.

Throughout this book I will talk about taking care of yourself by utilizing the supports available to you. Use them to deal with your stress, too. Basically, these strategies consist of

- activities that deflect your attention or give you a break
- eating and sleeping well
- exercise
- socializing and support.

In my lectures and seminars, I often describe caregiving as being like a watering can. You start off with the can full. If you water a plant every day, and you don't refill the can, there will come a point when the can is empty, and the plant will die. You have to fill the can before you can water the plant.

Put yourself first on the list of whom you take care of. If you don't, you will have a tendency to leave yourself out. By the time you figure out what is wrong, you will have some habits and behaviors that are destructive to you. Paradoxically, putting yourself first will make you better able to respond to your wife's needs.

How do you put yourself first? Make a list of options that will lower your stress, and build them into your schedule. Plan caregiving activities around them. If caregiving competes with what you have scheduled for yourself, find someone who can take over for you. Your caregiving schedule should be like trying to balance a checkbook: if you make a withdrawal, make sure that you make a deposit.

When a Parent Chooses to Live at Risk

Several times when I have been on the staff in a nursing home I have offered a room to someone who declined it despite the fact that she or he had fairly serious memory loss and/or physical problems. On occasion, I will then hear from a stressed-out son (or daughter) who has been the primary involved caregiver. "She just won't go," he tells me. I hear the exhaustion in his voice and the resignation of knowing that he will be continuing in this stressful situation with no relief in sight. When I look at the relationship, I find that he has been at the beck and call of his mother for years. Anything that she needs, he will go out and get; anytime she calls, he will rush over. The mother has been able to survive on her own because he has not been able to set limits or boundaries. Of course Mom is not going to move! She is all right living on her own; she has a personal, twenty-four-hour attendant!

If Mom is alert enough to make a decision, then I suggest to the son that he start setting some limits on what he will do for his mother. Let her "sink or swim" on her own until she makes the decision. This can be painful and frightening. He then has to step back until something happens to his mother. For instance, she will walk without a walker until she falls and breaks a hip, or she will prepare meals inadequately to the point where she becomes malnourished and has to be hospitalized. Then the mother has no options, but she knows it and acknowledges it. The son has to have the courage to let things progress naturally and on his mother's time.

Your mother has the right to make her own decisions, even bad ones. You are not responsible for her bad decisions. She is an adult. If she wishes to live at risk, that is her right. It does not matter whether you like it or are worried. But then it is also not your fault when something happens. Along with her right to choose comes responsibility for her choices. You need to allow her the rights and responsibilities of being an adult. Just because she is elderly does not mean that she should have any fewer freedoms or responsibilities than anyone else.

There is a payoff for you in stepping back and allowing your mother to take the risks she wishes. It allows you to know that you have truly respected her as a person. You have given her a gift of love that says you will handle your anxiety in a way that does not interfere with her. Your responsibility is then to learn to deal with that anxiety effectively.

It may be that your mother has been dominating and controlling throughout your life. If that is so, your inability to set limits in being a caregiver is probably characteristic of your relationship with your mother in general. If this is your situation, then you may want to buy a book or take a course on assertiveness training. You may want see a therapist to look at the relationship you have had with your mother. Even when you are fifty or sixty years old, you can still have a dysfunctional relationship with a parent.

How you handle this situation can ultimately have a strong positive effect on your life in general. Learning to assert yourself and learning to hold back from asserting yourself inappropriately over your mother are examples of learning about personal boundaries. It will give you a sense of freedom and of relief when you come to understand that you are best off when you try to control only yourself and that the only one who can dictate your behavior is you. Personal boundaries give you the ability to interact with others effectively. When you learn to assert yourself or change the dynamics of a primary relationship, such as with a family member, other relationships can improve.

Please note that allowing your mother to live at risk is an option only if she is able to make a reasonably competent decision. She must be able to understand the nature and consequences of her actions. If she is not, then you must find some other course of action. It may include having her deemed legally incapable. Usually, however, it does not come to this.

Making the Decision

There is often a kind of "gray zone" between being competent to make one's own decisions and being incompetent to do so. Sometimes people can make some decisions but not others. I had a ninety-year-old client who was perfectly clear about the fact she did not wish to give her freeloading son any money but who couldn't figure out why she couldn't hear her television (the sound was broken). Part of the reason for this is that the two capacities call on different parts and functions in the brain. This can be the most confusing and difficult time to have to make a decision.

If you have been caregiving for someone at home for a while, you know that the decision about moving can be like any other decision that is the result of an increase in care needs. It is like taking away a driver's license or getting someone to wear an incontinence product. It is like a little dance sometimes—you push, then pull back, then push again. Sometimes you just make the decision and know that it is the right one. This is why you need to have good boundaries; it will help you make the right decision.

Your Legal Right to Make Decisions for Your Relative: A Warning

If you have been your husband's caregiver, you may think that you are the one who should be able to make decisions about his care. In fact, you probably have been doing so.

There is a legal process for obtaining the right to make decisions for someone. This includes both financial decisions and decisions about personal matters. If you are totally exhausted from caregiving, or if your husband is impaired but refusing to go into care, you still may not have the legal right to have him admitted. Once he is admitted, you may want to sell your house and move to an apartment, but if his name is on the deed, you may not have the legal right to sell it. If you don't have the legal right to make decisions, someone in your family or elsewhere in the system may challenge you. This could make things slow, hard, and expensive for you.

You don't always need the legal right to have your husband admitted to a residence (see chapter 10). Some nursing homes and jurisdictions will allow placement without it. Assisted living residences will usually require it. Here I need to emphasize that if he (or someone else) says no, you may be out of luck, and the nursing home or someone else in the official or medical system may back him up.

FINANCIAL DECISION MAKING

There are two ways you can obtain the legal right to make financial decisions for your husband. First, if he is mentally competent, he can complete documents that give you that right. You may be able to do this through the bank or a notary public regarding financial decisions by obtaining what is usually called the "power of attorney." If your husband has given you power of attorney while he is competent, you will need to make sure that it is an enduring or durable power of attorney. This means that if he becomes incompetent, you still have the right to make decisions. If it is not enduring and he becomes incompetent, the power of attorney could become invalid. While he is competent, even if you have power of attorney, he still has the right to do his finances, and he can revoke your power of attorney whenever he wishes.

PERSONAL CARE DECISIONS

To make personal care decisions for someone else, you need to become the "committee of person" or "medical power of attorney" or "health care proxy" (other terms might be used in your state or province). If your husband is competent, he can give you the right to act for him if he becomes unable to act on his own behalf.

If your husband is no longer competent to make personal or financial decisions, you will have to go to court. The court will want evidence that he is not competent to handle himself or his affairs. This can entail several lengthy and expensive interviews with a psychologist, physician, or other professional. In all states and provinces, there is legislation regarding financial and personal competency.

There are many gray areas when it comes to competency. Even though you may believe that your husband is competent, or even if a lawyer witnesses a document that your husband signs, these documents are sometimes challenged through the courts. I have seen families engaged in horrible battles both over funds and over what to do with a loved one because there was no agreement about a relative's competency or ability to have signed documents. If you think that this may become a problem, have a physician or psychiatrist or other professional, such as a nurse or social worker, perform a competency exam and send you a report. It is more expensive in the beginning, but it can be worth it in the long run.

Even if you don't think this will become a problem, plan for it anyway. If you think, "My children wouldn't fight like that," well, my dears, let me tell you . . . conflict around money and decision making for parents happens in families where you would least expect it. Is this possibility a legacy you want to bequeath to your children?

Advance Directives and Medical Decisions

Advance directives are a series of documents that relate to the question of caring for a person if she becomes disabled to the point that she is no longer able to make decisions for herself. These include the power of attorney documents as well as (although sometimes using different names) living wills, care agreements, degrees of intervention, representation agreements, and do not resuscitate (DNR) orders. They all answer the question "What do you want done if . . . ?"

Advance directives documents vary throughout the United States and Canada. They may also vary from residence to residence. You need to ask the residence what its policy and procedures are regarding end of life, terminal illness, or disability. Aging with Dignity (www.agingwithdignity.org) and National Hospice and Palliative Care Organization's (NHPCO) Caring Connections (www.caringinfo .org) have documents and information that deal with these issues and that are legally recognized in most states. Note that the laws and regulations governing advance directive documents vary among states and provinces.

LIVING WILLS

A living will, which sometimes incorporates some of the same directions as the medical power of attorney, is an overall document that describes what you want to have happen in various situations, such as if there is a question of needing life support, if you have a heart attack, or if you need pain medication. If you have a terminal illness, do you want to be given artificial feeding and hydration through tubes? Do you wish only comfort care, or do you want all the intensive care that is available? A living will is sometimes limited to the time when the principal has a terminal illness. Depending on where you live, a living will without certain guidelines may not have legal validity, and another document may be needed.

ADVANCE MEDICAL DIRECTIVES

An advance medical directive is broader than a living will. It talks about a range of medical and care decisions that are sometimes made when a person is not able to make them himself. Besides the kind of decisions you want made and how you want them carried out, it asks you to name a medical power of attorney, health care proxy, or committee of person to make sure these decisions are followed. The document may have to be a durable or enduring type, which gives this person the right to make decisions when you cannot tell them to take over. Advance medical directives describe the circumstances under which you want your medical power of attorney to step in. It also describes the limits on that person's decision-making rights. These issues may also be part of legislation in your area—for instance, in your state you may need two physicians to say your husband cannot make his own decisions before you are legally able to start acting as his medical proxy. The advance medical directive may include the same information as a living will. Make sure you check with a lawyer to find out the legal terminology and the correct legal documents for where you live. You do not have to choose a family member to be your medical power of attorney, and you can have different people be your medical power of attorney and your financial power of attorney.

Issues that may be dealt with in advance medical directives include:

- Whom do you want to make decisions for you if you become disabled?
- Would you like a second person to make decisions for you? Whom?
- What kind of decisions do you want your representative to make (legal, financial, medical)? Do you want different people to make different ones?
- If there is a dispute in the family or between representatives, how do you want it settled?
- What process do you wish to be used to decide if you are disabled (physicians' or psychologists' assessments)?

- If you become disabled and are in a coma, what do you want (or not want) done? Artificial respiration? Feeding tubes? For how long?
- If you become disabled and your representative deems that you have a poor quality of life, and if you have a heart attack or stroke, do you want to be revived?
- How do you want someone to decide when to take you off life support?
- If you are disabled and are dying, what kind of care do you want? Comfort care and pain control only? Intensive care? Care at home? Do you want to be transferred to a hospital?
- If you are dying, do you want pain relief even if it reduces your alertness or makes you unaware?
- Do you want someone with you when you are dying? Whom?
- What kind of funeral and burial arrangements do you want?

DO NOT RESUSCITATE ORDERS

Do not resuscitate (DNR, or "no code") orders are instructions on your medical chart or in your will that guide the attending medical personnel not to perform CPR or otherwise try to revive you if you have had a heart attack, stroke, or other incident (for instance, a motor vehicle accident). It says that you want them to let you die naturally.

DEGREE OF INTERVENTION

You may hear the term "degree of intervention." This is a guide that allows you to choose, from among several options, what you want to happen if you become ill in a residence. The degree of intervention chosen should reflect what is in someone's advance directives. It often consists of four levels (or degrees):

Level 1: stay in the residence and be kept comfortable, but not be given antibiotics or other medications to cure you
Level 2: stay in the home and receive all medications and treatments possible within the home
Level 3: be transferred to a hospital but not given CPR or taken to intensive care

Level 4: be taken to a hospital and given all possible medical interventions.

The advantage to choosing level 1 or 2 is that they allow someone to die naturally in familiar surroundings.

Before or after admission, a nursing home (and perhaps an assisted living residence) will present you with documents that ask you to decide some if not all of these advance-directive-type questions. The home will use them as a guide in the provision of care. Any home receiving Medicaid or Medicare funding must inform you of your rights regarding advance directives. Make sure you discuss these issues carefully with them. A home that is religiously based may not be willing to carry out some of the wishes you have; they are supposed to tell you this.

There has been at least one case in the United States in which a home was successfully sued because they did not follow the advance directives that were set out in a resident's living will. However, it is important that you keep in mind that there are times when a decision must be made quickly by the staff, and it may not be black and white. Also, remember that the staff are *people;* that means that sometimes they may act from their own moral bias or from their hearts. Finally, remember that in assisted living residences, they may not have the staff or monitoring procedures to implement CPR.

Ideally, you and your husband will have talked about these questions previously. If not, do it now. You may want to have a family meeting in which anyone who has a stake is given some input. (See chapter 3, "Family Decision Making.") If you don't discuss these issues beforehand, you can end up in conflict later because different members of your family will have different feelings. It also saves you and your family from having to make painful decisions, because your husband has already told you what he wants. It gives you permission to do something that you might feel is too painful to do otherwise. For example, an advance directive can say that if your husband has dementia and develops pneumonia, he is to be kept in the home, given fluids, and kept comfortable only. That saves you from having to decide if he should be sent to the hospital and/or given intravenous antibiotics. He has already told you that he doesn't want that.

I once worked with the children of a woman who had had a stroke. They were trying to decide end-of-life issues. The daughter wanted her mother to be allowed to die in the nursing home with just comfort care. Her son wanted her to be brought to intensive care and to have everything possible done. His reason? Her estate wasn't settled in terms of power of attorney, and if she died before that was settled, it would be difficult to settle her estate. His concern was not what was best for his mother, it was for his inheritance.

Discussing advance directives can be as difficult as the decision for a loved one to move into a care facility. People do not like to talk about death. Use the same approach I discussed earlier, in the section "How to Talk about Care." Another approach is to say, "I'm afraid to make a decision you might not like," or "I'm afraid we will all fight about _____ if you don't give us instructions."

Make sure you understand the implications of the documents you sign and the decisions you make. For instance, if you have questions about the conditions under which a DNR order will not be carried out, ask. If you have signed a form saying that you don't want heroic measures, does that mean the nursing home will never transport your husband to a hospital?

The decisions you make now are usually reversible—you can always change your mind. However, documents that your husband has signed and are legally recognized may be irreversible, despite your wishes. The problem is that if you have not given any instructions or signed any documents that give the facility some guidance, the facility will probably do what it needs to do to protect itself legally. The home may err on the side of caution, but the decisions it makes may be different from what you or your husband would choose.

Check with your ombudsperson, health department, office on aging, Alzheimer Association, coalition for people with disabilities, or lawyer for the legally recognized advance directives form where you live. You can also use Aging with Dignity's Five Wishes document (www.fivewishes.org). This is recognized in most states and is widely distributed in the United States. You can view the document online, and it will give you an idea of what you need to cover.

Lydia Jean

It had been at least five years since I first suspected that my sister was losing her mental faculties. I live more than five hours' drive away, and we have no family members in the city where she lives. Lydia Jean was good at hiding her declining abilities. I believe some of her friends were unaware for a long time that anything was wrong. She didn't think she was getting old and objected when any family member suggested she go into a home where she would be well taken care of. Her response was always, "I can take care of myself."

No one could talk to Lydia Jean about her memory. She became angry and blamed others when she forgot things. She would claim that nobody had told her. She once complained that a niece had stolen her teacup. None of us was able to convince her otherwise. I found that cup, broken, carefully wrapped and hidden away. There were many of these instances. One time she told us that Tiny, her dog, came to visit her. But Tiny had died several years before. She was hallucinating, and I knew she was not taking any medication. Call it dementia or Alzheimer disease, the progressive stress made my life a torment as I tried to cope with the suspicions, anger, and obsessions that were obscuring the personality of my sister.

Finally she received a letter from the Motor Vehicle Department saying that because she was diagnosed with dementia, her license was revoked. She could not understand why, because she had never had an accident. She was unable to understand the meaning of dementia. She said she wouldn't drive but wanted the car to stay. We said okay, but she forgot and drove nearly every day. When the mental health worker phoned me and said the car had to be taken or they would take action themselves,

I had no alternative. Lydia Jean was bitter and I bore the brunt of her rage.

I had many sleepless nights wondering how I should handle the situation as her memory got worse and she got more frail. A concerned neighbor kept an eye on her, and one day found her in the bathtub unable to get out. She was cold and confused.

I knew she had to have someone with her twenty-four hours a day, but she would not allow this. Another sister came from out of town and stayed with her for months; at times she found Lydia Jean intolerable. She had to leave.

After that, Lydia Jean fell three times that I am aware of. The last time was outside in her empty carport. A friend was driving by and saw her lying on the cement and called an ambulance. She was taken to the hospital and diagnosed with a fractured hip. Under the circumstances, this was a blessing. After a lengthy stay in the hospital, she was transferred directly to a nursing home. They would not discharge her home. Finally, I knew she would be well taken care of.

Lydia Jean has been in the home more than six months now. She is adjusting well, no more eating alone and no more lonely evenings. I am not familiar with her medication, but it is calming her while not changing her personality. My nieces who live out of town went to see her. They took her back to her house for a visit, then out to lunch. They reported that they had never had a nicer visit with their Aunt Lydia Jean. She wanted to go back to her house after lunch, but they had no trouble returning her to the nursing home. When they told me that, it was the first time I had had a good feeling about her being in a nursing home. It helped convince me that the right decision had been made.

I love my sister, and it has been a painful process. I know she is too sick to be alone in her own home, and good care will improve the quality of her everyday life. I truly believe she is in a good care facility.

CHAPTER 3

Family Decision Making

Family Relationships and Care Decisions

It may be that more than one family member is involved in making the decision that your mother needs care. This can lead to a good deal of family stress or conflict. The conflict may be a continuation of ill will that has been overt or covert since long before Mother needed help. Often, however, conflict arises even in families in which relationships have been good.

I saw one family with an elderly father over a period of two years. Originally, I saw the oldest daughter, Miriam, who was the one who lived closest to her father in the city. She had one sister in the suburbs, a brother who lived a couple hundred kilometers north of the city, and a sister who lived even farther north. Miriam was the take-charge one, but she was burning out and frustrated with her siblings. She felt she could not go out of town or on vacation for more than a few days because no one was able to look after her father. They always depended on her for information, updates, and knowing what to do. A couple of months into my work with Miriam, the other siblings came into town, and we had a family meeting. The younger sister said that she wanted to help but felt that Miriam wouldn't trust her. "You always treat me like I can't do it." The other siblings were also willing to do what they could and come to town when necessary. They had different feelings about what should happen. The brother thought maybe a nursing home was best because of the strain on Miriam. Eventually, Miriam had to confront her own role and actions: a part of her didn't want to give in, didn't trust her siblings, and was afraid that if she left, her father would die. She found that if she wanted some relief, she had to open up, let her siblings help, and consider other options.

Miriam's family is not unusual. Conflict often arises because of family dynamics and family roles. Even though you all are adults, as soon as you have to start dealing with your siblings in a decision-making process, especially one in which your parent is involved, it is easy to revert back to behaviors and roles you used when you were children. The older sister becomes the older sister again, the younger brother becomes the baby again. This is a stressful and emotional situation for all of you. When we get into that kind of situation with people from our past, we tend to deal with them and the situation as we did in the past. We tend to act in this way because we have no other model to use.

You also may still be carrying around the feelings toward each other that you had when you were children. Although you don't like to admit it, maybe there is jealousy, maybe there are feelings of inadequacy, maybe you felt that Mom loved your brother best. (I've seen families in which each child thought Mom loved another one best. It was amazing how she had managed to divide all her children, setting them against each other for life, until they realized what she had done.)

Even though you are all going through the process of having Mom move into a residence, it does not mean that you are all emotionally resolving things at the same time. One of you may be ready; one of you may not be able to bear the fact that she is getting older. One of you may feel guilty; one of you may not. You have all had different relationships with your mother. You also all face different personal, work, and financial stresses. These differences will affect how you evaluate a situation and how you feel about it. They will have an impact on what you think should happen and when it should be done. It does not mean that any one of you is right or wrong. It means that you are different people with different lives.

When you are thinking about your family roles, also think about the current role that Mom is playing. Her role affects the rest of you. I dealt with a family with three adult children who were incredibly angry with each other. Each had an idea about what was best for their eighty-four-year-old mother. When one talked to her about it, she agreed with him. Then he would leave, and another would talk to Mom, and she would agree with that one. The mother had been a conflict avoider throughout her marriage, which is how she survived with a physically abusive husband. She was basically pitting her children against each other because she was afraid of hurting or disagreeing with them. The result was that her children ended up in conflict as they tried to figure out what was best for her, combined with their own needs, values, and issues.

Families in which one person lives out of town are particularly vulnerable to conflict (see chapter 15, "Out-of-Town Caregivers"). Your brother, living far away, may not realize Mother's true condition. When he comes into town to visit her, she will be able to rise to the occasion, hiding the extent of her disability or masking from him how much care she needs. Sometimes the out-of-town child (particularly if it is a son) is Mom's golden boy. She has idealized him, and they have a relationship that pairs them together, leaving the in-town caregiver outside. Or he may come into town, be involved for a weekend, then leave you to pick up the pieces. As he is involved for only a weekend, he does not experience the full burden of the caregiving process or the full scope of what is needed over the course of a month or so. So he can go home and think, "Where's the problem?" Despite his best intentions, this can leave you feeling angry with both him and your mother.

If you are the one in town, you may feel that you have more right to make a decision than your brother who lives out of town. After all, you are doing most of the work. You may be dismayed that he is calling you and giving suggestions. It may even feel like he is criticizing what you are doing. Whereas you want his support, you may feel that he is making things more difficult for you. You can end up feeling resentful. If you don't say anything, you can end up boiling for a long time.

How to Make Family Decisions

Caregiving and decisions about housing may call on you and your family members to work together, requiring ways to behave and communicate that are unfamiliar to you. It is like you are starting a business together, or you and colleagues have a new project or product to produce and launch. In your business or work setting, the decision-making process is already established and the roles are assigned. You are at the start of a long-term project. But in a family, this project arises out of family history and is developed haphazardly.

Step back and try to look at the structure of what you are doing, the "big picture." Identify the patterns and actions you are all taking and try to verbalize them and how they are functioning. As early as possible in the caregiving process, everybody who is involved should define roles by deciding who will do what. This includes what out-of-town siblings will do. List the tasks and divide them up. The earlier you are able to develop a system that works for all of you, the easier it will be.

If you are the primary caregiver, begin keeping a journal such as the "Event and Action Log" in appendix 2. Describe the process of decline and record the things that your mother has done that indicate her need for care. Also record the tasks you perform as the caregiver. Include the doctor's visits, phone calls, shopping, and so on. You are not doing this to score points with the others. You are doing it so that they have a clear understanding of what is happening with your mother, what her needs are, and what your role has been.

When keeping a journal, making decisions, carrying out caregiving responsibilities, you may want to use online help, such as www.myfamily.com or www.carepages.com, or a private blog through a site such as www.blogger.com. This way, everyone always has access to what has happened and who has done what. You can keep anything you want on this site—changes of medications, what happened in a visit to the nursing home, when you bought shirts and underwear. It will give everyone a true picture, and they can add what they wish through comments on the site. If you want to go any further with technology, you can set up an online webcam that the others can watch. This raises privacy issues about your mother, but it can help to give family members an objective picture of what is happening.

It may help if the out-of-town relative takes care of your mother for a couple of weeks or up to a month. Even if Mom can hide her condition for a while, she probably will not be able to do so for more than ten days. This gives him an opportunity to go through her cycle of care needs. Once he has had that experience, there is a common framework for understanding and planning.

Also, be clear about what everybody expects from his or her contribution. If you expect to be given the family house in exchange for living with Mom and taking care of her, everybody else should know that. If your out-of-town sister is contributing money and expects to get it back from the inheritance, you should know this now. Depending on the circumstances, you may want to write up what is called a private-care agreement that is binding to all of you. This sets up who is doing what and what each person will receive for it. Remember, too, that there may be provisions in your mother's will for the dispersal of effects and property, which have to be kept in mind when making these agreements.

Family Meetings

Often it is helpful to have a formal family meeting to discuss the caregiving situation. The type of meeting you have and who will be there may vary according to where you are in the caregiving process, how you are already dealing with each other, and where Mom is in her ability to participate.

You may want to have a more or less formal meeting. If you are beginning to look at more complex issues such as finances and housing, it may be more formal; if you are looking at who does what, it could be less formal.

A formal meeting has several advantages. It allows you to go through issues in an orderly and concrete manner. It will help you do some good planning and review. It can help clear up misunderstandings. If there are a few people involved, it will decrease the need for Tom to call Gladys, who will call Fred, who will call Tom, who will then do such and such, which ends up not being what Gladys thought was going to happen. If you do decide on a formal meeting, these points may help:

1. Have it in a neutral place.
2. Come prepared. Bring the documents and information you will need.

3. If your mother is not going to be there, someone should ask her about what she would like regarding the issues to be discussed.
4. Make up an agenda.
5. Set some goals, such as defining the problems, finding resources, or coming up with solutions.
6. If there is a lot to discuss, schedule several meetings, rather than pushing yourselves to finish everything at once. It is better to have several meetings when people are not pressed for time to finish or feeling exhausted.
7. Start with some basic rules for good communication, below.
8. Remember to keep the focus on your mother.
9. This discussion is not the place or time to work out your own relationships.
10. Take minutes or notes.

If you get stuck, you might want to back off and have a discussion about your family and how it has functioned in the past. What was your family like as you were growing up? Discuss the roles you think you played. See if you can verbalize the family rules. (See an explanation of the concept of family rules in chapter 4 under "Adult Children.") Look at the communication patterns in the family. See how parental relationships affected you all. This kind of discussion can help you understand each other better and move forward when you are stuck. It might bring you all closer.

It may help to remember that sometimes people come into conflict because they have different goals, positions, or agendas. But underneath these are people's needs, wants, and fears. To move beyond conflict, you need to find the common interests—the needs, wants, fears that are creating them. The way to accomplish this is through basic and good communication techniques; using them will aid you enormously to have a successful meeting. They are the skills of empathy and listening.

Good empathy and listening can be difficult when it is your family and you have different needs, wants, and fears. Listening means suspending what *you* need, want, or fear, to focus on *your brother's* needs, wants, and fears. It means biting your tongue when you want to say, "Yeah, but . . . " If you do that, you will be able to understand him. Tell him what you heard by reflecting back what he said. Try to tell him you heard those needs, wants, and fears. The only way you and he both know you have heard is to keep trying until he says you got it. You should all have a turn to speak and be understood. A good meeting agenda will state a problem that takes in everyone's needs. An optimal outcome finds a way to meet as many as possible.

Basic rules for good communication in a meeting are:

1. When talking about yourself, start with something like "I always thought," or "It looked to me that."
2. When talking about others, use a question: "What did it look like to you?"
3. Do not tell anyone else what his or her experience was growing up.
4. Understand that each person is talking about what it was like for them. This does not mean they are right or wrong. They are describing what life looked like for them.
5. Don't interrupt. Listen to *all* of what someone is saying. When we become upset or stressed, it is easy to interrupt and jump in.
6. Wait five seconds before you start talking.
7. Show you understand by repeating back the ideas and feelings others have stated.
8. Before moving on to the next topic, ask if there is anything more to be discussed about the current topic.
9. Stick to the present.
10. Keep to the facts of your mother's situation.

You may want to hire an outside mediator of some kind to help run your meeting, especially if you anticipate some conflict. Someone who is not emotionally involved can help to keep you on track and resolve or contain the conflict. Having a family meeting is not something most people are used to doing; this alone can be stressful. You can choose a family therapist or a geriatric care manager (see chapter 15, "Out-of-Town Caregivers") who is experienced in dealing with these issues. A good mediator will help you all come up with decisions and talk to each other by focusing on interests and not on outcomes. A good mediator will have experience dealing with families and groups. The money you spend will be worth it if you end up saving your family relationships. A geriatric care manager will also be experienced and knowledgeable about geriatrics and services in your area. When you are trying to make decisions, this knowledge will be invaluable.

One of the goals in a family meeting may be to understand what everyone is thinking and feeling about the current situation. (This is different from working out your relationships.) The first thing that you may want to put on the agenda is a round robin in which everybody has a chance to say what it is like for him or her. What are they feeling as they watch Mom decline? How are the tasks that they are doing affecting them? How is it affecting their spouses and children? How does it feel to be an out-of-town relative while someone else is more involved?

Remember the communication techniques. The task for everyone who is not talking is to listen. Wait for everybody to have a turn. At the end, there should be no comments, arguments, or crosstalk. There should be no attempt to talk someone out of what she is thinking or feeling. She is not right or wrong; it is what is true for her. This part of the discussion is also not about winning, it is about understanding. You are not contestants on "Queen for a Day," where the best of the bad luck stories wins the new washing machine. If you are all trying to win, you all lose.

Make sure you put finances on the family conference agenda. Does everybody know what the financial situation is, where assets and finances are, and what is available to be spent on care? Does everyone agree on how finances should be handled? If finances are a "hot topic" in your family, you may want to have a separate meeting to make decisions about them.

If there is conflict around money, it is especially important for everyone to have an understanding of your mother's diagnosis and where a disease or disability is leading. Everyone should also understand the costs of responding to the disease and of care. This knowledge can lead to a natural decision on finances.

In the end, if you can't reach an agreement on finances, maybe the best answer will be a trustee from the bank who can oversee money issues as they relate to care. A trustee costs money, but this solution ensures that finances will be handled fairly by a neutral party for the benefit of Mother first.

There is nothing wrong with wanting an inheritance. I know we all say we shouldn't count our chickens before they hatch. However, if you have been promised something or have known that there is a certain amount of money in the family and then find it is not going to be there for you, that can be a disappointment. Feeling disappointed or resentful may not feel "right" to you, but many people experience those feelings even though they won't admit it. What is not acceptable is when the feelings translate into adverse actions. It is not all right to deny care or opt for a lower standard of care because you want an inheritance or because you have debts to pay off. That is financial abuse.

Make sure that you feel comfortable with the agreements you make and that the rules are fair. If you do not feel that way, try to identify why not and continue problem solving until you do feel the decisions are fair. Remember to watch out for the family dynamics. If someone is acting as the older sister and not as an equal, bring that up and see if you can work around it. She may have unintentionally slipped into her role as easily as you might into yours (but it is easier to see when she does it than to recognize when you are). Be aware of yourself as well, your feelings and sense of self. Even though she is the older sister, she may still be right. Give yourselves time to work things out. If you have to have several meetings, allow yourselves to do so.

Finally, remember to keep your eye on the ball (or, in this case, your mother). She is the one who is important here. Remind yourself that what is best for her is the solution you are looking for. That is how everyone wins the washing machine.

At the end of your discussion, everybody should be able to write down what he or she is doing and why it is best for your mother. Everyone should also write down what he is giving, what he expects back, and in what form or amount he expects it. Compare what you have written. From this you can develop a single document that will be a clear contract. Make sure that you feel comfortable with the document and that it is fair. If you don't, don't sign it.

Your written agreement may be an evolving document. As Mom becomes more disabled, there will be new tasks that need to be taken care of. Problems that you hadn't thought of can arise, and the document may need to be revised. There may also be changes in the circumstances of those who are party to the agreement. Review it once a year or once every six months.

Keep Your Relative Involved

Inherent in caregiving is the gradual taking on of tasks and responsibilities that your loved one has always done for themselves, or at least directed for themselves. So in some way, caregiving is a process of change in independence. Independence is often not about doing—it is about deciding about the doing. For this reason, to every extent possible, the care receiver (especially if it is a younger person) should be actively involved in arranging or knowing about the arrangements that are being made around her. If she is not, anything that is decided can meet with additional resistance as she tries to maintain her sense of control, pride, and self-worth.

The earlier in the caregiving process you begin to have meetings, the more your mother will be essentially directing the meeting. With assisted living becoming a more and more common option, this means you have to have meetings earlier. You are not deciding between home and a nursing home, you are deciding among a number and range of options.

Keeping your mother involved means giving her the opportunity to understand what things are like for you and what the future can look like. It may mean telling her that you are calling your brother who is out of town to ask him to do some of the things you have been doing. It may mean explaining that you cannot do all the cooking you have been doing. Your mother will need to understand why the circumstances are changing.

You will need to stand firm, especially if she asks you if she is becoming too much of a burden or if you do not want to bother anymore. Keep track of your "guilt meter." It can go over the top and make you back down. This can result in more resentment, exhaustion, and, ultimately, earlier admission of your relative to care.

Your mother can be involved in a family meeting whether it is informal or formal. If her cognitive impairment is more progressed, she might not understand all the issues but will be able to sit in on the meetings that she will understand. If it doesn't work out, then you can schedule a separate meeting without her. If she is in the meeting, make sure things are worded so that she understands that she is not the problem; the problem is the situation. This is another instance in which it can be helpful to have a professional involved. He or she will help moderate the emotions and can act as an advocate for your mother so she does not feel ganged up on.

If your mother has dementia, she may still be able to accurately tell you what she wants or what is important to her. Dementia is about more than loss of memory. It is about loss of reasoning, or judgment, or planning, or expressive ability, and more. She may have capability in one area, but not in others, so everyone will need to be aware of what her abilities are. Her abilities can also vary due to other factors (see chapter 11, "Settling In").

Mary

The constant and intense nature of Mom's behavior finally made me aware that life was becoming difficult for her. My concerns had already been growing: for her safety, her inability to prepare meals, the danger of kitchen fires, her vulnerability to theft and mugging, her inability to handle medications. I was receiving repeated worried phone calls from her throughout the night.

Mom's obsession with bowel movements finally resulted in her referral to the university Alzheimer clinic. My sister Faye came to the coast to be with us for the tests. After they were finished, the doctor, a kind and compassionate man, assured Mom that she was healthy and had performed the puzzle tests very well. In private he told Faye and me that there was no evidence of stroke or accidental trauma to the brain, so in all likelihood Mom had Alzheimer disease.

We were to do the following immediately: arrange for power of attorney, prevent Mom from driving her car, and put her in a safer living environment. We were not to tell her she had Alzheimer disease, correct her mistakes, or argue with her. We were to try to prevent confusion as much as possible.

Power of attorney was surprisingly easy to obtain. Faye and I calmly approached Mom on the premise of being able to look after her affairs if she ever needed our help. The first two attempts were met with a definite "No." The next day Mom was more agreeable, so off we went to see a lawyer. I'll always remember the guilt I felt when I signed my name on the power of attorney form.

Then came the letter from the Motor Vehicle Division requesting that she appear for a driving test. She failed but was given a learner's license.

She drove on her own anyway! We were finally able to get her to stop driving by taking her car in for servicing. We delayed returning it for as long as possible.

This time in our relationship can be described only as ugly. Mom was livid about the car. Her accusations of theft and her threats to commit suicide, to involve police, and to buy another car were relentless.

Her threat to buy another car opened up a new worry. We appealed to her bank to curtail her withdrawals. They were sympathetic but would agree only to red flag her account. I would be contacted if a large amount of money was being withdrawn—but they reminded me that it was her money. To take more drastic action, I needed to get a committeeship. Then I would have the legal right to control her finances. So we began our expensive visits to a lawyer to declare my mother mentally incompetent.

The Health Department became involved with us when Mom was diagnosed with Alzheimer disease. The caseworker assessed Mom in June. She advised us that Mom needed more structure to her days but was basically managing well on her own. We got her a companion and found her an adult day center to go to a couple days a week.

During that summer I took the caregivers course put on by the Alzheimer Society. This was invaluable. I now realized why Mom acted as she did. I was given strategies to ease Mom's agitation and, for the first time, I was given a clear picture of where we were heading with Mom. They said it was imperative that she be placed on a waiting list for nursing home care immediately.

We set out to find a room that would please Mom. We toured several homes, each one being met with great resistance from her. She repeatedly told us, "I have no intention of moving. I am perfectly safe and happy where I am." But I eventually got her name on a list.

This was the first time that Mom had let us see her account books. It was probably the clearest picture I had that her disease was progressing. It also showed me what a struggle Mom was having. I realized it was only a matter of time before I'd have to assume full control of her financial affairs.

Finally there came a time when I knew I was no longer going to be able to supervise Mom's daily routines. Every Sunday she came for a visit and dinner. Every time I would have a good ten-minute cry after Mom returned home in the evening.

The moment we'd been both waiting for and dreading finally arrived. Mom was to go to Bayview Manor Center. We chose a day when she would be at her day care. My husband and I went to her apartment in the morning to pack and label her necessities. We gathered a few treasures to help her like her new home, such as her comforter, a TV, and a cozy chair. We took these to Bayview and got her room ready.

Mom's companion picked her up at the day care and brought her to Bayview at 1:30 in the afternoon. The companion said her good-byes and the staff took over.

Mom was most anxious. She knew what we were up to and she knew she was powerless to stop us. We took her to her room and pointed out her clothes, her dresser, her chair, and her TV. We told her she would stay there only until I returned from summer holidays.

Mom was not to be dissuaded. She paced the floor. She ripped her name off the door. She shouted.

I will never forget Mom's phone calls and her constant attempts to escape in the beginning. She'd try every door and gate. Finally she turned to me and said, "This is a terrible thing you did to me."

I still dream about that first day. But then I only have to think about the next day when Faye and I packed up her apartment to realize it was the only thing—and the best thing—that we could do for Mom. I had had no idea about the kind of filth Mom had been living in. Envelopes of uncooked rolled oats were stashed all over the place. There were bugs everywhere. Mom had been the most fastidious person I knew. To see that she had been living in such filthy conditions was heart wrenching.

I view the first year that Mom was in Bayview as a time of adjustment for both of us. Her TV became a problem, so we took it home. She had lost the ability to concentrate, anyway. She insisted on wearing glasses that were the wrong prescription. They were weak and, as she no longer read, I realized it didn't matter that they were not the proper ones.

Bayview did its best to make families welcome, but it's hard to feel like a family when you have no living room setting in which to socialize. But a living room was our way of socializing, not Mom's. We slowly accepted it.

I've had to learn how to visit. I worry about Mom's jealousy and possessiveness with me and the other residents. She becomes angry and vocal if I socialize with them. I am constantly trying to think of things I can do with her. She can no longer visit, so we must be where there are distractions to comment on. I realize that, to be successful, everything must be done in short intervals: half-hour car drives, short-order restaurants, picnic lunches, and outings for an ice cream.

Mom is content just to walk the halls at Bayview—up and down, around and around. I have tried crocheting, playing cards, crossword puzzles, photo albums (all things she used to love), but found these activities bothered her, so I try something else. The important thing is to keep trying.

The most difficult part of visiting is saying good-bye. Rarely does Mom say good-bye without putting up a fuss. She wants to come home with me. I find it helps to reassure her that I'll be back in a couple of days. "Give me a kiss, Mom. I must go." Then I turn around and leave. It's difficult; I won't pretend that it isn't. I have no easy solutions.

I am losing my mother. Every month this loss becomes more apparent, and I have to attempt to replace her in my own memories to make the pictures of my family fit.

My greatest comfort is knowing that Mom is safe. She is cared for by knowledgeable and compassionate staff members. Programs are numerous, especially music therapy, art therapy, and look good/feel good programs. I appreciate the coordinated effort of many: the social worker, administrator, program coordinators, nurses, and nurse's aides. I am made to feel that they care about her and that her needs are special.

Through all of this, my sister Faye, although living a great distance away, was an immense help with Mom. We were always in complete agreement as to Mom's diagnosis and care. Faye, too, joined the Alzheimer Society. We phoned each other at least once a week. She flew out to be with me on the tough days. Family support was so important because it helped me share my guilt.

Joining the Alzheimer Society and taking the caregivers course were essential. They matter-of-factly talk about the disease and let you know where you are now and show you where you are headed. They offer strategies to cope with your loved one's needs. They discuss your individual situation and advise you on not only what must be done but also how to go about doing it.

I found that my feelings of isolation diminished when I talked to others. I would advise other people in this situation to find someone who has been a caregiver or is going through similar experiences. Friends who do not share your experiences can be of only limited help. They don't understand the depth of the disease, the constant worry, and the ever-changing and ever-present challenges. You think you've conquered one hurdle, only to come up against another.

I had to learn that my feelings of guilt are normal. I was making decisions for her that caused everyone much distress. I often worried, "How do I know this is the right decision?" I kept a diary and recorded unpleasant incidents and also the accompanying emotions. I had a desk calendar on which I recorded every contact that had been made with Mom that day. This record keeping allowed me to transfer my feelings to paper. It also showed me how increasingly dependent and frightened Mom was becoming. It helped ease my guilt because I could see how we had no choice.

Life goes on. I am coping no longer as a caregiver but once again as a daughter. Believe me, this is much easier.

CHAPTER 4

Guilt, Loss, and Grief

For many people, one of the hardest things they have ever done is walk out of the nursing home on admission day and leave behind their loved one. They will never forget saying good-bye at the door, turning their back, and walking away. It is the culmination of a turmoil of emotions they have been feeling for many months or even years. Chief among those are often shame and guilt. Mixed with the shame and guilt, however, are many other emotions: fear, anxiety, confusion, anger, resentment, sadness, and grief. This chapter discusses guilt, grief, and loss separately because they are about your relationship. The fear, anxiety, and confusion often relate more to the home and what will happen there. They are covered in chapter 10, "Moving Day."

It is often easier for families, as well as Mom or Dad, when the housing being chosen is assisted living. There is less guilt for family members because assisted living units often look like small apartments, and people have more independence and usually more choice about going in. They often can go in as a couple too. However, there is still grief and loss, and it can be sad; there may still be high anxiety.

What Is Guilt?

"Every time I think about my mother needing to be in a nursing home," one of my clients once said to me, "I think about how I promised my father before he died I would always take care of her. If I put her in a nursing home, I would be letting him down."

Guilt is like a little voice in our heads. It tells us how we should act and behave and criticizes what we have done. It is the voice of standards that we have set for ourselves or, sometimes, that we think society has set. Sometimes it is the standard that our parents have set. Sometimes it is our fears about how other people will think about us. Guilt is your inner voice (or that of people in your social group or family) criticizing you for putting a family member in a home. In a sense, guilt tells us that we are letting ourselves down.

Sometimes guilt serves a positive purpose. Think about what a society would look like without guilt (for me it would be a lot of chocolate cake and several extra pounds). It would be a world where people had little consideration for others. Guilt gives us the opportunity to go back, look at, and review or take responsibility for what we have done or said. However, with caregivers, I am going to assume that you do not need to review your actions yet once more. Most of you have hung on a long time and run the same racecourse too many times. I think that if you really feel the need to review something, you could watch some reruns on television.

One of the problems with guilt is that it leads to shame. Shame is the voice that talks to us about who we are. It is often the eruption of beliefs we have about ourselves, with which we grew up. Shame is incredibly destructive, more so than guilt. It destroys the possibility of feeling good about yourself. For example, if you "put" your husband in a nursing home, the message can become, "There is something wrong with me." It defines you as a defective or weak person. The belief blocks your ability to listen to a reasoning voice, either your own or that of someone else who tries to help you see yourself or your situation differently. It is as though you see the sky as red and everyone else sees it as blue. You "know" the truth because you can see it, and no one can convince you otherwise.

In a more humorous vein, think of guilt and shame as your conscience on steroids. Your conscience is that part of your personality that is useful and necessary to help you live a moral and ethical life. But when it becomes unresolvable guilt, it has ballooned out of proportion and gotten way out of control. When it becomes shame, it convicts you. If guilt is the jailor, shame is the jail.

No matter where they come from, in the end, the guilt and shame that we feel are something that we do to ourselves. No one can make us feel guilty. Someone can apply pressure, but ultimately, it is our voice, our belief, our judgment. The bad news about this is that we are often much harder on ourselves than anyone else is on us. The good news is that because we make ourselves feel guilty, we don't have to depend on anyone else to forgive us. Because shame is our belief, we can change it.

Conflicts That Give Rise to Guilt

No matter where your mother is in the process of moving, you may feel that you are abandoning, or have abandoned, her. You may see her as being at her most vulnerable, and yourself as the one who has protected and taken care of her when she became less and less able to do so for herself. You may begin to question yourself and who you are. "If I were stronger," "If I were willing to _____." Along with that may start to come the shoulds: "I should have waited longer," "I should have been stronger." When the guilt becomes strong, you may start to blame other people: "If my brother/sister were around to help more often," "If the doctor had ordered more home support for her, . . . " When you are having these feelings, look underneath to see what else is going on. Often there are feelings of helplessness or failure: "If only I were different, then this would not be happening." These are the messages that you use to convince yourself that something is wrong with you—the shame messages. Don't blame yourself; there is nothing wrong or defective about you. It is not your fault that she is sick or disabled. At the same time, the blaming guilt can be focused outward at a sibling who has not supported you or your mother, or at your father for being too selfish. Be ready to understand this blaming and anger as the same pain of loss.

You may have always thought of yourself as a strong person. To place your mother in a nursing home proves to you at some level that you are weak. This sets you up for a powerful conflict: if I am so strong, what does it mean if I do something that means I am weak? This makes you an awfully harsh judge of yourself. Even strong people are allowed to say that they cannot do something or do not want to do it anymore. That doesn't take away your strength; it allows you to be realistic by acknowledging your limits. Sometimes it takes more strength to set limits for yourself than to give in to guilt. It is okay to say no.

I remember one man I talked with who had placed his wife in a nursing home. He had resolved to be strong until the end when she was first diagnosed with Alzheimer disease. But as the years went on, he was becoming overburdened. His children were all telling him he had to place her, because it was becoming too much for him and he couldn't keep doing it. I told him that I disagreed with his children; I thought he could have kept on going. He looked at me, startled that I would say that. Then I said, "But what would it cost you?" He looked at me for a minute, and then he understood.

After placement, you may feel a great sense of relief. Even the relief can lead to some guilt. It is almost as though you are thinking, "If I really cared, I wouldn't be feeling relief. This must mean I don't care enough." (Isn't it interesting what we go through to make ourselves miserable?) It is okay to feel relief from a burden. It does not mean that you love your mother any less. You can love her and not want to keep doing what you have been doing. People sometimes have conflicting feelings at the same time.

Families and Guilt

Sometimes husbands and wives have an especially hard time. "I married him 'for better or for worse, in sickness and in health, till death do us part' and now I am doing this to him." It is helpful to remember that most of the time, this is not something you want to do. Think about what you would do if your spouse had a terminal disease. If he would be better off in a hospital, would you keep him at home? Probably not. Placing him in a nursing home when you are not able to provide the care he needs is no different. You are not abandoning him, you are choosing care for him.

Husbands and wives can also see their situation as one of having to choose between themselves and their partner. Placing your spouse may feel like you are choosing yourself over him, leading you to label yourself as selfish. "Selfish" is a word dripping with judgment; but what it means is "about the self." There is good selfish and bad selfish. By the time you are seeking placement, you probably have been putting your husband first for a long time. Nowhere does it say that you need to exhaust yourself or impair your health in your role as spouse or caregiver.

Another man who came to me one day had been his wife's caregiver for many years. He was worn out from watching her and not sleeping or eating well himself, but he could not bring himself to bring her into care. He was wracked by the fear of abandoning her (and his fear of being alone). He was also wracked by guilt because he felt he should be bringing her into care. I finally suggested to him that if he chose to kill himself being his wife's caregiver, he should make some good plans for her for when he was gone because then there would be no one for her.

For many women of the generation that is now seeking care, it was the husband who made the family decisions. For them to make the decision that their husband has to go into care can be frightening because they are not used to making big decisions. They may not have the confidence in themselves to make such a decision. They may feel that they are doing something wrong, and that they are taking over from their husbands. It is one more painful piece of evidence of the changes in him and their relationship that they are being forced to acknowledge.

Almost harder still is the placement decision for younger people. If you are in your thirties or forties, there is no role model because it is a relatively infrequent occurrence. There is often no appropriate residence for your husband. It may also mean that you are placing the father of young children and are facing explaining to them why Daddy has to go live somewhere else. Underneath all of that, you, like your husband, may be struggling with anger and resentment at having "this" happen to you. The difference is that you also have the guilt about placement and then guilt about your anger and resentment, and no support for expressing it. I can tell you these feelings are common.

Adult Children

If you are an adult child who is a caregiver, you are probably painfully aware of experiencing the difficult and anxiety-producing "role reversal." You feel it when your father is no longer able or willing to make decisions for himself. You have to tell him to see the doctor, which bills to pay this month, when to change his clothes, and what to eat. Finally you may end up having to tell your father that he needs to go to a home. The person who was always strong and capable and there for you now needs to be taken care of. It is a little like a death. Making decisions for your father is a clear indication to you that the person you loved is, in some ways, gone.

I would suggest that you are not "parenting your parent." It may *feel* like you are. This is often the expression that is used in the media. But your parent is not a child. He is someone with a disability. You are the caregiver for someone with a disability. The difference is that this says to you that you are both still adults.

Whatever we call the situation, a change in behavior between parent and child is hard because we grow up with what are called family rules. These are the guidelines that taught us how we behave with each other: who says what to whom, who makes decisions, how we talk to each other, what we talk about. In some families, for example, the rules can be "We don't talk about sex," or "Nobody criticizes Dad." The rules are usually unspoken and learned since childhood. They feel natural and normal; we don't even realize that they are there, governing our behavior. (One way to understand your family rules is to compare the behavior in your family to the behavior in the family of your spouse or friends.) When you can no longer handle the caregiving and must tell your father what needs to happen, you are breaking the rule: "We do not tell our parents what to do, or set limits with our parents." It feels wrong and uncomfortable.

Sometimes the rules must change because the circumstances change. Although telling your father what is best does not feel comfortable to you, that does not mean that it is wrong or you should not be doing it. It means that the behavior feels different. Like any new habit or behavior, it takes time to learn it, and it may never become comfortable.

For some children, guilt, shame, and the feeling that they are abandoning their father are worse because they promised that they would never put him in a nursing home. He may have remembered doing that to his mother or father. The terror of what those older homes were like was something he never got over. You think to yourself, "I promised him I would never do this. It was his worst fear and now I am making it come true."

You may feel that your father took care of you when you needed him. You look at yourself and feel like an ogre of some sort because you are "refusing" to take care of him. This is especially true in the split between immigrant parents and first-generation children, for whom the cultural values of the old country still have a hold on both generations. In some ways, cultural values are like family rules on a larger scale. They are equally or more powerful, because often there is a community that is involved. Everyone in the community will know what your father's children "did" to him. What your father and the others learned in the old country—children take care of their elderly parents—and therefore what is expected of you, is somewhere in the back of his mind. It is unfair of you to compare yourself to your father, to your father's country, or to that culture. Yet he may be doing that and you may be feeling the pull. It is also perhaps unfair that the community holds onto the same, but they do, and every time you go to the church or synagogue or mosque, you may feel the elders looking at you.

If you are an only child or a spouse or partner with no children, the guilt can be especially hard because there is no one to share the decision-making process with you. Friends can help and they can listen, but you are the one with the emotional attachment. You are also the one with the responsibility. If something goes wrong, you see yourself as the one and only person responsible for what happened. Much of your decision-making process happens in your mind and in discussion with yourself. This makes it easier to be hard on yourself. There is no one around to help you put limits on your self-criticism or pull you out of it. Internal dialogue like this can make you feel crazy, and it is fertile soil for your conscience on steroids.

Guilt, Culture, and Society Today

At a general level, you as a caregiver are dealing with the many cultural and social changes that have occurred in the last sixty years.

First, today less support is available from extended families—brothers and sisters are separated, children move out of town. Second, more women are working outside of the home, so do not have the time to assume the role of caregiver in the way that they may have done in the past. Third, society is more transient, so there is less support from informal sources such as neighbors and friends. Also, people are living longer with more frailties. They need more care, have more complicated needs, and need care longer. The result of these changes is that people can no longer look after elderly relatives the way families used to. Both the options available and the pressures on you are different from the ones that were present years ago. The needs have changed, but the cultural values change more slowly. This creates the gap between what you think should be possible and what is actually possible. This gap is a partial instigator of the guilt and shame.

When Guilt Has Other Purposes in Your Life

I once admitted a woman to a nursing home whose son and daughter-in-law had cared for her at home for ten years. The daughter-in-law especially was wracked with guilt and shame. Their background included an unhappy marriage and a small, closely knit Christian community. Keeping the mother at home had served to help the couple avoid the problems in their marriage and bring them admiration from the community for their "sacrifices." Putting her in care meant that they had to face their marriage and lose the admiration.

Sometimes guilt and shame serve a psychological purpose. Although they are painful, they tell us and everybody else that we care. Without them, it may look to us or to others as though we are cold and uncaring. Other people at some level want the admiration that comes for all their hard work. You need to accept that you do care or that placement was necessary. Nobody knows your situation better than you do. Others are not living with it in the present, and they did not live with it in the past.

Guilt can also sometimes be a signal about something deeper. Sometimes guilt is not about the actual event or decision about placement in seniors housing, it is about something that happened long ago. You may need some help in sorting through issues of shame and guilt. If you do, you can talk to the social worker in the facility (if he or she has time) or ask for a referral for private counseling.

Not All Relationships Were Ideal

I had a very wealthy client a couple of years ago with three daughters, none of whom were involved in helping him in a consistent manner. He was a strong-minded but open man who shared a lot of his pain with me. I liked him very much. But it was only after a chance meeting with his grandson that I learned how abusive he had been to his daughters as they were growing up. Then I understood how remarkable it was that they were there at all when he had a health crisis.

Not all marriages were happy and loving, and many children did not have supportive, loving parents. To end up being a caregiver for someone with whom you did not have a good relationship or who was abusive may divide you between doing what you feel is your duty and doing what you would like to do. That is, part of you tells yourself that you should be the caregiver, and part of you says that you shouldn't have to have anything to do with this person. As I mentioned above, a part of you is angry and resentful at what you have had to put up with in your life from your spouse or parent. A part of you wants to tell this person to go to hell, and a part of you may see a frail and pitiful old man. You may tilt back and forth, pulling yourself two ways. The anger and resentment are normal and common feelings but may make you question why you are placing your relative in a home. The guilt you feel can help you mask or handle feelings of anger and resentment, powerful feelings that make you wonder if you love your mother or husband. For those of you in this situation, placement becomes even harder.

Despite your anger, resentment, and bitterness, you can still have legitimate reasons for seeking care for your parent or spouse. You have a right to set your own limits. You have a right to your life. You may be considering care earlier than someone who had a close relationship with their family member might. In some ways, it helps to think of relationships as being like bank accounts. Over the years, we make withdrawals and deposits. Emotional deposits are the love, caring, and support we have given. Withdrawals are hurts, abuse, neglect, or lies. All relationships are made up of both withdrawals and deposits. In some relationships, withdrawals are larger and more frequent, in others deposits are. If your relationship is in a deficit balance, it will affect your ability to be a caregiver. Caregivers who have had a loving relationship with their spouse or parent generally have money in the emotional bank, which contributes to what we could call emotional stamina.

Emotional stamina is the ability you have to cope with stress. It is personal and individual. That is why you cannot compare yourself to others to prove to yourself that you should not be placing Dad in care. When the relationship previous to the caregiving situation was good, emotional stamina can be stronger. The love, caring, shared experiences, trust, and respect that you built created strong bonds and commitment. When those things did not happen, less of a bond was built.

Emotional stamina is complicated. It depends on internal strengths; some people handle stress better than others. It also depends on external situations, the pressures on you. Maybe you have growing children; maybe you have your own health problem. You may have a job that demands too much of your time. If your external situation is stressful or demanding, fewer emotional resources are available for the added burden of caregiving.

For many people, emotional stamina depends on the extent of their social or family support network. You may be a sole caregiver or the only one of three children who is involved with your father, as opposed to a family in which all the children are sharing a burden equally. If you receive less support, you may be able to give less support.

Beyond the differences in emotional stamina, there are also differences in caregiving situations. Even though two people may have cared for their mothers for the same length of time, the needs of the two mothers may be very different. One may be wandering out of the house and the other may be afraid to walk out the door. One may be incontinent but sleeping and the other may be continent but not sleeping. Don't compare yourself to someone else; you cannot really know what he or she is going through.

Not everyone experiences guilt or shame when she has to place a relative. (Please don't feel guilty about not having guilt.) This may be because it was the relative's choice to enter a facility. She may have been lucky enough to have had conversations with the relative before the need arose in which she got emotional permission for placement. Or she may just be able to realize and accept that she has done all she can do for her relative.

Some people do not experience caregiving as a burden. For whatever reason, they experience it as a special time and part of the relationship that they have had. Not that they would have chosen it, but they can take it as a gift that is both bitter and meaningful. I remember one man who told me he had cared for his father in his home for three years before the father died at age ninety-three. "It was hard," he told me, "because we had never gotten along. But we grew closer, and now I would not have traded that opportunity for anything." It does not mean that someone is somehow "better" or stronger than you because you experience the caregiving as too great a burden. It is all right for you to decide for yourself when you cannot do it anymore. You do not have to apologize to anyone. It also does not mean that you are less of a caregiver; you aren't. It doesn't mean you love your wife less than someone else loves theirs. But, as I said in chapter 1, you are allowing the role to change.

Guilt and Dementia

Even though it is ultimately you who has to forgive yourself for your actions, people often tend to ask for forgiveness from someone else, usually from the person who has been "harmed." When your father with dementia is angry with you for suggesting that he needs to move or when you visit him and he is angry with you for leaving him, you may find yourself trying to explain over and over again why things are the way they are. Don't try to reason with him or make him understand. Don't try to seek his forgiveness. One of the effects of dementia is that people lose what is called executive function—the ability to plan and reason, for example. *Your father is not able to reason things out, he doesn't have the capacity to forgive you.* Agree with your father, tell him it is not fair, then change the subject or drop it and don't say anything. It will be hard for him to argue with someone who isn't going to argue back. He is right: it is not fair, for either of you. If you continue to disagree, explain, or ask for forgiveness, you will be on a treadmill, unable to get off. If his reasoning and understanding are not intact, you need to turn somewhere else to ask for forgiveness.

The truth is that you may be a better caregiver after your father has gone into care than in some of the time preceding. You will not have the anger or resentment or frustration. You will be getting a full night's sleep. You will not have the fear of a telephone call that Dad has fallen and cannot get up. Assuming he is in a good home, you will know that he is clean, not wearing clothes soiled from urine, taking medication as it has been prescribed, and eating three meals a day. When you don't have these worries or feelings, you can have a better relationship with your father and you can go back to being a son.

If Dad is not in such a good home, you need to remind yourself that he is there because that is what is available. Most likely you did not say to yourself, "Gee, this place smells terrible. Let's put Dad in here." You will do what you can to make it better.

Dealing with Guilt

You do not have to be a prisoner of guilt. In this section are a number of actions that can help you. Read them and choose a few to try. You will have to work at them consistently over time. They do work if you allow them to.

Over the past few years, the fields of counseling and psychology have developed an approach called mindfulness. Mindfulness comes from a meditation and Buddhist approach to life in general. Instead of trying to "get rid of" guilt, mindfulness would teach you to notice it in your life, experience it, and let it go. Instead of fighting guilt, you are disarming its power over you. Because the situation of being a caregiver and having a loved one in a nursing home or seniors housing is an ongoing one over which you have no power, a mindfulness-based approach is well suited to handling the emotions you experience about it.

Briefly, to get a feel for what this is like, try the following. Find a calm and relaxing place in your home or outdoors where you will not be disturbed. Sitting up, close your eyes and start to breathe in a slow and rhythmical way. Pay attention to your muscles and body. Gradually do a body sweep, head to toe, and relax all the muscles in your body. Then concentrate by counting your breath: breathing in, one; breathing out, two. As you are doing that, notice your thoughts; do not try to change them, manipulate them, or get rid of them, just notice them as they come up. Then go back to your breathing. When feelings and thoughts of guilt come up, notice them, too. The noticing is similar to the way you would notice something in the countryside as you drive past it in your car: you cannot change what you notice, you can just see it and let it go as the car moves on. If this approach appeals to you, look into it further. A good source for mindfulness is *The Mindful Way though Depression*, by Mark Williams et al. It contains a CD with exercises. Jon Kabat-Zinn, one of the authors, has also written several books and put out some audio recordings on meditation and mindfulness.

Many of the following techniques fall under the description of what is called cognitive or cognitive-behavioral restructuring. This assumes that feelings arise from thoughts that are developed from people's history and experience. To change your feelings, you can work on changing your thoughts. The trick is that you have to work at it. You have to become committed to doing the work until the changes take place in your thinking. It does not happen overnight.

> *Technique 1, part A:* Make a list of what you have had to change in your life and how caregiving has affected you. Most people have good and valid reasons for placing their relative, especially in a nursing home. In fact, most people hang on too long before doing so. You know why you are doing what you are. What did you sacrifice? How much of your own life did you give up? How much sleep did you lose? How has worry changed you? How much did you neglect your spouse and children?
>
> *Technique 1, part B:* Look into your future. Take a look at the total picture of your life from the list you wrote. Ask yourself

what it would be like to keep doing this every day for another year, not just when your father is having a good day. Do you find yourself getting short-tempered with him? Can you keep depriving the rest of your family or your wife of your attention? Are you ready to keep driving to his house every day? Can you go much longer with your sleep disrupted? Are you willing to end up in a situation in which you become abusive, in which your family is suffering, or in which your emotional or physical health is impaired? Are you willing to do a disservice to everyone, including your mother, for whom you are trying to care?

Technique 2: As in technique 1, develop a two-column cost/benefit analysis. One column is costs, one is benefits. Will the benefits outweigh the costs? If you are part of the "sandwich generation," as you write down costs and benefits, you might also want to include the costs and benefits to your wife and children. It might make the balance sheet different.

Technique 3: Keep a journal either daily or a couple of times a week. In it, describe your caregiving journey. This will help to release your feelings as they occur. Reread it every now and then. If you are writing in it honestly, you will see what caregiving is doing to you and your family and the cost to you. It can help you decide when you have done what you should.

Technique 4: If you have not kept a journal (or sometimes even if you have), it helps to write out your caregiving story. Write down from the first minute up to right now what you have been going through and the reasons you are proceeding as you are. This helps you see what you have been through and acknowledges all you have done. You will find it is a lot more—and a lot more difficult—than what you give yourself credit for.

Technique 5: If you are willing to be rigorously honest with yourself, you can start to examine what the gains might be from guilt. Is there a payoff, something that encourages you at some level to hold on? Take a piece of paper and just start writing whatever reasons come into your head. You may discover something that is holding you back and that you need to think about to move on.

Technique 6: Pretend that you are a friend of yours, and write a letter to yourself. Would you forgive someone else in your shoes? Sometimes the standards we set for ourselves are higher than what we would expect from others.

Technique 7: This is best done with a guide such as a therapist, but you can try it on your own. Set out two chairs. You sit in one, and imagine your guilt sitting in the other (or use a doll you have labeled). Talk to the guilt. Have the guilt talk back. (I know you feel foolish doing this. Do it anyway, okay?) Enter into a dialogue with your feelings. As you do this, listen to what both are saying. Notice how you feel and what you think about what you are hearing. At one point, you may want to switch chairs and be the guilt talking to you. Listen to how the guilt talks to you. If you can, record the conversations and listen to them. You can also do this with a friend, where the friend plays you or your guilt and you play the other. Then switch roles.

Technique 8: One of the most effective actions you can take is to find a support group. See if there is a group in the nursing home. Call the Alzheimer's Association, the Heart and Stroke Foundation, or the Parkinson Foundation, for example. Many communities have caregivers' groups offered through a hospital. A support group helps you form a reference outside yourself that can help you to forgive yourself. It is like an external conscience. I have had people tell me that they do not wish to sit around and listen to a bunch of people talk about their problems. Most support groups also talk about solutions, both practical and emotional. They tell you what other people did and how they did it, so you don't have to reinvent the wheel. They also let you know that you are not alone and that your guilt is manageable. Sometimes they are fun. You can meet some wonderful people and make some close friends.

Technique 9: If no support group is available, try to find an individual you can talk to. Sometimes just saying things aloud to someone else can help you see the situation in a new light. Find a peer who has been through what you are going through. See if the nursing home has a social worker or other counselor available. On a more formal level, find someone you can ask to be your coach. Talk to him or her regularly. Make a commitment to listen to the person.

Technique 10: If you are a religious person, ask God for strength, help to heal, and forgiveness. God has a better grasp on life than you do, and has been doing it longer. Let God decide if you should be forgiven. Most likely, God will be easier on you than you are.

Technique 11: If God is temporarily unavailable, you can talk to your pastor, rabbi, priest, imam, or other religious or spiritual advisor. Not only are these people excellent sources of strength and comfort, but also they can stay by your side as you are making a decision about placement and for the whole journey afterward. They often are experienced with seniors residences and aging and understand what you are going through. As one woman said to me, "I couldn't have done it without [the pastor]. He was helpful in a way no one else could be because religion has always been such a part of our lives." Even if religion has not been a big part of your life, it is there when you need it. If you choose to believe in God, God is there for you when you need to turn to God.

Technique 12: Books and Web sites. John Bradshaw's book *Healing the Shame That Binds You* is an excellent resource for examining the more deep-seated aspects of shame in our lives. He looks at how shame develops in our formative years, its meaning, and how it carries on into and affects us in our adult life. There are several Web sites that have caregiver stories, support groups, and approaches. Become a member of those Web sites (see Resources, p. 349).

Technique 13: If none of the above techniques works, write the word GUILT on a large piece of paper. Go to the broom closet and take out the largest broom you can find. Put the paper on the floor. Raise the broom high over your head. Then whack the heck out of the GUILT as hard as you can. Do it as often as you need to. Break the broom. Brooms are cheap.

Some people absolutely refuse to let go of their guilt. If this is you, I have one more option.

Technique 14: Start rearranging your house. Empty out half the drawers in your dresser. Clear out half of the coat closet, set an extra place at the table, put a set of fresh towels in the bathroom, and make up a fresh bed in the guest bedroom. Dedicate all of that to Guilt. If Guilt is going to live with you, you might as well make it comfortable.

In the end, you need to realize that you cannot save your father. Life is how life is, no matter how painful it can sometimes be. You are not a superpower, and you are not God. You did not make the situation he is in, and you cannot make him better. This means that it is not you who needs forgiving, because you are not responsible for the situation.

In summary, to heal from guilt and shame, you first must want to heal from it. You will not love your father any less without the guilt. You must allow yourself to heal by forgiving yourself for your actions, decision, and feelings. You may have to work at it, but you can do it. Be kind and gentle with yourself. Allow yourself to say when you have had enough, and allow yourself to set limits and boundaries for yourself. Forgiveness does not come in a box that you unwrap; it is more like a piece of music that takes time to hear. Try to forgive yourself a little bit every day. At the end of some time, you will hear the melody.

Letting Go

If your husband is going into care, you probably have already experienced to some extent the feeling of having to let go of him. You have let go of the image of who he used to be. You have let go of the hope that he will be able to do the things that he used to do—talk to you the way he used to, love you as he did. When he goes into a nursing home, the process of letting go may intensify or recur.

As you let go of who he used to be, you let go of the relationship you had. You may even feel that your marriage is ending or has ended. Partly this happens because the things you used to do for and with each other change. Those actions made up the relationship that was your marriage. You replace them with actions that create a relationship of caregiver and care receiver.

When your husband enters the nursing home, you may feel like you are having to let go of the caregiver's role. Someone else will be taking care of your husband for the most part. You will be allowing someone else to help wash, feed, bathe, and dress him. You may find yourself wondering what that will leave you. You may feel bitter or resentful at someone else doing what you used to do, even if you were tired and worn out from doing it. Letting someone else take care of him is also like coming to terms with your own limitations and doubts, knowing that you cannot protect him any longer.

Changes of this magnitude in a relationship can be frightening. Partly this is because in some ways we define ourselves through our relationships. I am a wife, a father, a brother. When there is a change in your primary relationship, it can lead you to wonder, "Who am I?" and "How or to whom am I important?"

If you are an adult child, you may feel that you are losing your father when he goes into a seniors residence. If you have already lost one parent, this can be especially hard. Even though you may be an adult, the feeling of having a parent is like having a psychological protector. Losing a second parent may in some way leave you feeling abandoned or all alone. This can be frightening at your very core. With the loss of a second parent, you become the "Older Generation" of the family—another new role and position. Even if you haven't felt for a long time that you "needed" your protector, just the knowledge in the back of your mind that he was there provided a kind of security. You don't know it is there until you don't have it anymore.

An only child has it harder still. Only children tend to have more intense relationships with their parents than do children from families of more than one child. So letting go can be harder. Also, as an only child, you are losing the primary family link you had with your past: what made you, for better or worse, who you are today. You are losing your only intimate history and the only person who accepted you unconditionally and nourished you since the day you were born. People have this feeling even if their relationship with a parent was troublesome.

Younger people have a difficult time in another way when they have to move a spouse into care. For you, placing your husband means letting go of a future that you had planned and hoped for. It means rewriting the script that you had created for the rest of your life. So you are losing not only your husband but also your future.

When one half of a younger couple goes into care, it also shifts child rearing more onto the spouse remaining at home. In some ways, at times, this makes it easier. If you did a lot of the caregiving, then there is just less work, but there is also not the other parent there to support you.

So you may feel cheated. It may feel to you like you are being abandoned by your husband, and you can feel angry and bitter. As if that isn't enough, a lot of times people feel ashamed of having those feelings (remember "the shoulds"). So instead of being able to reach out and talk about what is going on, they hold it in. It is okay to talk about grief, but you may think, "I can't tell someone how angry I am at him." You can stay with those feelings, and they will pass.

When your husband enters the residence, you will be letting go in the physical sense—he will no longer be in the family home. You will have to face what can be painful loneliness. Sometimes this is what makes people hang on. Their fear of being alone is greater than their fear of burnout or the next step. The emptiness of your house can be a concrete reminder of the reality of your situation. It says that this probably is not going to get any better; if anything, it is going to get worse. You are letting go of some hope. It is an emotional letting go.

As you go through the process of letting go, your husband is going through it too. He is letting go of his independence, his home, and his marriage. Often he is letting go of much of his decision-making rights. He is letting go of his responsibilities around the home. This is in addition to the other losses to which he may or may not have already adjusted: the ability to dress, walk, do his own banking or shopping, go out by himself in the larger community, or even think and remember clearly.

People may experience this process of letting go even when a parent is going to an assisted living facility. For certain, when a couple is in one complex but in separate rooms or parts, they go through it. It is not about the place so much as the gaps and meanings that are given to the situation.

The most difficult periods in relationships are often when both parties are going through stressful situations at the same time. If it were just one of you, the other would be able to rally and be supportive. When it is both of you, you are both needy. This is the reason you may be experiencing increased friction with a parent or spouse as he goes into care. For you to support your husband can mean having to put aside your own needs for a time. Even though you may not mean it, you can end up feeling angry and resentful that your needs are not being met. That was not part of the agreement.

Grief and Loss

Letting go is a process of grief and loss, the resolution of which often takes up to a year. To come to acceptance means ups and downs. It involves anger and rage and sadness and depression. You will have many different feelings and thoughts that come and go. You will have good days and bad days. If it is your mother in care, she may have bright days when it seems she could have still lived at home. Then you start to be hopeful that she will "come back," and you will wonder if you have done the right thing. If it is your husband in care, you may have days when your loneliness is overwhelming and your house feels huge and empty. Your resolution will waiver and you will want to take him back home just for a week.

Remind yourself firmly about your husband's prognosis. Reread your journal or notebook about what you went through while he was at home. Often what he has is progressive: despite the ups and downs, he will get worse. Let your hopes guide you to enjoy what you can, not delude you into thinking that things will get better. It is so easy to allow yourself to hope, but your hopes can end up letting you down over and over again if you are not realistic.

Sometimes what changes is the nature of hope. You hope for good days, to see some happiness or joy in your husband's face. You can hope to see him doing an activity or making a friend. You can hope to see him receive some tender care. You can hope to find some joy and peace on your own.

AMBIGUOUS LOSS

The grief process can be more difficult in the circumstance of placing your husband in a nursing home than in losing him to death. Death has some finality, but someone in care is still alive but also gone. This is a kind of ambiguous loss. If your husband is in a home, you realize on one hand that you are still married, and on the other hand you may feel like you are less than married because the parts of what made up your marriage are missing. If it is your father who is in a home, you may feel when you visit that the person who stands in front of you is not really your father—he is not the person you knew, and yet he is. In a way he is gone, but in a way he is not. It is hard to resolve the grief over someone who is only partially gone. It is hard to let go when you can change your mind and take someone home or when her condition goes up and down.

RECURRING LOSS

Similar to ambiguous loss is recurring loss. This is the process in which you get used to your husband being at one stage of his disease, and then he slips to another. I remember as my mother was dying over two years, at first she was just tired, and then she was weak, and then she needed help doing things, and then she went into the hospital but came out, and then there was the last time, when she went in, and I knew she wouldn't come out. Each time, I had to get used to losing a little bit more. Your husband may be able to play cards, then he can't, and then he can't walk, and you lose him again, and then he can't recognize you, and you have lost another part of him. Then you grieve that also.

ANTICIPATORY GRIEF

Before the actual time of placement, you may be experiencing what is called anticipatory grief. That may be one of the reasons why you are holding back from placement. The grief—or fear and reluctance to feel it—can be so overwhelming that you try to avoid it by not allowing your husband to go into the home.

About the time you are placing your husband and have to turn him over to the care staff, you may start feeling intense pain, because this is the time when you are letting go. It is also the actual event: what you feared or avoided is happening. The pain can be physical as well as emotional—upset stomach, anxiety, sleeplessness, irritability. Remember the explanation of stress in chapter 2.

You may be surprised at the feeling of anger when it comes. It may be directed at yourself, your husband, the care staff, God, or some or all of these. You may find yourself lashing out at your family or at the cashier in the grocery store. If you are not used to being an angry person, this can be confusing and frightening. Be assured that it is a normal part of grief. The anger is a way to help protect yourself from fear and emotional pain. If you are able to continue through the grief process, the anger will subside.

If your husband is in a home where the care is poor or suspect, you will have an even harder task. You will have to figure out how to let go, yet how to remain involved to the point that he is not at risk. Partly this will mean more closely overseeing care than providing it yourself. You will have to learn how the home functions or is deficient and see what you can do to meet those deficiencies, short of moving in yourself.

There are many ways at looking at the process of grief. Best known in the literature is Elizabeth Kübler-Ross's seminal book, *On Death and Dying*, in which she identified five stages of grief: denial, anger, bargaining, depression, and acceptance. Other people have labeled stages with other terms, describing the first one as shock. Be aware that these are only descriptions of emotional processes. They occur differently, and they often do not occur in order. Often people move back and forth, especially in situations of ambiguous and sequential loss.

Handling Grief

To let go, you need to be willing to let go. Hanging on will not change the situation; it will only prevent you from making the best of it. Letting go does not mean you are abandoning your husband. It means that the nature of the relationship will change. It doesn't mean that you will no longer love or care about your husband, but the nature of loving care will change.

It means being willing to face your feelings of grief and loss going through it. You cannot hide from them, or try to be so strong all the time that you do not feel them. There will be times when you do not want to face your feelings, when the pain is too great. Be gentle with yourself. Distract yourself with an activity or something else, and come back to them when you are able.

If you are not willing to face your feelings, they can surface in other ways, such as depression and ill health. In my counseling practice I have seen many people who shut themselves up emotionally after the death of a loved one many years before, after being sexually assaulted, or following some other trauma. They chose marriages they should not have, they entered into addictions, they limited their education, and they distanced themselves from other family members. The tragedy is that not only did they not grieve, but also they did not achieve what they could have, because they never dealt with what happened. In the long run, the price you pay will be higher because you will be having the feelings longer. It is a little like the choice between short-term pain with relief and long-term pain.

Use supports and resources that are available to you. Despite what you may think, there are often many people available to you if you look. Find a support group or a competent therapist. Maybe there is someone from the health department who arranges nursing home placements. If the home that you are looking at has a social worker, helping with grief is often part of her job. Talk to another daughter or son or wife or husband who has been through the process. Use some of the techniques I mentioned for dealing with guilt.

Supports will help you meet those needs that you have put aside in responding to those of your husband. Now is the time to respond to yourself. If you don't, you will deplete yourself faster. Again, think of yourself as a watering can: if you keep watering the plants without filling up, the can will eventually be empty.

Remember that even though someone else will be taking care of your husband, you are not replaceable. In some ways, your role is even more important than it was. You may not be doing the physical care that you used to, but you are still the primary caregiver in the emotional sense. Even the best staff can never replace the loving relationship and feelings that exist between family members. Staff members will never be able to validate a resident's importance and individuality the way you do. Staff members will never be able to let a resident know that he counts the way his family can. When your husband goes into care, you can concentrate on the emotional aspects of your relationship. Ultimately that is what creates and maintains love.

Marjorie

I would like to put into words how difficult it is to watch a much-loved and capable parent floundering in the confusion of her mind from insecurity and frustration. You fight so hard to keep things going as they were. It is difficult to accept the changes and the reversal of roles. It is also frightening from a personal point of view and makes one feel vulnerable. Writing this down gives me some sense of release and is therapeutic.

We had been the grateful recipients of varying degrees of assistance before Mum went into the home. She received home care from the province and an assessment at the hospital. The staff at the hospital treated us with empathy and appreciated the stress that caring for Mum was putting on my husband and me. They directed us to other channels of assistance and advice.

Mum started attending adult day care for two and then three days a week at the nursing home where she was going to go to live. She also got two hours of home support services on the other weekdays. It afforded her the opportunity to mingle and enjoy the company of her peers in a safe, pleasant, and friendly environment. It also gave her a chance to perform mental and physical activities such as crafts, quizzes, discussions, and exercise. After a few months of attendance, she changed from being nervous, shy, and clinging to more her former self. It also gave her something of her own to talk about with us.

The day care and home care enabled my husband and me to have some free time together, which we urgently required. There were many other benefits, most of all a terrific relief in not having to worry about Mum's happiness and welfare twenty-four hours a day. We could *not* have carried on as we were without this day care.

Before Mum moved into the nursing home, she had a week of respite care there. That week helped her to see what it would be like when she actually went to live there permanently. Even though she might not remember, we could remind her that she had already been there and enjoyed it.

The transition of moving into the retirement center went smoothly and pretty well stress free for my mother. It just seemed like a natural progression. She already knew a lot of the people, both residents and staff, and was familiar with the building and the routines, so she did not experience the natural trauma of someone coming from her own home environment into "care." Members of the day care helped her settle in by paying a visit to her room and welcoming her.

I was the one who felt stressed. When I left Mum at the home that first day, I felt a sense of loss. It helped that I knew the day center staff would keep an eye on her. They and the staff of the home gave me positive feedback as to how she was doing. This was reassuring to me. It helped me feel I had made the right choice.

I still am finding the letting go difficult. Even though I know it is the best thing for us all, it is difficult. With the help of some counseling from the social worker at the home, I know I am getting to the point of acceptance. I am reconciled to redefining my role in Mum's future care. I can't do what I was doing. I have come to realize that I cannot and should not be totally responsible for my mother's happiness. With the help of the staff at the home, I can still be there to complement their good work and feel that I am helping my mother.

Just writing this has been therapeutic to me. It helps me see what I have been through. I know I have a lot further to go, but knowing I have come this far makes me hope I can keep on going and my feelings will continue to get easier.

PART II

THE RESIDENCE

CHAPTER 5

About Nursing Homes and Assisted Living Facilities

What makes a fulfilling life, do you think? It seems to me that it varies from person to person but usually includes having a pleasant physical environment, interesting activities, and loving, fulfilling relationships. It usually includes having found some meaning and purpose to life. People who have fulfilling lives have found contentment through a healthy psychological adjustment. They have an acceptance of who they are and what they have done, are doing, or hope to do in the future. Ideally, you could find a seniors residence for your father where he would be able to achieve this kind of life.

The nature of meaning, purpose, passion, and interests changes as people age. They vary from person to person. What they are for you might be different from what they are for your father. What was true for him five years ago might not be true now. I remember one woman who told me that she believed that God had a purpose for her. "What is that?" I asked her. "To be nice to other people," she told me. That was it, but that was enough for her. Other people have told me they want to live because they have a family who loves them.

Unfortunately, your father may not have had a fulfilling life before moving. It may have been a personality issue or the result of circumstance. It is unlikely that any residence would make up for that. They cannot change your father into someone he wasn't, and they cannot change the things that have happened to him. Also, even the best residences rarely meet the ideal that can make a life fulfilling. This is especially true in nursing homes; life will not be perfect in care, and a nursing home will never be like someone's own home. But there are ways that a residence can try.

What you need to remember is that you also cannot "give" your father a fulfilling life. You cannot make up for what he has lost or is losing by giving up his home and going into a residence. You cannot bring back his eyesight, his health, or his wife. You also cannot be everything to him that he needs. If you think you can and you try to do so, you will be lost in an ongoing struggle that you cannot win. Or you will end up giving up your own life. He has to find fulfillment, meaning, and purpose on his own to whatever extent is possible for him, given his psychological and financial resources. What you can try to do is maximize the potential for fulfillment. Partly that is done through your ongoing relationship with him. Maintain your relationship, but be aware of your limitations and boundaries. Another way you can help to do this is by choosing the appropriate residence.

Keeping Your Relative at Home

You have probably used all the options available to maintain your father at home. In Canada all the provinces have subsidized systems that include home care, adult day care, and respite beds (in which a person goes into care for up to four weeks a year). Adult day care will often pick up your father at home, provide a full-day program, maybe give a bath once a week, pack meals to take home, and monitor medications and health. The various parts of the system are integrated with the residential care systems. This means that once someone is in the system, he can progress as his needs become greater.

In the United States, all of these options are available, but generally you must find means to pay for them privately, and the care system is not integrated. In both countries, it is possible to put together a plan that will help someone stay at home for a long time. If you do not have the time or knowledge, this is another area where a geriatric care manager has expertise. In recent years, the federal and state governments have begun to offer funded programs such as PACE (Program of All-inclusive Care for the Elderly) that will help to keep people in their homes. These programs are often aimed at the frail elderly most at risk for institutionalization. Through a combination of programs and services, they attempt to meet the needs of the people in their homes. Their services are subsidized by Medicaid and Medicare (see Resources, p. 352).

If you do take the route of caring for someone in the community, it is essential that you develop a plan to help you cope with the emotional and physical burdens that you will experience. Part of this plan includes social support and relief from caregiving duties for yourself. A couple of studies have indicated that people who take advantage of this kind of support are able to continue caregiving longer than those who do not.

The practical part of the plan should include organizing your caregiving. This means lists. They will include a

- list of medications, including prescriber, dosage, when and how often taken
- list of medical people involved
- list of appointments coming up
- list of documents and professionals, such as accountants, who are involved
- list of medical history, treatments, and allergies
- list of expenses
- list of your lists
- list of each time you take a drink while you try to keep track of the other lists.

A number of books and Web sites have information to help you keep someone at home. Books include *The Baby Boomer's Guide to Caring for Aging Parents*, by Bart Astor; *The Complete Eldercare Planner*, by Joy Loverde; *Keeping Them Healthy, Keeping Them Home: How to Care for Your Loved Ones at Home*, by Ellen M. Caruso; and *Therapeutic Caregiving*, by Barbara J. Bridges. Canadians can read *The Complete Canadian Eldercare Guide: A Handbook to Caring for Your Aging Parents*, by Caroline Tapp-MacDougall.

Web sites and books can help you decide if keeping your father at home is something that you are able to do. In theory, you may want to; in reality, it may not be practical. They will also give you a picture of the difficulties you may encounter and guide you in planning so that these difficulties don't become problems. Plans and knowledge will help you minimize the stress and anxiety that can lead to exhaustion and burnout. Take a look at these; there is no reason for you to have to waste your time and risk your health by finding solutions on your own.

Use books and resources to help you until you have to take the next step. Do not use them to convince yourself you can avoid using a nursing home. If you do, you may be setting yourself up to fail, and you will make your next steps harder. Do not use them to push yourself, to find "the answer," or somehow to increase your guilt because you eventually have to use outside care.

If you decide to care for your father by bringing him to your home, remember that you are deciding about something that is not static. It is likely that your father will deteriorate in some way. This means that the burden on you will become increasingly difficult. You may not be able to do it for very long. This will mean that your father has to move again, suffer another loss, and feel "not wanted" by you in your home.

Be prepared for how the decision to move a parent into your home will affect you and your family. The expectations that your parent has on you may not be what you have in mind. Even if your partner or spouse agrees to have an in-law move into the home, it can be difficult. There will be a shift in your relationship. There will be a loss of privacy. There will be increased demands on you that will pull you from your spouse. It will also have an impact on any children living at home. It may be hard for them to cope with a grandparent with behaviors resulting from grief or dementia. Your attention will be taken away from them at times, and they may feel resentful. Having a parent live with you can also bring up many of the old conflicts that you may have had with the parent, which may have been in abeyance since you left the family home.

Even if you move a parent to your community but not into your home, it can be difficult. They may expect to see you every day. They will be in a strange community with different stores, different views, different temperatures maybe. It will not *feel* the same. Unless there is a good reason, I usually recommend that people not move a parent to their community if it can be avoided.

If you want to give yourself an objective picture of your caregiving "career," ask yourself what you are willing to do or what you think you can put up with and what will "trigger" your decision to move Dad into a residence. Some of the tasks and problems you may have to face or hire someone to perform are

- bathing
- dressing
- putting on and changing incontinence products
- feeding
- wandering
- constant repetition of questions
- clinging behavior
- outbursts of aggression or anger
- loss of sleep
- marital or family tension.

You might also make another list. On this one, write down all the tasks you or your family perform for your father. Next to it, put two other columns and list the tasks that you expect to be doing one year and two years from now. This chart will show what your caregiving role is now and what it will become. It will enable you to match your father's needs with the options available. It will also reduce the chance that you will opt for one type of care only to have to make another move in the near future.

Still there are trade-offs. My client whose father had moved in with him for the last three years of his life said to me, "I would never have changed it and I don't regret it. We became closer than we ever were." For some people and families, having Dad live with them is a joy and brings a wonderful quality to their lives. It teaches their children compassion and gives them beautiful memories of Grandpa that will last for the rest of their lives.

Where to Start Finding a Nursing Home or Assisted Living Facility

In the United States, both state and federal regulations govern nursing homes. All states have area agencies on aging that are responsible for seeing that nursing homes are meeting regulated standards. These agencies handle complaints and do yearly surveys of nursing homes.

The area agencies on aging all provide a range of other services that will help you find resources to allow someone to stay in his or her own home. Each state also has an ombudsperson, mandated under the Older Americans Act, whose office is responsible for protecting the rights of residents of care facilities. Although the area agencies on aging may not be able to recommend one specific place, they are excellent resources for general information.

The ombudsperson or the state agencies have lists of nursing homes and assisted living residences. They also have copies of the survey results on nursing homes and often on assisted living facilities. You can find them through www.eldercare.gov, in the phone book in the government sections, or by calling directory assistance. Be aware that the names of the area agencies on aging differ from state to state. Other sites to look at include www.ec-online.net, www.seniorhousingnet.com/seniors, www.gilbertguide.com, and www.assistedlivinginfo.com. They all have additional information on care, caregiving, and topics related to aging.

To find information on the quality of nursing homes, you can look at Medicare's Web site; www.medicare.gov also has extensive information on homes and surveys by state. The surveys list the deficiencies noted when the home was inspected. If you look at these, make sure you check the deficiencies, rather than just comparing how many there are. Some types of deficiency may be more acceptable to you than others; for instance, the rate of flu vaccination versus the rate of pressure sores. The Centers for Medicare and Medicaid Services has a "Special Focus Facility List." This is a listing of facilities that have a history of serious quality issues and that are included in a program to improve their quality. Lists of government surveys of nursing homes by state can be found at www.memberofthefamily.net. They also have their own "Watch List" of homes that is interesting if a bit frightening. You will have to decide for yourself, after looking at the surveys and deficiencies, if they merit passing up a home. When you do finally choose a residence, use the deficiencies, if there were any, as a guideline when monitoring care to know where to pay particular attention.

Assisted living is regulated by the individual states. The regulations governing them vary enormously. In some states they are almost as regulated as nursing homes, in other states much less so. As noted, they are not uniformly inspected and the ratings made available, as is the case for nursing homes. This makes the process of choosing one more difficult and the services more open to problems.

In Canada, nursing homes are regulated through provincial legislation. The regulations may be enforced at the provincial or the local level, often through the health department or Health Authority. Local health authorities may also have specific guidelines and regulations. Look in the government (blue) pages of the phone book to find the numbers of the health department, or see appendix 1, "Accessing Care in Canada," at the back of this book. You might be lucky to reach a worker who will give you the real information on which homes are better than others. Often they are not able to tell you this, as they work in the system. You may have to ask a question like, "Where would you want your father to be?" Assisted living is at this point much less regulated than are nursing homes. There may be a separate agency through the provincial government that is responsible for them. Ask your local health authority about what agency regulates and oversees assisted living in your province.

The Resources section at the back of this book lists several other Web sites you can use. Often you can find names of homes through the Alzheimer's Association or other caregivers' organizations. Ministers, doctors, social workers, and hospital discharge planners usually have knowledge about facilities. In the United States, and to a limited extent in Canada, you can engage the services of a geriatric care manager (National Association of Professional Geriatric Care Managers, 520-881-8008; www.caremanager.org), who will help you sort through the maze of options. The advantage to going these routes as opposed to government routes is that people will often recommend which places you can trust and which you should stay away from. Government agencies will not be able to do that, or not directly.

Several companies purport to be experts on referrals to seniors residences. They may have some information, but they also may be receiving a payment from the facilities for people they refer who actually end up living in the residence. They also may not have a complete list, meaning, if a facility does not offer them a referral fee, they will not refer to them. This may limit your finding a residence that would be right for your father.

In some areas, the staff in hospitals may know less about assisted living than about nursing home options. They tend to discharge less to assisted living because often if someone is in the hospital and cannot go home he or she needs the care of a nursing home or rehabilitation center. There are also fewer assisted living choices, and they may not be government funded or accept Medicaid.

You should do some networking among your friends, people you know at church or in your workplace, and so on. Try to talk to more than one person with experience of the same facility, and compare what each says. Talking to other people helps you understand what the nursing home is like. You can fine-tune the questions you need to ask at the particular home. It can also help you figure out what is realistically possible as opposed to what guides like this one tell you.

A word of caution: if someone you know has had a bad experience with a particular home, this does not necessarily mean that the home is not a good one. Assess the person you are talking to. If she is deep in grief, denial, or resentment, then no place may ever fit the bill. Also, even the best homes are not perfect, and there can be glitches.

When you are first considering a nursing home or other care option, you should begin to formulate an understanding of the care system in your state or province. Each state or province, and sometimes each home, has its own rules for eligibility, for waiting lists, for payments, for Medicaid. In the United States, national standards have come out of the Older Americans Act. When I have been on the staff of nursing homes, I have often spent a good deal of time with people explaining to them how the system works and how they can make it work for them.

One tactic to make sure you understand the system and how it works is to call two or three different offices of the same agency and ask the same question. If you are given the same answer two or three times, then you can probably trust it. If different people give you different answers, keep digging and asking questions. Sometimes there is more flexibility in a system than it first appears. Regulations are often not straightforward and can be open to interpretation by the staff person applying them.

Applying for Seniors Housing

In the United States, you generally must seek out each home and apply individually on your own. If you are in the hospital, the social worker or discharge planner may initially contact potential homes for you. In some states a standardized process or form must be completed before you can apply. In some states you must have a doctor's referral. You will have to find out the requirements in your state.

In Canada, most provinces now have a single-point entry system of care for elderly persons. "Single-point entry" means that one public agency will follow your father from first contact, when all he may need is care in his own home, up to and after placement. This agency will assess your father and decide how much care he needs. They will help him and you decide if he can manage at home or if he needs a residential setting. If he needs a nursing home, they will assess what kind of home can best provide it. They manage waiting lists for public facilities that often offer high-quality care. (See appendix 1, "Accessing Care in Canada.")

Remember that when you are applying for and viewing a home, the home is also checking out you and your father. A home wants to know whether you will be able to pay or if payment such as Medicaid or long-term care insurance has been arranged. Homes that depend on Medicaid payments may be looking for more impaired residents because their funding may be based on the amount of care a resident needs—the more care, the higher the payment. Some homes limit the number of Medicaid residents they will accept because Medicaid payments are often less than what they charge privately paying clients.

A residence will also want to know whether they can provide the care that your father needs. This can be especially true in independent living or assisted living residences, where the staff may be smaller and services are limited. Each residence will do an assessment, which can include looking at your father's ability to feed, wash, and dress himself; his ability to walk or transfer himself, for example, from his bed to a wheelchair, or on and off the toilet; and his memory and other cognitive functions. They will also look carefully at his behavior.

Aggression, alcohol abuse, and sexual disinhibition are triggers that make residences wary about admitting someone and often will lead to outright refusal. Legally, it can be hard for a residence to get your father to move once he is there, so they want to screen to make sure they won't have the problem.

It does not do you any good to minimize the behavior or habits that your father has. To be fair to the residence, they need to be able to know if they can provide the necessary care and supervision, and they need to be able to protect the other residents. If you are not honest about some aspect of Dad's behavior, you may be setting him up to fail, which will mean another move.

I had a friend who was the director of care in a campus-of-care facility. She told me frankly, "Peter, I cherry pick my residents. I have a lot of people who want to live here. If I have some concerns about a resident, their behavior, or their family, I will not admit them." Most facilities realize that they are admitting a whole family, not just the individual resident who will live there. They know that they are not just working with your father, they are also dealing with you: your feelings about him and about his going into a home and the other stresses that you and your family have. They will want to figure out if they can handle you. If they feel that you will be extremely litigious, argumentative, demanding, or verbally abusive to their staff, they will think twice before admitting your father. I am not trying to tell you to put on your best party dress and shoes and "act like a lady," but remember that they are trying to figure out what their future will be like, too.

About Good Care and Good Caring

A nursing home can provide good care, good caring, or both. There is a difference between good care and good caring. You can have one without the other. The staff can have the best training in the world but still not be providing good caring. They can also provide good caring without being able to provide good care. You want both.

Good care means up-to-date and competent professional practice from all the staff members in a home. It can come only from people who have training and knowledge in the field of geriatrics. Registered nurses should have training in gerontology. Nurse's aides should have been through a certified training program. The recreation staff should be headed by someone who has a degree in recreation therapy and experience in geriatrics. The director of nursing should have multiple years of experience and training in geriatrics. The home should have educational programs for its staff.

What do the staff learn in geriatric training? Depending on the role, they learn about how to provide direct care to fragile, impaired elderly persons and about the psychological and behavioral issues that come up with aging, dementia, and care. Practical skills they learn include feeding, lifting, changing, and bathing. They learn about medications and pain relief. They should learn about family issues and dynamics (but often do not). They learn to be at the front line of identifying symptoms and behaviors that call for investigation.

Good care also comes from the consulting and backup that is provided to the home. This means that they have access to geriatric physicians and geriatric mental health providers. Their pharmacist should be knowledgeable about medications for elderly persons. These are the people who are the specialists on whom the staff can fall back when there is a complex medical or psychosocial concern. This is essential, because often with elderly people problems that come up encompass both concerns.

Good caring means that the staff understands and responds to the emotional needs of the residents and behaves in a manner that meets those needs. It comes from people who are warm and loving. Good caring comes about when staff members treat residents like people, with respect and dignity. It occurs when the housekeeper talks to the resident as he or she makes the bed or cleans the bathroom. It occurs when the care aide talks to your father as he or she bathes, feeds, and dresses him. Good caring comes about through the building of good relationships between the staff and the residents and among the staff members themselves. Good caring also comes when there is a good administrative structure.

At the system level, good caring comes from a nursing home that is client centered as opposed to system centered. This means that to the greatest extent possible the system is arranged so that it meets the needs of the residents and their families; it does not try to make the residents and families fit the needs of the system. That said, this does not mean that when you say, "Jump," they should say, "How high?" It means that the men and women who work in the system can understand your point of view and make an effort to accommodate it. Remember that when they cannot, it does not necessarily mean that they don't want to.

In the United States, according to the statistics, it is hard to obtain either good care or good caring. Studies have documented that adequate care is provided in less than 50 percent of the nursing homes in some areas. Some studies put the numbers closer to 3 percent. I don't want to scare you—good care and good, caring people are out there. But you need to have your eyes open.

Models of Care

The way a residence functions derives from how the people in administration believe care and service should be provided. Partly this reflects their view of older people, partly it reflects how they see what they are doing. Partly too (and sometimes more than partly) it comes from financial considerations. Wherever it comes from, every residence is operating from some kind of model of care.

Client-centered care is one model. It means the residence involves families and residents in care planning and decision making as well as in policy development and, to an extent, the running of the home. This is especially true when they are accommodating a younger and more able client. Client-centered care asks, "What does the client want?" as opposed to "What do we think is best for the client?"

Asking what the client (or customer) wants is a key question. It indicates respect for the person as an individual. It puts the client in control of planning her environment. Asking what is best for the client puts the system in control and assumes that the client is dependent and unable to make decisions. This assumption entails an assumption about you, the family member, as well as about your father.

I have been working on a model that I call client- or resident-generated care. It goes beyond client-centered, which works from the outside, and instead views care as it would be if it were generated from and by the client, as though the person were designing the system for him- or herself. Resident-generated care looks at resident and family values, history, lifestyle, and other characteristics and asks how they can be replicated or instituted in the residence. It doesn't mean that the residents can do exactly the same things they did before moving to the facility. It means that they can, as much as possible, have a lifestyle that imparts the same satisfaction. A tall order, I know.

Many homes have developed and implemented a client-centered system on their own. Many have hired consultants or used outside models to help them (an excellent example of this can be found in William Thomas's *Life Worth Living: How Someone You Love Can Still Enjoy Life in a Nursing Home—The Eden Alternative in Action*).

Many homes "talk the talk." They may talk to you about making the facility a home or maximizing every resident's dignity and self-worth. They may talk about the client being the team leader and about partnerships with residents and families. Unfortunately, many homes do not operate under the philosophy that they think or say they use (which may or may not be spelled out in a mission statement). Several residences where I have clients post their mission and philosophy statements in full and plain view. Every time I read them I shake my head in disbelief because the actual service that they provide is nothing like what they have posted on their walls.

In the beginning of this section, I asked, "What makes a satisfying life?" and mentioned meaning and purpose. Ideally, whatever model or philosophy a home has, there is an opportunity for people to have some meaning and purpose. That is also where the family comes in—you provide meaning and purpose to your loved one just by virtue of the relationship you have. This is something that can never be taken from you or replaced by the staff.

People need to feel needed and wanted, that there is some reason to get out of bed every day. As people age, a lot of the meaning and purpose is lost—we give up our jobs, we are not raising children, we can't ski or drive anymore. In a sense, sometimes, we give up who we are, or it is taken from us by age, well-intentioned family members, society, illness, or disability.

Ask yourself why you get up every day. Then ask yourself what life would be like if you didn't have those things to make you get out of bed (vacuuming doesn't count). Then ask yourself how you would begin to replace those things if you were somehow disabled. Can a nursing home or assisted living facility provide meaning and purpose? Maybe the people in them can start.

It is hard to figure this out when you are looking at a home before placement. The only thing you can do is watch and listen while you visit. When you are taking a tour, ask if they have a mission statement or philosophy of care and ask how they put it into action. Listen for words and look for activities and opportunities that speak to meaning and purpose.

When you have found a residence that provides good care and good caring, ideally what you have found is a residence that also has the potential to create a satisfying life for your father. Your father may be going into a residence because of problems, but he is going there to live.

On Abuse

One of the greatest fears that you may have for Dad is "What happens when I am not here?" Your worst fear may be abuse. If your father goes into a home that is not very good and where you can see evidence of neglect, not only will this fear be worse, but also you can be overwhelmed by anger and by a sense of helplessness as you try to figure out what to do or how to encourage the staff to pay attention to him. It is beyond the scope of this book to do an in-depth examination of senior abuse, but we can take a look at when and why it occurs, what it is, and perhaps how to prevent it.

WHAT IS ABUSE?

There are several forms and varying severities of abuse, and any of them can occur in a care facility. Abuse can be hitting someone, holding the person roughly, or the inappropriate use of restraints, chemical or physical. It can be coercing the person into making decisions against her will.

Abuse can be emotional, in that residents may feel frightened of or threatened by the staff, or otherwise insecure in their environment, and become sad, lonely, and withdrawn. If a resident is mocked, laughed at, or humiliated, this can be abusive.

Abuse can be sexual—anything from inappropriate touching up to sexual intercourse without consent.

Financial abuse is spending the money of a dependent person on yourself or others when it is needed for her care, not providing enough money for her to receive adequate care, or even not buying her whatever extras she could afford. Financial abuse is using someone's money or resources for any purpose for which she would not approve.

It is abusive when a resident is overmedicated or on the wrong medication because someone has not checked if it is appropriate to the person and their situation. It is abusive when a resident's condition declines because the home has not adequately investigated a problem or made adequate attempts to correct it. It is abusive when a resident becomes incontinent because it is easier to keep her in diapers than to help her to the bathroom; or when she loses the ability to walk because it is easier for the staff to push her around in a wheelchair or let her stay in bed than to walk with her to the dining room or to recreation programs.

Whereas abuse is an action perpetrated on another person, neglect can be seen as a lack of action—when something is not done. This can be when someone is left on the toilet too long, or when he hasn't had his toenails attended to by a podiatrist, when he hasn't been changed from soiled clothing, or when bed rails are not locked when they are raised for the night. It can be when a resident is left in a room by herself for most of the day because there is not the staff to bring her to activities or out into the sunshine. Although these things may not be legally considered neglect, as they are not intended to be so, they are neglectful, and they should not occur.

Physical and sexual abuse do occur in seniors residences, though the incidence is difficult to measure. Much abuse is unseen and unreported. Residents and families can be frightened to report what has happened. Staff members sometimes can be intimidated by threats that they will lose their jobs if they complain or report abuse. Or they can be fearful that if they report it, the home will close. Some residents are disabled to the point that they are incapable of reporting. The result is that accurate statistics are hard to come by. However, there have been estimates that abuse and neglect occur systematically in 30 to 97 percent of U.S. nursing homes.

Abuse is also about intent. Accidents happen, no matter how good a home is. This includes dropping someone and medication errors. They are not acceptable occurrences, but they happen. The difference is the rate of incidence. If accidents or mistakes happen often, in some ways this may be seen as the result of neglect or abuse at a systemic level and is about the home, not the personnel.

SIGNS OF ABUSE

Is your father suffering from neglect or abuse? It will help if you know the signs:

- Are there pressure sores (decubitus ulcers) on his body?
- Does he have unexplained bruises or injuries?
- Do any of these injuries or bruises happen just at one time of day?
- Is he clean? Are his clothes clean?
- Has his physical state or ability declined for no apparent reason or for unacceptable reasons?
- Is he having falls?
- Has he become incontinent all of a sudden?
- Has he become depressed or agitated for no apparent reason? Is there rocking, sucking, or mumbling behavior?
- Has he stopped eating?
- Is he suddenly being restrained or having medications added?
- Are his equipment, hearing aids, glasses, or dentures broken or in poor repair?
- Does he seem afraid of the staff or of a particular staff member?
- Is he saying that someone has hit or pushed him?
- Do you feel the staff or administration are taking your inquiries seriously?
- Do you have the feeling that the staff or administration are trying to hide something?

WHY ABUSE OCCURS

Often, abuse is about power or control on the part of the perpetrator. This person has the psychological propensity to abuse. He puts himself in a situation in which he has power over someone. The other person is already vulnerable and unable for whatever reason to stand up for herself. Usually the abused person is dependent either physically or emotionally on the abuser. A nursing home is a prime situation for this kind of perpetrator because the clients are frail, vulnerable, and dependent on the staff. The situation can be rectified only when a home discovers the perpetrator.

I recently saw a woman in my office who had been married for twenty-five years. It was a second marriage for both the woman and her husband, a wonderful marriage according to her. In the last five years, her husband had been gradually deteriorating due to dementia. At one point, he hit her, and she tied his hands together because she was exhausted and alone and she didn't know what to do. Was that abusive? Yes. Was she a mean or nasty woman? Not at all.

When abuse is not about power, it is often about feelings of inadequacy or helplessness on the part of the caregiver. Anyone can be an abuser. Even the best caregivers, whether in the home or in a nursing home or assisted living residence, can become overwhelmed. I have known many wonderful people, like the woman I described above, who ended up emotionally or physically abusing an elderly person. Remember the section on stress and burnout? Abuse happens when a caregiver feels that nothing she is doing is working or she is so tired that she can't go on. She is isolated and has minimal support. She sees no way out and no way to relieve the emotional pressure. Anger, irritation, and depression occur, creating the potential for an abusive situation. Whereas being overwhelmed by a *feeling* is acceptable, the action of abuse is not.

Think of what it is like for you in your work when the staff is being reduced and you are supposed to do the same work or more with less help. You may try to cut corners, or you may stop doing the extras. If you can never finish the work, are exhausted, and feel you have no choices, you can become lethargic and uncaring. You may feel overwhelmed, stressed, and inadequate. You may have a feeling of resentment toward the boss, but on whom or on what do you take it out? This is what happens to nurses and nurse's aides. Sometimes they are victims of the system also. One advocate for elderly people told me that she receives as many calls from nurse's aides who are upset about conditions in a nursing home as from family members.

Often the staff members do not intend to neglect a resident; it happens when they are too busy. Sometimes they have to make a choice, a kind of on-the-spot triage. Are they going to change Mr. Smith's dressing, take Mrs. Carino's blood pressure, turn Ms. Matin in bed, or make sure Mrs. Eckel is drinking her vitamin supplement? Sometimes they have to do all at once: a care aide may help Mr. Smith out of bed and onto the toilet; from there she will go to help Mr. Giattis brush his teeth; and then to Mrs. Morgan to help her choose her clothes, and then back to Mr. Smith on the toilet. If Mrs. Morgan cannot choose her clothes fast enough, Mr. Smith can end up on the toilet for a long time.

In some homes, staffing is so poor that only the first few priorities will receive attention. The nurse's aides are not to blame; it is the home, the company that owns it, and the system that allows for poor staffing. In some assisted living residences, the needs of the residents have gone beyond what the home was designed or staffed for.

Neglect should not happen, and you should not excuse it when it does occur. You need to be aware that it has happened and address it with the staff immediately. However, the time to become alarmed with the home is when you see that it is happening regularly, throughout the system, and when several staff members are involved. This is an indication of problems with the home and the care as a whole.

In some ways, nursing homes in a for-profit system are set up to have abuse and neglect occur. If there is a squeeze for profit, they will have to find more money from somewhere. More revenue can come from cutting the food budget or the cleaning budget. It sometimes comes from charging for services that have not been performed or for equipment that has not been used or ordered. But the prime place to save money is on personnel, because staffing is the largest share of the budget. A residence may either reduce staffing or hire minimally qualified people. Economizing on the staff is possible because the minimal standards of care in the United States are woefully inadequate. Standards for education or hiring nurse's aides are often minimal, allowing homes to keep wages low. In the for-profit sector, profit and care can be competing forces. It is easy to see how management and ownership systems can give rise to the conditions under which abuse occurs.

Large nursing home chains can be set up so that ultimate, legal responsibility is difficult to pin down. That means instituting legal action is difficult, and thus allows the homes to function below optimal standards.

The U.S. system of funding and the size and organization of the bureaucratic systems of monitoring are factors that allow abuse and neglect to occur and continue. When a complaint is lodged with the authorities, it is supposed to be investigated within seven days. In fact, it can take months. Because standards are so low, a complaint about care may not make an impact. When fraud and abuse occur, the homes and the companies that run them are given minimal slaps on the wrist. Fines are low, and can be appealed. They are told to clean up or improve their practice. Unscrupulous owners are permitted to keep running homes. Rarely are they closed down. An October 1997 *Time* magazine article noted that in one year more than 95 percent of the homes that government inspectors recommended not receive funds got them anyway, more than 97 percent of the homes recommended to require special staff training did not have to follow through, and more than 90 percent that were recommended to be fined for violations paid none. When inspections do not lead to effective action on problems, there is no incentive to make the provision of good-quality care more important than profits.

In Canada, the vast majority of facilities are nonprofit and/or charitable organizations. Wages are much better than in the United States. The system is smaller, which makes monitoring easier. Many of the homes are unionized, so the management treats the staff better. This is not to say that abuse and neglect do not occur in Canada; they do. If you find problems, it will often be neglect rather than abuse. Lately more for-profit homes and chains have been setting up for business. Some of these do provide good and competent care. But when I look back at the homes and systems that I have known in Canada, many of the best ones were the nonprofits and many were in the publicly funded system.

To look at it from another point of view, handling complaints about staff abuse can be difficult for an administrator. All complaints need to be taken seriously. But sometimes residents can misconstrue things, forget things, or simply be seeking attention. I have seen many residents who accused staff members of stealing, only to find the "stolen" item somewhere that the resident had hidden it and forgotten. An American nurse's aide once related to me a story about a nurse who held an agitated resident's hands at her side until she regained control, rather than administering a medication to her. This action could look like abuse, until you understand the situation and have some trust in the staff. I have also known residents who said a staff member was rude or hit them when clearly it did not occur.

Handling complaints can also be difficult in a unionized facility. I have seen unions that protected their members from termination even though it was clear that neglect or abuse had occurred. I have seen homes that did fire staff members for neglect and abuse but could only do so by buying out the person, which cost several thousand dollars.

The difficulty for families in monitoring care is that sometimes what looks like abuse can be the result of a fall or the natural bruising that happens to older people's fragile skin. Sometimes people stop eating, or it is difficult to get them to take liquids. Sometimes people do fall. Conversely, even if you rightly suspect abuse, the home can tell you that, for example, your father had a fall, fell out of bed, or refuses to eat.

PREVENTING ABUSE

No matter how much legislation, education, and monitoring we have, there are always going to be people who abuse, so there is always going to be abuse; we cannot monitor the whole world closely, just as we cannot monitor child abuse out of existence. You should be able to expect that the system and homes would not be set up to foster abuse, but unfortunately this is an unintentional result of the present U.S. system. Abuse can happen in the best of facilities, but is less likely in a good home if you have done your homework and if you pay attention and stay involved.

The potential for abuse is reduced when the staff, especially nurses and nurse's aides, are well supported by the management of the home. For starters, this means adequate staff, which will allow them to have a feeling that they are able to do their job—that it is not a losing battle. This is why it is important to look at the ratio of nurses and nurse's aides to residents when you are considering a facility for your family member.

Support also means being treated with respect and adequate financial compensation. It means that the management pays attention to the staff so that they are not overwhelmed or under undue stress. A system in which people do not feel they have any input or control over their environment is one that leads to a sense of helplessness. One way for a home to support its staff is an Employee and Family Assistance Program (EFAP) through which employees can access counseling. You can ask if the facility has one for their staff.

The staff also need to know that the facility will back them up and support them where and how they need it. (This does not mean protecting them when there are legitimate concerns or inadequacies.) They need to know that the management will not let them be unfairly harassed by families or residents and that they will not be placed in dangerous situations because a home is more interested in revenue and resident numbers than in staff safety.

If you think physical and verbal abuse of staff do not happen to nurse's aides, dietary personnel, and other staff members, let me tell you they do. I recently encountered a gentleman whose mother was admitted to a home where I do some consulting, one of the best in the province. Within a week he had yelled at three or four staff members. The first time I came in after his mother's admission, a care aide, a nurse, and the nursing administrator all warned me independently about the man's rudeness and attacks. We were all aware of his anxiety, depression, and isolation, but the way he handled it was not appropriate. Yes, sometimes the staff has to be called on the carpet because of neglect, but sometimes they are unfairly harassed by people who are unable to handle their emotions in any other way or by residents who treat them like servants. Sometimes they are attacked by residents who should not be there in the first place because the home is not equipped to handle them, but who are there because they can pay the fee.

Adequate training and ongoing education will help avoid or decrease the incidence of resident abuse. The staff should be adequately trained to do the jobs for which they were hired. If they are not, the home should either provide the training or let them go (or not hire them in the first place, but hiring good staff members who are well trained is not easy). Training should include information about not only physical care but also the aging process and cognitive decline. They need to know how diseases such as dementia and stroke affect people.

The staff need to understand the meaning of violent and aggressive behavior from residents and family members. They need to know that some behavior is not aimed at them personally. In the example of the gentleman above, it was about the emotions and situations of the family member. With residents it may be part of their illness or emotional condition. The staff need to know skills to avoid aggressive behavior and to defuse it if it does occur. This information and these skills can be taught. It is not fair for the staff to be placed in situations for which they are unprepared, and it is not fair to the residents.

A nursing home with open communication that confronts issues such as abuse directly is less likely to create conditions under which abuse would occur and is less likely to shield people who are potentially abusers. Does the home talk to the residents about abuse? Do they encourage open communication and input from the residents and the family? Do they take complaints about the staff seriously? Is information about abuse part of their ongoing education guidelines? A strong family council (see chapter 16, "Making a Home Better") can be instrumental in mitigating the causes of abuse because it provides support to the staff. This can decrease their sense of isolation and feeling overwhelmed by a difficult job. In a home that is not so well run, it also lets them know that many pairs of eyes are watching.

My experience has been that most staff members in nursing homes are incredibly good and caring people. This is true whether they are laundry, dining room, or nursing staff. They go out of their way, beyond their job descriptions, and spend out of their own pockets because they care about the residents. They are troubled by the inadequacies they see and frustrated by their helplessness to fix them. There is often a genuine closeness between some staff members and residents. I can tell you that the relationships I have had with many residents (and their families) have touched my heart and my life in ways for which I will always be grateful.

RESIDENT-ON-RESIDENT ABUSE

There are occasional instances of abuse of residents by other residents. This may be between two cognitively aware residents, between an aware resident and one who is not, or two cognitively impaired residents (although due to the impairment, as they are not able to form intent with reasonable judgment and understanding, it is hard to call this "abuse"). It happens for a variety of reasons.

There is a large incidence of depression and "institutionalization" in nursing homes. Depression can lead to aggressive behavior. Often residents never get out of the building or away from the home. There is sometimes overcrowding; too many people in a space not designed for them (think of prison riots). With cognitively impaired residents, they may misinterpret one another's actions, feel threatened, or hit out in confusion. They may be suffering from pain or be overmedicated and not have those concerns addressed. Sexual acting out may occur because a resident thinks another resident is his wife. The issues need to be addressed by the system. Each incident has to be understood for not only what happened, but also its meaning, and through an understanding of the needs and abilities of the residents involved.

In the end, there is only so much you can do about abuse of any kind. Visit at different times during the day and evening. Get to know the staff and try to treat them with respect and understanding. Get to know other families and the verbal residents and be aware of what their experiences have been. Make sure the home is taking your concerns seriously and investigating. You can follow some of the suggestions I list in chapter 16. You will have to decide if the signs that you see are the result of abuse or part of a physical condition or something that has been misconstrued, or simply an accident.

You need to be aware and take precautions (which may include setting up a video monitor). Once you know the home and have some trust in it, start to relax, bit by bit, and see if it is justifiable to allow your trust to grow. If abuse does occur, you will need to begin either to remove your relative or to start another process (see chapter 13).

Specialized Dementia Care Units

The 1980s saw the creation of special care units, or dementia units. You can now find SCUs in assisted living residences as well as nursing homes. These are usually sections of a residence dedicated to residents who for some reason would be at risk in a general population. This may be because they would wander away, because their behavior would put them or the other residents at risk, because they need a smaller and lower stimulating environment, or other reasons. The units are usually secured so that residents cannot leave without knowing a code or having a passkey. Ideally, there is particularly low stimulation (not low activity) so that agitation or upset is minimized. These residents should have a separate dining area. There should be some room to wander about in and access to the outdoors. There should be consistency in the staff members who know the residents well. Consistency of caregivers is important to elderly persons; it makes them feel safe. It is even more important with confused people.

There is a wide variation in how dementia units have been designed and function. In some homes, it is an area that has been specifically built for people with dementia. The hallways are shorter, and the physical space encourages interaction and orientation to the environment. In other homes, it is nothing more than a locked unit that has been sectioned off from the rest of the home. In some, the care is warm and loving and meets the needs of the impaired residents; in others, the staffing and care is no different from that in the rest of the building.

The residents in an SCU may or may not have nursing care needs; what they do have are high needs for direction, reassurance, orientation, and help with their personal care. When you are comparing SCUs, compare the number of actual nurse's aides.

Just because your father has dementia, however, does not mean that he belongs in a special care unit. Does he need a low level of stimulation? Would he become lost or frightened in the larger facility? Would he try to leave and then get lost? Would he be socially or physically invasive to other residents or their space? If he does need a special care unit, make sure you view it specifically before admission.

You may have a strong reaction to dementia units—even stronger than to a home in general. It can be upsetting to think that your father is at "such a bad stage" that he needs this type of unit. Some people, however, function well in these units, much better than they would in the general population. Often the staff is better trained and more focused on providing care for people with dementia. There is less pressure on the residents to perform to a social standard that they can no longer meet. It is acceptable for them to wander into another resident's room, wear someone else's clothes, or be dressed somewhat bizarrely. Residents do not get lost as much, and they tend to feel more secure because the spaces are smaller. They can make friends among people who are similar. I have seen some touching companionships take place here between residents.

Costs

The costs of care can vary enormously, depending on where you live. In the Canadian public system, for example, someone can have a private room with sink and toilet for less than forty dollars a day. In private facilities in Canada and the United States, costs can go up to seven thousand dollars a month. Costs of care often increase as a person's care needs increase or as a person moves from one section of a complex to another.

MEDICARE AND MEDICAID

In the United States, the Department of Health and Human Services' Centers for Medicare and Medicaid Services (CMS) are responsible for the Medicare and Medicaid programs. Benefits through these programs are often available to help defray costs of skilled nursing care facilities.

Medicare is a federal insurance program that is basically the same throughout the country. Under certain conditions, Medicare (Part A) may pay full coverage for the first twenty days in a skilled nursing facility and eighty additional days minus a co-payment (that is, the portion of the costs that you would usually have to pay to receive the benefits). To receive payment, the resident must have been discharged from a hospital stay of at least three nights within the past thirty days. Medicare Part A pays for residents who need skilled nursing services, as defined by the legislation. It also pays for some therapy, and can pay for it even in the event of a plateau if there is a reasonable expectation of some improvement or if therapy is necessary to maintain the progress achieved. This last is particularly important because it can mean the difference between ongoing therapy (and a much improved life) or not. You can dispute a decision that says your father has "plateaued" by gathering evidence and independent, outside opinions.

Medicare (Part B) may pay for doctors, therapists, and other services not covered by Part A. However, the amount paid for a particular item, such as physical therapy, may be limited. Once someone has had a certain number of treatments, he may be ineligible for the rest of the year. Benefits under Part B must be applied for separately. The premiums are relatively inexpensive and are valuable because of the range of items covered. Apply for Medicare within seven months of eligibility, usually at age sixty-five. If you wait longer, premiums go up.

Medicaid is the assistance program jointly funded by the federal and state governments which will pay for nursing home care when Medicare is not applicable or when Medicare benefits have expired. Medicaid is administered at the state level. To be eligible for Medicaid, you may have had to "spend down," that is, dispose of the majority of your assets first. This means that you will have had to pay the initial costs of a nursing home or assisted living until your assets are below the required level. A spouse still living at home may keep a home, a car, and a limited amount of cash.

The rules and regulations of Medicaid vary from state to state. Make sure you understand what you have to do in your state and how to handle assets. Do not assume that you cannot keep them; learn the rules. You will have to do some research in your area. Find out what kinds of documentation you will need to enable you to benefit from subsidies. This can include several years of income tax statements, bank statements, and receipts for medical expenses, for example. As I mentioned above, some states have received a waiver from Medicaid so that they are able to fund people in assisted living facilities that do not qualify as skilled nursing facilities.

Applying for Medicaid can be a daunting task, and there are some lawyers, social workers, and geriatric care managers who have made it part of their business to help people through the maze. The rules governing Medicaid can also be confusing. Spending down your assets, what you may keep, and how to pay off bills are all complicated issues. If you know the rules, you will avoid making costly mistakes or having to give up some benefits and therapies. In general, you should carefully examine any kinds of costs you are presented with. If you have questions about them and about what Medicaid or Medicare should be funding, refuse to pay them until you have gotten some advice.

Some homes want you to have approval for Medicaid in place before admission. Others will help you apply for Medicare and Medicaid benefits. If you are turned down for either, you can and should appeal the ruling.

SUPPLEMENTAL INSURANCE (MEDIGAP AND MEDICARE ADVANTAGE PLANS)

You can also buy Medigap or Medicare Select insurance policies. These are policies, numbered A through L, that are bought through a private insurance company but are government regulated. They were designed to help with the costs that original Medicare does not cover. All except Plan A cover the Medicare hospital deductible (what you must pay before Medicare starts paying). They also pay for most co-payments. Some pay for other Medicare deductibles. Some of the Medigap policies will pay the co-payment fees for days twenty-one through one hundred in a skilled nursing facility. Some may also pay for items that Medicare does not cover. They, like Medicare, will not pay more. There are varying restrictions and benefits in the policies and eligibility times.

Another option is the Medicare Advantage Plans. These are health insurance plans purchased through private companies that have contracted with Medicare. They must provide the same benefits as original Medicare, but the specifics of coverage may vary. They are most often health maintenance organizations (HMOs) but may be preferred provider organizations (PPOs) or private fee-for-service plans. You pay a certain rate to the HMO and they provide your Medicare benefits. You will still have to pay your Medicare Part B premium. There are advantages and disadvantages. There may be some increased coverage, but there are limitations on which services and service providers you are allowed to use. If you choose Medicare Advantage, your Medigap policy may not pay for benefits. Remember too that these are through private companies, and their profit motive may conflict with your getting the care or service you want.

Figuring out the appropriate Medicare option is complicated. The Centers for Medicare and Medicaid Services (CMS) puts out excellent guides to help you understand Medicare. The basic one is called "Guide to Health Insurance for People with Medicare." They also have guides that explain Medicare Advantage Plans, Medigap policies, and Medicare Part D (see below). These are available by contacting 1-800-MEDICARE or at www.medicare.gov. The Web site has many other features, including a guide to nursing homes and addresses of your state ombudsperson. Both the guides and the Web site will direct you to information sources and counseling regarding Medicare and Medicaid in your state.

AARP (www.aarp.org) puts out excellent guides that explain Medicare, Medigap, and the various other Medicare options. They explain how to make some rational choices for what is right for you. Get all these guides before acting. The Medicare Rights Center (www.medicarerights.org) is an independent organization dedicated to helping people find the information and assistance they need regarding Medicare. They can also direct you to information about Medicaid in your state. They have a telephone assistance line (800-333-4114) staffed by trained counselors. They also have newsletters you can sign up for. I recommend you get the newsletters, as they can help you prepare for changes and information you may need in the future.

MEDICARE PART D (DRUG BENEFITS)

Medicare's drug benefit (Medicare Part D) program went into effect in 2006. Under this benefit, you may choose among plans to provide insurance that pays, or helps pay, for medications. The plans are provided through private companies. You do not have to have the drug benefit, but it can be a good idea to do so if you do not have another prescription drug insurance policy. You can get either a stand-alone policy if you continue with the original Medicare, or a drug plan can be a benefit of a Medicare Advantage program. You will pay a yearly deductible as well as a monthly fee. You will also pay a portion of the cost of each prescription. Also, there may be a coverage gap: this means that after you have paid a certain amount, you will have to pay all the costs of your drugs up to another amount, after which you reach a point where the insurance starts again. If you have limited income or are on Medicaid, you may be eligible for Extra Help, which may pay the monthly fee and the yearly deductible as well as some more of the drug costs. If your family member is in a nursing home, you need to make sure that her home's pharmacy is covered under her insuring company's plan. You also need to make sure that her company's plan covers the medications she is being prescribed. If not, you can either change plans (no more than about one a month) or see if her physician can change her medication to one that is covered by her company's plan. Note that some medications and circumstances are covered by Medicare Part A; these might not be covered under your Part D plan. If you do not check, you may end up with a bill.

In Canada, provincial costs and subsidies vary. All provinces fund homes, and all provincial health care programs cover basic health care costs. A home's daily fee always totals less than someone's pension income. In some provinces there is a ceiling on fees to residents, regardless of assets and income. A couple of provinces require you to deplete your own resources before they will provide for you. Your provincial medical plan may pay some, but will not cover all, of the expenses incurred if you end up in a U.S. nursing home, so be sure to buy additional insurance if you are traveling to the United States. Canadian residents should look at appendix 1 of this book, "Accessing Care in Canada."

OTHER PAYMENT OPTIONS

There are at least three other options for nursing home payment. These are reverse mortgages, lines of credit, and long-term care insurance.

A reverse mortgage is a plan in which a bank lends you money based on a percentage of the value of your home. The bank pays you either a lump sum or a specified amount over a specified period of time. There may be initial costs, interest charges, or processing costs.

The money is paid back, along with accrued interest, on sale of the property or death of the recipient.

Be careful about using a reverse mortgage. A reverse mortgage is not free money. They are heavily advertised on television and print as being the best thing since sliced bread. The truth can be very different. People can end up with few assets. Here is an excerpt from an article on my Web site, www.diamondgeriatrics.com, written by a family member of an elderly man who had taken out a reverse mortgage:

> I recently have been helping my uncle sell his condo and although he had said that his reverse mortgage was awful, I was not prepared for the tremendous bite a reverse mortgage takes. In the 12 2/3 years that he had the mortgage, the debt rose by 4 times! Plus, in the small print, it was stipulated that he had to pay an additional amount that turned out to be 84 percent of the original loan.
>
> So, say his original loan was for $10,000, he paid back:
>
> - 4 times original: $40,000
> - Additional amount: $8,400
> - Total owed: $48,400
>
> This total debt is close to 5 times the original amount borrowed in just 12 2/3 years.

If you are going to consider this option to pay for nursing homes, you might also want to consider using it to help keep your father at home with in-home help. For more information on reverse mortgages, contact the National Center for Home Equity Conversion (see Resources). Their Web site is a great source for you.

The second option is a line of credit on a property, which can be a better option than the reverse mortgage. To examine this option, see your banker or financial advisor for the specifics for your state or province.

The third option is long-term care insurance. These policies vary enormously in coverage, policy costs, elimination periods, and benefit periods. Options to inquire about include

- What kind of care does the policy cover (home care, nursing home, assisted living)?

- Does it pay sufficient benefits over a length of time (three years minimum)?
- Does it pay all the expenses, wherever you receive care?
- What conditions does it cover (Alzheimer disease, other dementias, etc.)?
- What are the conditions under which the benefits will start to be paid?
- Is there inflation protection so that the policy is valuable when you need it?
- How many payment days are you responsible for (the elimination period) before the policy comes into effect?
- Are the premiums a set price, and are they waived when you receive care?
- Are benefits ongoing, or is there a dollar limit?

Long-term care insurance can end up costing you more than your savings, and the monthly premiums can be expensive. Buy it if you are trying to protect your assets and if your circumstances are such that Medicaid coverage will not be available to you for a couple of years. Try to assess whether the payments will end up costing you more than the benefits. It does offer you flexibility and a range of options that you would not have if you had no insurance and no savings. For instance, you might be able to move into the residence of your choice faster, or the quality of the residence you can afford might be better.

The Administration on Aging (AOA) has an excellent Web site called the National Clearinghouse for Long-Term Care Information. There is a specific section on paying for care and, within that, one on long-term care insurance (www.longtermcare.gov/LTC/Main_Site/ Paying_LTC/Private_Programs/LTC_Insurance/index.aspx).

Long-term insurance should also be an option if it covers assisted living and/or home support and home health care. The vast majority of people say they want to remain in their own homes as long they can. As we are living longer, general frailty, incontinence, mismedication, social isolation, and dementia are the primary factors that are going to affect someone's ability to stay at home.

Canadian residents will want to look carefully to assess the benefits of long-term care insurance because provincially funded nursing homes and assisted living residences are often adequate to excellent in the care that they provide. However, the government is the gatekeeper for nursing homes and many assisted living residences. They decide what you are eligible for, when you can enter, and where you can enter. There is no need to go to a private home except if you are waiting for a space in the publicly funded home of your choice. However, that option of choice can be important. It also gives you choice about when you can access nursing homes or assisted living. There are and will most likely always be limits on what the provincial health authorities will provide in terms of home care support. Long-term care insurance will be invaluable to help make up the difference between what is offered and what you need to stay in your home. If you are spending time in the United States, you may want long-term care insurance that covers you in case you need nursing home care on an emergency basis until you are well enough to return home.

Spouses need to find out how having a relative go into a nursing home will affect their pensions. In Canada this situation is called an involuntary separation, and when it happens, both members of a couple are allowed to apply for full Old Age Security and Guaranteed Income Supplement benefits. In the United States what a spouse is allowed to keep varies from state to state.

OTHER CONSIDERATIONS REGARDING COSTS

In the United States the costs of "qualified" long-term care and home care services are tax-deductible medical expenses if they exceed a specified portion of gross income. In some cases you may also claim a relative as a dependent. Premiums for long-term care insurance may in some instances be tax deductible. Some costs are tax deductible in Canada as well. You may have to have a doctor certify that you are disabled to have certain deductions kick in. There are various benefits available to caregivers also. Consult an accountant for the specifics of your situation. Alzheimer's Association chapters are usually knowledgeable in this area also.

When you are considering a home and again when your father has been admitted, find out all the costs of care. In the United States, nursing homes that receive Medicaid funds are required to tell you all costs. They should tell you what is covered under Medicaid and Medicare and what you will be responsible for. If something is covered under Medicaid, make sure you are not charged extra for it. You should find out about charges for extras such as toiletries, bus outings, and additional care. If you are suspicious about what you are being charged, call the local area agency on aging to find out what charges are allowed. Make sure your father has received what he has paid for also.

The various styles of assisted living facilities have different costs and payment structures. These can include an initial large payment that would pay for an apartment and then monthly maintenance living charges. There may be a monthly rent but an additional charge for each extra service, say for help with dressing, monitoring someone taking medication, and help with a bath. If you are considering assisted living, be especially diligent about finding out all costs and limitations before you buy. Unlike for nursing homes, there are no regulations concerning the disclosure of costs and services for assisted living facilities.

Nursing Homes and Legal Responsibility

Nursing homes are concerned with legal issues in general, although with all the lawsuits for neglect, abuse, and fraud, it appears that many need to be a lot more concerned. Abuse and neglect are legitimate reasons for lawsuits. Sometimes lawsuits are frivolous and malicious and are the result of people inappropriately dealing with unresolved grief or other feelings. I can't tell you how many times over the past few years people have threatened to sue homes I worked in despite the fact that their relative had received good care. The potential for lawsuits affects many areas of life in a nursing home. This includes how care is provided, whether and how restraints are used, what furniture is allowed in people's rooms, and what activities are provided. It affects who will be admitted or allowed to remain as a resident in the home. It means the staff spends a lot of time in meetings and keeping documentation.

The way any residence may try to skirt its responsibilities to provide care and service is through the admission documents that they will ask you to sign. That is why you should (a) read those documents carefully and (b) understand your rights under the law. You could ask your lawyer to read them also. In the United States, an admission document cannot take away the home's responsibility to provide the care the law says it should. This means you cannot sign away your rights.

The result of the threat of lawsuits is sometimes better care, but unfortunately it can lead to more restrictions, less flexibility, and less hands-on care from the staff. This means that when you ask for something to be done or for a variation in some rules, a home may say no. It may seem like a simple request to you, but behind the negative response may be legal concerns the home has.

Mildred

The first thing you notice is the smell. It's a soapy, antiseptic smell that lets you know you are someplace where soapy, antiseptic smells are necessary.

I had the unfortunate duty of having to tour nursing homes recently, trying to choose one for my mother. At age seventy-three, after three strokes and with advancing kidney disease, she needed round-the-clock professional care, much more than could be provided at home.

My brother and I were given a printout of Medicare guidelines, a listing of seventy-six Detroit-area nursing homes, and a week's time to make a decision. We made a few choices that looked promising and began touring the different facilities.

Medicare has a Web site called Nursing Home Compare (www .medicare.gov/NHCompare/home.aspx). It has a searchable database that shows comparative information about individual nursing homes, including annual inspection results and health status reports. For anyone anxious about finding a suitable facility for a loved one, such information is indispensable. I checked it daily as we began our tours of nursing homes.

We were led on these tours by nervous, talkative admissions counselors who rapidly walked us through their facilities, doing their best to put a positive spin on a dreadful circumstance. It was astounding what some counselors considered the selling points of their facilities. We were told the solitary 2' × 2' window in all the residents' rooms allowed residents to "keep in touch with the outside world." Confused residents in wheelchairs sat alone in hallways outside their rooms, some crying, some mumbling to themselves, creating a time that, according to the admissions counselor, allowed them a "sense of freedom and independence." While some areas such as a pristine dining room and a vacant exercise room were proudly displayed, we were not allowed to tour the kitchen, and we were given a discourse on how the "importance of the nurse-to-patient ratio is a myth."

Most residents' rooms looked like potential nightmares. Two people were assigned to each room, which threw any pretext of privacy out the two-foot window. The rooms were exceedingly cramped, with every square inch of wall space taken up with beds, bureaus, wheelchairs, oxygen tanks, large lights, and clothes baskets. Each resident was allowed to bring a television from home, and the accompanying din caused by two televisions loudly tuned to different stations in such a small room was nervewracking.

Subsequent visits to other nursing homes revealed that two people to a room was a luxury. Many times there were four and sometimes six people to a room. One coordinator commented that six to a room was a positive environment, as "one person usually acts as a 'mother hen' for the rest." This seemed odd as I looked around the room and saw all the people lying in their beds, most wearing oxygen masks. It looked like a barracks in purgatory.

Most nursing home facilities had buzzer systems that were activated anytime an outside door to the building was opened. These were used as a kind of reverse burglar alarm, not so much to keep people out as to keep people in. The buzzer was going off with the regularity of a junior high school changing classes. Those few residents who were able to walk definitely wanted out.

Anyone who has an aging parent and thinks Medicare will cover any nursing home stay that might be needed is in for a terrible shock. Medicare covers only the first twenty days in a nursing home, or "skilled care facility." For days 21 through 100, the patient must pay the first $95.00 per day. After day 100, the patient is responsible for 100 percent of the nursing home charges. For any long-term admission, this can quickly become financially suffocating for any family.

As the Baby Boom generation struggles through its fifth decade, their parents are struggling through old age. As of 1997, there were 1.5 million Americans in nursing homes, with three-quarters of them women aged 65 to 84. With medical advancements, new prescription drugs,

122

and emphasis on personal fitness, Americans are living longer than ever before. The question for Americans seems to be, Now what do we do with them?

Good nursing homes do exist, but they must be sought out using all the resources that one can muster. One great and immediate source of information is the Internet, where numerous protective agencies, watchdog groups, and family members can instantly voice an opinion or throw up a red flag. The Medicare Nursing Home Compare site promises to be an invaluable resource. The Michigan Consumer's Guide to Nursing Homes (www.hcam.org) has the latest scores from state inspections and what violations were cited.

Many times after visiting the different nursing facilities, I would come home physically ill. Nausea and dizziness would overcome me, brought on by the stress of making such a choice. By the time we had finished making all the tours, I had not slept or eaten a complete meal for days and was filled with dread at the problems and complications I knew life had in store for my mother and me.

We toured eleven homes in all and found only one that was marginally acceptable. That particular home had an admissions coordinator who seemed to care about individuals, not just resident files; she was more concerned with people than paper. And the home had a head nurse who sat down and talked to us about Mom's condition. The rooms still had a miserable quality to them, but trade-offs had to be made. The week's time we were given was almost up and we had to decide.

A few days before the transfer from the hospital to the nursing home, Mom died. While death is always a sad occasion, I believed that it was God's blessing that she did not have to make that last terrible move. I would never have gotten a night's sleep, constantly wondering about the care she was receiving.

Sometimes I remember all the other elderly moms and dads I saw on my tours, and I wonder if they are getting the care they need. And I wonder if their families get any sleep at all.

It is good to be young and strong in America. But the images I saw on my nursing home quest would have even the most robust American pondering: What will my room look like as my journey winds down?

CHAPTER 6

Viewing the Residence

If you are not careful, searching out the right residence can be almost a full-time job. If you were to ask all the questions that you find in some lists (and what I have listed below) and do all the things that are suggested, visiting each residence could be a marathon. It might work better to gain a feel for a few of the homes you visit, then choose a couple for more in-depth visits and interviews.

Be aware of who is giving you a tour. In a for-profit residence, often it is a marketing person. This does not mean that he will give you a false image of what the residence is about, but, as the job title implies, his job is to sell, and to sell you *his* residence, not the one down the street. This can mean that his primary interest is not in helping you decide if his residence is or is not the best fit for you. Also, a marketing director may not know about how care is provided or about geriatrics and the needs of elderly persons.

Be aware of who or what company owns the residence. Is it a large chain, a small chain, or a single owner? Find out what their record of care has been, including their compliances with regulations and whether they have had fines, convictions, or other actions taken against them. You can find some of this information when checking the Nursing Home Compare site www.medicare.gov/nhcompare or by searching the Internet for the company name. A small chain or individually owned home or a nonprofit may be more responsive to you or your father than a larger one with a corporate culture that is directed from far away.

Balance what goes on in the residence with how close it is to where you live. Even if you will be there to visit for a couple of hours a day, the home has to be adequate for your husband for twenty-four hours every day. Think realistically about how often you will visit. You may come in every day for the first two weeks, but then only once or twice a week after a few months. If you have friends who already have a relative in a residence, go with them to visit. They can point out details that you might miss, and it will give you an opportunity to go beyond the person who officially gives tours.

The most important thing in visiting a residence is how the place feels to you. Does there seem to be kindness in the atmosphere? Is there an energy in the air? Is there kindness in the staff's voices or smiles on their faces? Watch for how the staff interacts with each other and with the residents. Watch how the residents act with each other during programs. Listen to how much noise there is. Notice the colors and the furniture.

Depending on your schedule, you should be able to visit several times. Go for a meal. Visit during some of the activities. Have a drink at happy hour. Would you buy shoes without trying them on and walking a bit in them? It's the same with a seniors residence.

Take a look at the residents you see. For nursing homes: Do they appear well dressed, groomed, and washed? Do the women have on any nail polish or makeup? Is their hair done nicely? If any residents are using equipment such as a walker or a wheelchair, does it seem to be in good repair? If they have on bandages or dressings, are they clean and well put on? These things tell you that the staff members are doing their jobs, indicating good care and good caring. You may see a few residents who do not present a good picture; people are sometimes incontinent despite the best staff effort, and sometimes people do not want to wash or groom themselves. But the majority should appear well cared for physically.

For assisted living, you might also look at additional indicators of quality: are residents busy? Are they talking to each other? Are they participating in offered activities? Are they friendly, warm, and welcoming as you tour? Pay attention to the mix of people in the home. Do the people appear to be functioning at an appropriate level, or are a lot of them needing more care? What happens in the dining room; how are people seated together? Are the activities and recreational opportunities appropriate to assisted living, or to what your husband and you need and will need in the future?

A gauge of the quality of care in nursing homes is the incidence of pressure sores (see chapter 12). You can ask about this during the tour. (Whether they will give you an honest answer is something different.) You can also review the official inspection report, which will mention whether sores were discovered. However, it is a random inspection, so just because they are not mentioned in the report does not mean there have not been any. A good home will have had a low incidence of pressure sores.

When you are touring residences, develop a comparison chart for yourself such as the one in questionnaire 1, "Guide to Viewing Nursing Homes," in appendix 2. For each home, rate each item 1, 2, or 3, or write yes/no or good/fair/poor, or use a check mark. Write a few notes after the visit to each home. This comparative chart will be helpful to you after you have seen several homes and you can't quite remember how one measured up against another. Many Web sites have charts and questionnaires you can look at as well. When you are asking questions and looking around, be aware that you may not find your ideal facility. That is the reality of the situation. If your husband is being discharged from a hospital, there will be pressure on you to make a quick choice, which may not be what you would otherwise consider. You may have to accept less than the optimal in all areas of good care and good caring. You will have to pick out what is important and what is less important. This can vary according to your husband's needs—he may benefit most from a home that has good access to physical therapy. If he is blind, he may want a small home. If he has reduced mobility, he may want short hallways. He may not want to use elevators (which tend to get backed up during meal times). If he is able to assist in the viewing process, consult with him about what is most important and highlight those points on your list of questions to ask.

Staffing

Ask about staffing. For nursing homes especially, compare separate ratios of nurses to residents and nurse's aides to residents. Make sure they tell you the number of *nurses and nurse's aides* to clients, not the number of staff members to clients. The latter can include the housekeepers, laundry personnel, and so on. You might want to ask about how the ratio varies according to shift. Nursing home staffing is much lower during the day than at night, when residents are sleeping. How does the home make sure it has enough staff members to help change incontinent residents during the night?

What kind of turnover in staff has there been? A high turnover can indicate problems (or it can indicate that the home is cleaning up problems). Do they use a lot of casual or agency staff members? Agency staff are not bad, but they generally do not know the residents as well as those who are on the regular staff do. That means that they are at a disadvantage in recognizing whether anything is different in your husband's condition and could miss warnings that something is wrong.

If you are looking at assisted living, is there a registered nurse or a licensed practical nurse? If so, is a nurse on duty all the time or just during the day? What are his or her responsibilities in terms of providing actual nursing? Who is available if there is an emergency: if someone has had a fall at night, or needs to go to the hospital, or needs to see a physician?

When you look at staffing levels, make sure you also understand the degree of disability of the people for whom the staff is caring. If their clientele contains a number of people who have high care needs, then they need a better caregiver-to-client ratio. If the clientele has only lighter care needs, then there can be fewer nurse's aides and nurses for more clients.

Find out who is on the staff beyond nurses, nurse's aides, and recreation staff. Is there music or art therapy? Is there a dentist or dental services? Is there a social worker? Is there a podiatrist who comes in regularly? In the United States, nursing homes that receive Medicaid funding must provide access to physical therapy, occupational therapy, and speech therapy if it is not provided on site.

Programming

Look at the programming in the home. Diverse programming should be available to meet the different needs and abilities of the residents. Assisted living may be more limited in terms of the recreation staff than are nursing homes, again because people are supposed to be more independent. However, even assisted living residents have a range of cognitive and physical abilities. How does the residence meet those various needs? How many recreation staff members are there? What is the scope of their job? Will they remind people about a program or are residents expected to be able to remember and go on their own?

Is there programming that fits your husband's needs? If you like a small facility, remember that one of the trade-offs for the intimacy that a small home provides is that usually the recreation schedule is smaller. Ask for a copy of the monthly recreation schedule. Pay attention to how much is scheduled on the weekend. Are there any programs to which families are invited? Are families welcome at all programs? How involved is the community and, more important, how involved can your husband be in the community?

You can also sit in on some of the activities to see how they are run. This could include the residents' council, which most homes have. See if you can talk to some of the residents and/or some of the family members to see what their experience has been. If there is a family council, call someone on it or go to a meeting.

Find out what the home's attitude is about physical activity. Will they encourage independence and rehabilitation? For instance, will they encourage your husband to walk to the dining room, or will they put him in a wheelchair because they don't have time to help him walk? Will they help him to dress or will they dress him? Help him to shave or shave him? All of these small activities are important for maintaining independence and emotional health.

When you are looking at activities and recreation, try to find out about resident life and how it is encouraged. If you think about it, we all have activities that we do every day that make up our life. We water the plants, read the paper, make the bed, have tea, walk over to visit with the neighbor, go shopping, and so on. These are activities that we do aside from "recreational activities," such as going to a show or having a party. Find out how the home encourages residents to have an everyday kind of life.

Policies

All homes have policies and procedures. Here are several you should try to find out about.

What are visiting hours and policies? According to U.S. law, nursing home residents may have visitors at any time of the day or night. Can you have a meal with your husband in the dining room? Can you celebrate special occasions? Is there a resident kitchen where you can cook a meal together? In your own home you come and go as you wish, have visitors, serve coffee. You should be able to do all this in a residence as well. What is the policy on roommates and room changes? If your husband has to have a roommate, how does the staff handle conflicts between roommates if they arise? Do they encourage residents to stay up at night for activities, or do they try to get everybody in bed by eight o'clock? If you are able to, you might want to do an evening visit before admission.

What are the policies and procedures concerning abuse? Find out if they have had incidences of alleged abuse and how they have dealt with them. Do they do criminal background checks on the staff? What kind of screening do they do? Later, call the licensing system in your area to find out about charges of abuse or neglect.

What are the safety policies and practices? Do they have an evacuation plan, and have they ever practiced it? Do they have fire drills?

One of the most important questions to ask is whether there are limitations on the care that the home can provide. If your husband's condition deteriorates, will he have to move? In what situations would that be? What are the requirements surrounding a move? Can you hire more help privately so he doesn't have to move? Does he have to take the first place available? Area agencies on aging report that some of the most common complaints about assisted living are about contracts and discharges. A residence may say they can't handle someone anymore and want to discharge them.

It is not legal in the United States to discharge someone from a nursing home because of Medicaid limitations. There are also regulations concerning transfers. A home must tell you the reasons for transfer, where your husband will be moved to, and the date of transfer or discharge. Residents have the right to appeal to the state and must be given the information necessary to contact the ombudsperson. Assisted living may or may not be covered by similar regulations, according to the state. In Canada, in some provinces, assisted living is now included in residential tenancy regulations, meaning that the facility must give you the standard notice to leave, for instance, one month, and you can appeal that legally.

You can ask about end-of-life care policies. If someone is dying, under what circumstances is the residence able to care for that person within the facility? Are they licensed to provide hospice care? How do they provide palliative care?

You will want to obtain a copy of the preadmission agreements. In some areas they are standardized; in some areas, homes have their own. This gives you a good idea of what the home expects and what you can expect. Remember, you are going to have to sign this document. Make sure you understand it, if it is written in legalese. Make sure you are willing and able to live up to the terms of what it says. However, as I mentioned earlier, a preadmission agreement cannot take away your rights or circumvent the Nursing Home Reform Law requirements on care.

Again, make sure you understand what charges are and under what circumstances that can or will change. Once someone is admitted to a residence, if you have questions about the legitimacy of charges, you may be out of luck, or you may be covered by state, provincial, or federal regulations. Remember that assisted living facilities are less regulated than nursing homes. In some areas they are not covered by the Nursing Home Reform Law.

Dining

After staffing, food is the primary area where a residence can cut corners to save money. This obviously affects what will be served, the quality of the item being served, and how often it appears on the menu. When you pay more for a residence, it may show up in the food budget.

Look at the meals and dining service. Appetizing descriptions can be written about pretty unimpressive food. How does the food look, and how is it presented and served? What happens in the dining room? Watch the service: are the food service workers interacting with the residents and listening to them, or are they talking to each other above the residents' heads? Request a copy of the menus for a whole month. A good question to use in comparing homes is "What is the budgeted cost per dinner/lunch/meals per day per resident?"

If your husband doesn't like what is being served, what happens? Will anyone notice? Will someone help him eat if he is unable to feed himself? Can you return another day with your husband and purchase a meal to try it? Can people bring their meals to their room or apartment if they don't feel like eating in the dining room, or have them brought to their room if they are too sick? Will there be a charge for that?

Physical Plant

Of course, a building should be in a good state of repair, but an old building does not mean that the care and caring within is not good. Even if the building is older, it should be well kept up. It should not have paint chipping, scratches all over, or a garden with more weeds than grass or plants. These things, rather than the age of the building, will give you a clue about the management approach and care. I had a client paying five thousand dollars a month in a relatively new facility where the garden looked like it was part of an abandoned house. It was consistent with the generally lower level of care provided by the facility.

When you look at the physical plant, look at lighting, equipment, and private space. Are fire exits well marked? Are fire exits accessible, or are they blocked by furniture or equipment? Is the bathroom equipped for a wheelchair? Are there grab bars around the toilet? How far are the dining room and activity rooms from residents' rooms? Are there single, double, or ward rooms? Is there a garden or other appropriate outdoor space? Are there stores or a coffee shop nearby?

Go over in your head how your husband lives during the day. Will the physical plant be able to accommodate him in the way he lives his life? Are the hallways long and convoluted? Is there sufficient public space? Does the layout seem to stimulate social interaction? Is the nursing station close enough to the rooms?

Surveys and Accreditation

Call your provincial health authority or state office on aging or state ombudsperson to find out if there have been any complaints about a residence you are considering. If there were, make sure you find out how they were resolved. In the United States, read the inspection report. Legally, it is available to you. The inspection reports do not always reflect what is truly going on in a home. It is easy for an inspector to miss problems and for problems to be misreported. Problem areas can be window dressed so they are not seen. Read them, but don't let them reassure you of something if your heart tells you that you are seeing or suspecting something different. Be aware, however, that there can be malicious and destructive complaints that are found to have no validity as well as valid complaints. For comparative information on rankings and surveys, go back to www.medicare.gov and look at their Nursing Home Compare section (www.medicare.gov/nhcompare). As noted earlier, you can also find survey reports on nursing homes and sometimes on assisted living through the area agencies on aging.

Many homes, especially in Canada, go through an accreditation process similar to the ones that hospitals go through. The national accreditation process is expensive and complete. Some homes are required to be accredited; others do it voluntarily. In the latter case, this is something of a commitment to care. However, homes know far in advance when the inspectors are coming and to whom they are going to talk. If the residence has been accredited, find out what the assessor found that was positive, what needed to be worked on, and how they are working on it.

John and Joyce

My father had been in St. Catherine's for four years before my mother had an aneurysm. They had no room for her at St. Catherine's, so for the nine months that remained of her life she lived at Sable Hill Home. We knew Dad was well looked after at St. Catherine's, but Sable Hill was a different story. The two facilities and our experiences couldn't have been more different.

Mom and Dad had both been Christian missionaries and priests. During their sixty years together, they were always a team. So when the signs of my father's Alzheimer disease were getting worse and worse, Mom was determined to take care of him. She was a woman of her time. It was her role to be responsible for everyone and everything in her family. She would have done it until she was dead. I watched her as she began breaking under the strain.

It started with the typical symptoms of Alzheimer disease. Dad was having trouble with word retrieval. Then he couldn't remember people. Then he was taking off in the middle of the night. Mom was always on edge, wondering when he was going to walk out the door. He would just say, "I am leaving," and she couldn't stop him. He was arguing. He was even getting violent, which he had never been in his life. We had to lock him in the house.

Finally we took him for a geriatric assessment. The assessment team members were able to give my mother some objective information and directions. She was still reluctant to let Dad go into a home. Finally I said to her that I was already losing one parent and I didn't want to lose two. That's what made her finally decide.

Even though Mom made the decision, the first six months were hard. She would go to see Dad every day. When we told her to take a rest of at least a day or two, she refused. She was afraid that if she missed a couple of days he would forget who she was. She was extremely critical of the care. She didn't like the way the staff did things; it wasn't the way she did them. I think underneath, she couldn't get used to having people do for Dad what she felt was her role. She felt pushed aside, like they were trying to take him away from her.

My brother and I tried to give her as much support as we could. We would come to the home, sometimes while she was visiting and sometimes when she wasn't there. It helped her to know that other people were coming in and she wasn't alone. We would call her every day to make sure she was doing all right.

The staff was extremely helpful. Just by doing small things for Dad, they returned some humanity to him. For example, they would say hello to him as they passed him in the hallway. Especially the chaplain. He had a way of letting you know that your family member was still a person, that he still mattered. I had been used to thinking that these old people were off in their own little world somewhere. But when it was my own family member, I felt differently.

After about six months, my mother came to see that St. Catherine's was a good place. She came to appreciate the care that Dad was getting and the staff. She could see how they served him tea, called him by his name, and held his hand. They also talked to us, let us know that they were interested in us too.

The staff, other residents, and family members became like an extended family for my mother. It was like she had a new life there. She would tell us which resident did what and which family member did what. She would go to birthday parties. She would tell us what was happening with the staff members, who got married, who had a baby.

A few years after he went into the home, Dad had a stroke. That was another crisis for my mother. Now there was even less that she could do for him. She couldn't help him to walk anymore. He couldn't speak. The words he used were unintelligible. It was heartbreaking for all of us, but especially for my mother. It was like she was losing another piece of him.

I tried to help my mother by looking for the hope and the positive that was still there. Music was helpful for us. When we gathered as a family or with residents to sing songs and hymns that were familiar to Dad, he would do his best to sing along. He would wave his arm as if he was the conductor of a great symphony. When he did this, we knew we had made a connection with him, and he with us. Dad still had a warm smile that engaged us and cheered our hearts. Sometimes when people asked him if he knew who I was, I would say, "of course." I knew he might not know my name, but he knew that I was someone who loved him. We read to him and we prayed with him beside us. Sometimes when we had a joke about something, we looked over at Dad and saw him chuckling to himself as if he were in on it too. All of these seemed to be ways to keep communicating with him.

Gradually, my mother adjusted to this phase of Dad's condition too. She continued to be a part of the St. Catherine's family. We could see she was adjusting.

Then she had her stroke. All of a sudden, everything changed. Mom had been driving, using e-mail; she was up and about and always doing things. In the back of our minds, we had always been preparing ourselves for losing Dad first. He was the one with the disease. It didn't seem right or fair.

Mom was first taken to the general hospital, and then later to the geriatric hospital. She became what they called a "bed blocker." They wanted us to find her a place right away. They said that she didn't need acute care, she needed a skilled nursing facility. At one point we had a meeting with the hospital staff. They proceeded to tell us that they wanted us to take her home that weekend. We told them that we couldn't. I was going away for a few days, the first vacation I had had in several years because I was always concerned about my parents. My brother had a flight out that afternoon. The social worker told us that the hospital was not a hotel. It was like they were just putting more and more on the family, and they weren't ready to listen to us. A couple of weeks later they took her to a facility. She was so sick that the facility sent her right back.

Finally, the hospital discharged her to Sable Hill because there was a bed available. The place was so big. The dining room held over one hundred people. When you went in the front door, the first thing you saw was all of these sick people being fed in this huge dining room. Nobody wants to see that as the first welcome into his or her home.

I hated going to Sable Hill. That was a horrible feeling to have. I felt so bad for Mom. I was just angry all the time. I was depressed and I felt hopeless because the care was so dodgy and so many things happened. I know how to be an advocate; I work in a large system. But there I always felt helpless. There were different staff people every day who never seemed to know or care about my mother. Once when I went to the nursing station, there were five staff members standing around talking. They ignored me until I finally said something to get their attention. One time they lost her wedding ring. When I reported it, no one seemed to care and no one tried to help us find it.

As all of this was happening, my brother and I had to become the primary people for Dad. It meant that we had to step in and begin to pay the bills, be aware of his care issues, etc. We were always in touch, but it had been my mother who was "command central" and the connection with the home. However, we had to kind of put Dad aside. We had confidence in the care at St. Catherine's. If something was on my mind, all I had to do was call the director of nursing and she would look after it. Sable Hill was totally the opposite.

I felt I had to go to Sable Hill every day. It felt like I was alone in having to watch out for my mother because it was so big and every day there were different staff members. Even when I left for the day, I didn't know what would happen later. I was upset by what I knew was going on. The staff would take their breaks during mealtimes. The food would be served in huge portions and it looked so unappetizing. If my mother got to the dining room, they would help her eat, but if she stayed in her room, she could be forgotten there. When you would ask for some assistance with helping her eat, the people who delivered the food would say that they were sorry, but it was not their job.

When I would come in to see my mother, I felt I had to check up on what had been happening. I was always upset because things wouldn't get done. It was like I had to be on guard. I would ask my mother things like, "Have you been to chapel?" I learned that I could not make assumptions the way I could at St. Catherine's. In the end, it seemed like the problem came from the fact that the staff had so little connection with the residents or the families. When you feel like the staff is connected to you or your family member, you feel that they will care. That is how they become your extended family in a way.

A lot of them did not mean to be mean or nasty. I knew how over-worked they were. It was not their fault, it was the system. The system seemed to exist for the system. I don't know why.

I tried to talk to the staff all the time, to see what could be done. I was as nice as I could be. I brought them chocolates. I let them know when I thought they had done some good things for my mother. You can't go in there and attack people. I knew if I lost it with them, then we would end up being labeled a "problem family."

I finally ended up having to talk to the people in charge. I discovered that the recreation people were good people to talk to. They would listen to what I had to say. They were willing to learn about who my mother was. I wanted them to know what a high-powered person she had been and how many friends she had had. Not that it made a difference maybe, but it made a difference to me. When Dad went to St. Catherine's, they asked us to write up a description of who he had been. They wanted to know.

I also learned that I would have to build a better support network for my mother. I called the staff chaplain and asked him to visit. I called other people and asked them to do the same. I also kept on talking to the staff. I made sure that she would get to the activities. If I hadn't intervened, they might not have taken her.

My mother had been at Sable Hill for only nine months when she died. The day she died, I went in to see her body. I was all by myself. There wasn't a single person who came into the room, not one staff person. I felt abandoned. Finally, out in the hallway I found a staff person. I asked her to ask if the chaplain could come. He did, and we said a prayer.

I guess we could have done better for Mom. If she had lived longer, we could have gotten her to a better place. Maybe I should have advo-cated more or talked to the ombudsperson. Even if I had, it might not have done any good—how would they change the system at the home? You don't know at the time. I tell myself that we did the best we could. If you know it will be for only two months, you can go all out, but if you don't know if it will be two months or two years, then you have to pace yourself. You have to save something for yourself and for your family.

Dad is still living at St. Catherine's. I play the piano for the teas at the home. He will sometimes call my name when I am playing a song that he truly likes. Other times he will grab my hand and hold on for dear life as if to say, "Be with me."

I still have many unanswered questions about the consciousness of people with dementia. What is it like if you have no memory and no awareness of most things? How can I make peace with my dad when the relationship is complicated by the changes he has had? What are the most comforting things I can do for him? Perhaps in time we will know more about these things, about where the soul resides, about what people with Alzheimer disease comprehend.

In the meantime, I guess I am more fortunate than most. As lost to me as Dad seems, he responds with a radiant smile that, to me, affirms his continuing love.

CHAPTER 7

Staff Roles:
Who Does What?

It may help you to understand the roles and responsibilities of the different personnel and departments in a residence. That way, you know who will be doing what for your father, who will be doing the things that you are used to doing, what you can expect and from whom you can expect it. It will also give you an idea of to whom you should talk if you need some information. Problems sometimes arise for family members when they are asking for help or information from someone who is not able or qualified to give it or who has a limited ability to comment.

The U.S. Nursing Home Reform Law requires each nursing home to care for its residents in such a manner and environment as will promote the maintenance or enhancement of the quality of life of each resident. Each nursing home is required to provide services and activities to attain or maintain the highest practicable physical, mental, and psychosocial well-being of each resident. The nursing home's goal, then, should be to hire staff members in a manner that allows the home to carry out this directive. How this actually looks, however, is a societal question. It will reflect what the government and people are willing to pay for it. At any rate, here are the staff members who should be working toward that goal for you.

Receptionist

In the first edition of this book, I left out the role of the receptionist. I don't know how I could have been so stupid. Neither did Pamela, the receptionist at a home in Vancouver who read that book and pointed it out to me. So, Pamela, this is for you.

In some ways, the receptionist has the most complicated and most difficult role in a nursing home or assisted living facility. He or she also has, in some ways, the most important (just ask Pamela). The receptionist is the person you meet first as you walk in the door. She or he sets the tone for the place and for you. There are some places I walk into where the receptionists looks up, smiles, and greets me warmly. In one home where I have a client, the receptionist has never done that in close to a year. Guess where I feel more welcome?

The receptionist usually knows all the residents and their visitors. She knows their comings and goings. The receptionist has a front-row seat on how other staff members interact with residents and family. It is often the receptionist who notices a behavioral or emotional concern with a resident. She can be the one who has to mediate arguments between residents and manage difficult behaviors. Usually she is multitasking: answering the phone, watching residents, monitoring the doors, accepting mail and packages, taking messages for the staff. She does this often without training and has had to learn on the job. In assisted living, the receptionist may be even more crucial because of the limited staff available to note some of the behaviors that would likely be picked up on by a larger staff in a nursing home.

Often the receptionist is the one to whom residents and family members, rightly or wrongly, choose to vent. Unfortunately, there may be little the receptionist can do except listen and pass concerns on. She or he is not part of care conferences or care planning and may have little say in how a home is run.

Administrator

The administrator is the person who has ultimate responsibility for the home. If the home is not part of a large chain or company, she is also the one who sets the tone for how the home runs. If she is an open, relaxed person, the home will reflect this; if she is rigid, the home will reflect her rigidity. The background of nursing home administrators varies tremendously. She could be a nurse, have an M.B.A., or have a social work or other degree. She will not necessarily have a background in gerontology. A good administrator will spend some time among the residents every day, maybe not visiting all areas and all residents, but being visible to the staff, residents, and families during the day. She will also be accessible within a reasonable amount of time. The administrator is the one you should contact when all else fails and before you go to a board of directors or an outside licensing agency. Try to get to know the administrator. This may entail having lunch or coffee with her once or twice a year or just stopping by for an appointment. It will help you feel connected to the home.

If a home is part of a chain or larger company, the administrator can be caught in the chain's system. The responsibility for profits and the policies of a company that has priorities other than good care can mean that an administrator is not able or willing to put the residents' care and well-being first. This is why it is important to know about a home's parent company.

Personal Care: Nurse's Aides

Most of the personal care in a nursing home is done by nurse's aides or certified nursing assistants (CNAs). The title will vary from region to region; in Canada they are often called care aides. These are the essential caregivers in the home. It is the nurse's aide who provides the "assist" in assisted living. In nursing homes they provide all of the care that is needed and not provided by the nurse. Unfortunately, they often have the least discretionary power or input into how the home is run. Ideally, they will have taken a course that teaches the basics of providing personal care for frail and fragile elderly persons.

It is the nurse's aide's responsibility to help a resident get up and ready for the day and to help her get ready for bed at night. They will also help with toileting and feeding. Usually they will help bring a resident to the dining room if the resident is unable to manage by herself. They also answer call bells. In a nursing home, nurse's aides usually do not give medication and they often do not record in residents' charts. In assisted living, they may give out medication or remind a resident to take his or her pills and watch while they do so. If they are doing this, they should have training to do so.

Nurse's aides are often the ones who know the residents best because they perform the most intimate personal care and they spend the most time with a resident. They know what a resident is or is not able to do. For the same reason, they may be the ones who have the closest personal relationship with the resident. Due to the frequency of contact, they are often a resident's primary social connection. They are also, therefore, the ones who most directly influence the resident's experience not only of the home but also of their life.

In assisted living the nurse's aides may have much more responsibility when there is minimal backup from a nurse. Supposedly in assisted living, residents are able to direct much, if not all, of their own care. In reality, of course, they often do not. This means that problems can be easily missed by a nurse's aide working without much support.

A nurse's aide can be responsible for a huge number of residents—up to fifteen or twenty during a day shift is not unusual in a medium-care facility. The night shift can be two or three times that many. In assisted living, they can have even more people to be responsible for, again because people are supposed to be more independent and need less help. This means remembering a staggering amount of information—who has a hearing aid, who wears glasses, who wants prunes in the morning, which family wants which resident dressed how, and so on. It means they must be aware of all sorts of changes in a resident's needs. Most important, depending on the acuity of the residents, it can easily mean that the nurse's aides do not have the time to do their work properly even if they want to. If you remember this, it will help you be more understanding of them and how difficult their work is. Many people, residents and families alike, somehow expect nurse's aides to be like servants, and they treat them as such. Please don't.

As someone pointed out to me, an assistant in a zoo sometimes earns more money than a nurse's aide. Although some wonderful people work as nurse's aides, the pay means that it will often attract relatively less educated people and lead to a high turnover. It also means that it is often immigrants who are the aides. If you stop and ask you will learn that in their own countries, these people may have been teachers, doctors, nurses, or other professionals. If the residence is in an affluent area, it can mean a long commute for these people at times when transit is not optimal.

Nurses

Licensed practical nurses (LPNs) and registered nurses (RNs) have training that lasts between eighteen months and four years of college. They oversee the physical care that is provided on the floor or the unit and often much of the emotional care.

It is in the area of nursing we see the major difference between nursing homes and assisted living. In the former, nurses are generally responsible for treatments and medications. They are the liaison between the resident and the physician. They are also responsible for doing initial assessments on admission. They do followup assessments when it appears that a resident is not doing well. They have primary responsibility for the physical health of your father, so they need to have good training in geriatrics (but often do not). The nurse on the floor is a good person to talk to when you have an initial question about some aspect of your father's medical condition or how he is functioning on a day-to-day basis.

In assisted living, the nursing may be much more limited. This varies according to the regulations of different states and provinces. Generally, the nurse in an assisted living facility is an overseer and does not provide direct nursing care on an ongoing basis. Many assisted living facilities have a nurse only during regular weekday work hours. There may be no nurses and no nurse's aides in the evenings and at night. When you are considering whether you need assisted living or a nursing home, you must take this into account. If you choose assisted living, think about what help Mum may need at night and how she will access it.

Many nursing homes use what is called a primary nurse model. This means that there is one nurse and one care aide who is your father's "primary" nurse and nurse's aide. They are responsible for your father's care plan and for routinely reviewing on a regular basis what is happening with your father. When the system is functioning well, it is kind of like an extra check to make sure that nothing is missed in your father's condition.

Most homes have a director of care who is responsible for nursing and nurse's aides. If it is a large home, there may also be one or more assistant directors of care who do the direct supervision of the nursing staff. She is also responsible for many of the policies and procedures regarding care. She should be well trained in gerontology. The director of care or assistant director of care is often the person who will resolve a problem that the floor nurse is unable to. She will have a good idea of which nurse is capable of doing what and how the nursing system is functioning in the home. The director of care is often responsible for other areas and professionals, such as recreation and other therapists.

Like the administrator, the director of care may have to keep one eye (or more) on the parent company's policies and priorities and try to balance those demands with the care needs of residents.

Dietitian and Food Services Staff

Most nursing homes have the services of a registered dietitian, who may or may not be head of the kitchen and food services. Even if she is not head of the kitchen, when there is a food- or eating-related issue, she is the one you can talk to. The dietitian does an assessment of each resident's nutritional needs. She will develop a diet and nutritional program that is appropriate for your father. This includes diabetic diets, gluten-free diets, and low-fat and other diets. Dietitians are also expert in the interaction of food, illness, and medications. Usually they are also knowledgeable about swallowing and eating difficulties. They will ensure that the food your father is served is the appropriate texture, such as pureed, minced, or cut up, if necessary to assist him in swallowing. The dietitian will monitor your father's weight and food intake.

Food services does the cooking and serving of meals. They carry out the instructions from the dietitian and/or the nursing department. They are also the ones who set up the dining room. If your father has disabilities such as arthritis that make it hard for him to open small packages or use certain utensils, for example, the food services staff have to have this information. They will then make sure that it is done for him. If he has certain likes or dislikes, allergies, or other concerns, they are the ones who need to know (more about this in chapter 13, "Communication and Problem Solving") because they are the ones who will actually serve him his food. They may also be the ones who can give you a picture of how your father manages in the dining room. Because dining is a main focus of many residents both as a necessary activity and as a social time, the food service workers are important to the residents' lives. Ideally, they interact with the residents while they serve them.

Food services may be the target of your father's complaints. While this may be valid, the complaints may really be driven by other issues, such as depression, anger, loneliness, or grief. Because it is hard to express those feelings, your father may be focusing on food or service, which are more concrete.

Social Worker

In the United States it is mandated that all homes have someone in a social service position, but he does not have to be a social worker by training. Usually this person is responsible for helping you with Medicare and Medicaid applications as well as other financial arrangements. In Canada, not all homes have a social worker. The social worker is a liaison with families and should be available to help people talk about the emotional or practical issues that arise. He is also sometimes like a detective. If there is a problem, he will help you figure out whom to approach and how and will help you see it through. The social worker will help you set up conferences and meetings to talk about your father's care. He will also help you to access outside resources and agencies that might be useful to you and your father. Often he runs support groups, family councils, and residents' councils. He should be able to provide information on community resources. Social workers are warm and wonderful people and you should probably take them out to lunch. Oh, did I mention I'm a social worker? That has no influence on what I just said.

Recreation Therapists

Recreation (or therapeutic recreation, or activities) is in some ways the lifeblood of a nursing home. The recreation worker's job is to provide stimulating activities that not only entertain your father but also enhance his capabilities and potential. Of course, not every activity or program is therapeutic, some are just plain fun. Generally a good recreation department will want to help your father maintain his skills, interests, personality, and social ability. Ideally, they are oriented to helping him with the issues of meaning and purpose in life. The idea is not to change him into something he never was, but to help him be all he can be. For example, if he never was a drinker, he probably isn't going to start having a nip during pub night (although, who knows—you may walk in and find him the life of the party with a lampshade on his head). The recreation department can help your father find companionship and a sense of individuality (but they cannot do it for him).

Recreation departments vary in size by the number of residents, and, like food services, according to budget. A residence may have several programs going on during the day, or maybe only one or two.

In a nursing home, programming supposedly takes in the range of abilities of the residents. The recreation staff will bring your father to programs that are appropriate for him if he cannot get there himself or forgets. The limit on this is their time. It takes a lot of time to set up a program and bring residents to it. Often a recreation worker will go to a resident's room and invite the resident, who will say no. Or he will say yes but then forget to go. After a while, the worker will know how best to approach your father to encourage him to take advantage of the activities.

In assisted living, the recreation department is usually limited. They will not provide the individual attention that your father would receive in a nursing home. They may not bring people to activities, or even remind them or call them. Also, the range of activities in assisted living may be limited. They may not have opportunities for people who are more cognitively impaired. This is another way for you to decide between housing options. If your father is not able to access recreation on his own, will he end up just being lonely in an assisted living facility?

In continuing-care retirement communities (CCRCs), you may be able to access the recreation programs in another part of the complex from the one in which your father lives. For instance, he may be able to use a program in the assisted living area even if he is in a nursing care unit. This is one question to ask about when viewing the facilities.

Most recreation departments produce a monthly calendar. It is a good idea to have a separate meeting with the director of recreation to go over the schedule and help the staff know what might interest your father. At the same time, you can let them know what you think is the best way to encourage his participation. Most homes have bus outings. Make sure you find out who gets to go on those, how often, and where they go. A resident may have to sign up for them, and if they cannot remember to do so, then they may not be able to go. Find out how you can be involved in recreation programs. What programs are there for families? Most activity departments will also keep statistics on program attendance. If you want to know after three months whether Dad is attending, they should be able to tell you.

Rehabilitation Staff

The rehabilitation staff can consist of a physical therapist (physiotherapist in Canada), physical therapy aides, occupational therapists, and speech therapists. Physical therapy is responsible for helping residents improve or maintain their physical ability. That includes improving the ability to stand up, sit down, or get on or off the bed. They help residents with walking ability, balance, maintaining muscle mass or flexibility, and, simply, exercise. Occupational therapists assist people in learning or relearning to do their ADL (activities of daily living), such as shaving, dressing, and washing. They (or the physical therapist) are also expert in assessing the equipment needs of a resident and recommending which kind of walker and wheelchair is best suited to the individual.

There is a wide variation between nursing homes as to the kind of rehabilitation programs that are available. As mentioned earlier, some nursing homes are also licensed rehabilitation centers. In some areas, the amount of rehabilitation staff is required by law for every certain number of residents. Other areas require no rehabilitation staff. In the United States, Medicare pays for some physical therapy services. All U.S. residents have the right to access physical therapy, occupational therapy, and speech therapy. If the home does not provide it, it must contract with an outside agency. The problem with this "one size fits all" approach is that, as one occupational therapist told me, "it means that lots of people who cannot benefit from these services receive them, so it becomes a factory approach. The people who could use the services the most don't benefit to their maximum potential."

Assisted living facilities may not provide rehabilitation services. They may have access to those services and even have a therapist in the building on a regular basis, but often rehabilitation is contracted out and usually is at an additional fee. If a resident needs physical therapy, occupational therapy, or speech therapy, it may be the responsibility of the family to arrange for it. In a CCRC, you may or may not have access to the services from the nursing units.

In Canada the provincial health programs subsidize physical therapy services up to a limited number of sessions. If there is no physical therapy in the nursing home, you may have to arrange for it or have your father brought to a clinic. (Often the physical therapists do not want to come to the home because they are not allowed to bill the government for transportation costs.) In both countries the amount of service is limited. Even without rehabilitation staff, many homes have a program that is designed to keep residents physically active, often through recreation.

Extended health plans often pay for rehabilitations services, as do sometimes long-term care insurance plans, or critical illness insurance plans. Check your policies, and know what is required to access the services.

Housekeepers / Building Maintenance Staff

Support services personnel, such as maintenance, groundskeepers, and especially housekeepers, may have many similarities with nurse's aides: poor pay, little education, harassment by families, and bigotry and racism on the part of residents. Housekeepers, who are in the residents' rooms frequently, often know the residents well and have developed close relationships with them. Housekeeping is done on a rotation, so rooms may not be thoroughly cleaned every day; but cleaning toilets and sinks and sweeping should be done every day. It is not the job of the housekeepers and maintenance people to dust a resident's personal items or fix the television or walker. They may do so, but it is generally not their job. You may want to ask what the home considers their responsibilities to be and how often they are to carry them out. Housekeepers are often the first people to be accused of stealing something from a resident. Theft may happen, but often a resident has simply forgotten where he put or hid money or an item.

Pharmacist

The average person at age eighty-five is taking about five to seven medications. A pharmacist is thus an important part of the care team. Different homes have different pharmacy arrangements. Sometimes pharmacists are at residents' care conferences, sometimes not. Sometimes one pharmacy provides medications; sometimes several.

Remember, the medications, potions, and treatments your father takes in his own home are his business. But the nursing home has legal obligations, and this can have an impact on its approach to medications. For one thing, the home will be much more cautious about interactions between naturopathic remedies and prescription drugs. If Dad is taking herbal or naturopathic medications, find out how the home will deal with these. It may be that they have to be obtained by prescription from a pharmacy. The assisted living residence may have a much more hands-off approach to medications, depending on the services they are providing and/or you are purchasing. They may provide medication reminders as part of the assisted living package but will not monitor whether there are interactions or whether your father is taking herbal supplements and other medications that may interact adversely.

Physicians

Some homes have "house" physicians; in others, people use their own doctors. In the United States, residents have the legal right to choose their physician. The advantage of a house physician is that she may be there more often and may know the staff and system better than a doctor who only has one or a few patients in the home. Conversely, she may be responsible for many patients and several homes and not be able to provide the care that your father needs.

In a nursing home, any doctor treating a resident must be willing to come see the resident in the home. The doctor's office should be close enough so that it is not a major inconvenience to do so. Usually if there is a problem, the nurse will contact the physician, but if you have questions, both you and your father have the right to contact the physician directly. Any physician working in the home should have an interest in geriatric medicine. She should also be available to you within a reasonable amount of time if you would like to talk to her. In assisted living, residents are expected to be able to make and go to doctor's appointments on their own. If they are unable to do so, it will be the family's responsibility to help with that.

Almost all homes also have a medical director. In the United States, it is required under law for all Medicare-participating homes. The medical director is at the facility for a limited number of hours or sessions per week. She is responsible for overseeing the medical care, medical standards and policies, and procedures. However, unless there is a problem, she may not know the individual residents. She will not become involved with the physicians unless there is a concern—it is not a preventative position in most cases. The medical director may not be a gerontologist or even have an in-depth knowledge of geriatric medicine.

Other Staff Members

A number of other disciplines are regularly involved in nursing homes. These include pastoral care workers (such as a priest or rabbi), music therapists, art therapists, and massage therapists. They are all valuable in helping residents have a fulfilling life. These people will often have insightful knowledge about how your father is doing and what his potential is. They can be valuable allies for you when you are setting goals and expectations.

Most residences will arrange for a podiatrist or foot-care nurse to come to the facility. Foot care is extremely important for elderly people. It can be critical for people with diabetes. The facility may or may not also have the services of a dentist, dental hygienist, and optometrist. If they do not, you may be able to bring in these services on your own. You will have to check to make sure your father is receiving the services or has asked to be seen.

Some nursing homes are bringing in or allow for a range of alternative health practices. These include reflexology, acupuncture, aromatherapy, massage, therapeutic touch, chiropractic, homeopathy, and other services brought in or provided in different residences. If you are interested in alternative or complementary medicine this is also an area you may have to investigate yourself. If you do wish to bring in complementary medical practitioners, especially in a nursing home, make sure you work with the doctor and staff so they know who is coming and what the person will be doing. Assisted living residents may have more freedom to arrange for these services on their own than do residents in nursing homes, which may be governed by corporate, facility, or government policies restricting or managing who has access to residents and what services they are allowed to provide. Some of this has to do with liability, sometimes it has to do with the attitude of the administration. I have found there is a wide variation among nursing homes regarding how open they are to having these professionals involved. Any complementary therapists should also find out if the residence wants them to note their activities in a resident's chart or file.

Some homes are developing models that give the staff fewer residents to work with but broader responsibilities. This means that instead of separate nurse's aides, housekeepers, or recreation staff members, one person will perform all of these roles. The same person who helps the resident get up in the morning and to the bathroom will help her in the dining room, make her bed with her, and then organize a card game with her and a couple of her neighbors.

Mabel

A year ago, we decided to seek a nursing home for my mother. She was on medication several times a day and on oxygen full time. She was unable to manage the medications and oxygen. I looked after her shopping, some cooking, paying her bills, and taking her to appointments. At this time, I was working four days a week. I went to her apartment every day around dinnertime to set out her medications for the following day and to make sure she was eating. Mom was requiring so much time that I had none left for my husband or children and grandchildren. We didn't go on any trips or even go out to dinner because we would have to rush home for the next medication time. The situation became a nightmare.

I requested a list of care facilities in our area from a local agency. Mom was assessed. I compiled a list of questions and made appointments with some of the places on my list. I toured a few and asked my questions. I then chose the one that seemed to address our needs the best, and Mom's name was entered on a waiting list. We were told that the wait could be as much as one year for her first choice.

As soon as there was an opening at one of the facilities, Mom and I went for a tour of the facility. She was not pleased with what she saw. She felt that it looked like a hospital. I reminded her that she required twenty-four-hour nursing and that it was set up to meet that need. She seemed to agree. She also noted that there were several people who seemed to just wander about, and this made her uncomfortable. The lady conducting the tour told her that "some people's bodies go and some people's minds go." She said that they did not feel these people should be locked up. Mom agreed. She also saw that there were several old people who needed wheelchairs. She was able to walk; she wasn't as infirm as they were. I reminded her that sometimes she was in a wheelchair to make it easier for her and that maybe many of them could walk, too.

At the end of the tour, we went into the office to fill out the admission papers. Mom seemed detached, as if it was not really going to happen. She said she didn't like it there and did not want to move. Then she started to cry.

When we moved her into the home, we tried to make things as familiar and comfortable as possible. We asked her opinion on where she would like things to go. We made sure she knew that if she needed anything, she would get it. We visited frequently so she knew we hadn't just left her there and forgotten about her.

Mom was used to the way she had been taking her medications and was insecure about the way the nurses were doing it. She complained that she had not received all her medications. The first few times, I checked with the nursing staff and they checked her chart and assured me she had. I assured Mom that she had received all her medications.

We had a problem with her oxygen equipment. I was told the staff knew how to operate the equipment. One day when I went in, Mom was upset because she had not been able to leave her room. She told me that the staff did not know how to fill her portable oxygen tank. I checked with the nursing station and found that to be true. I showed them how to fill it and that seemed to take care of the problem.

Mom complained about the food. I said that it was probably not what she was used to, but it was a balanced diet and that they were trying to please many different people. We made sure she always had goodies to eat in her room. There was a problem with some of the confused residents wandering into her room. I told her that maybe she should just ask them nicely to leave and if they didn't, then ring for the staff. If it got worse, then maybe she could close her door for a while or put a gate across it. She was afraid her laundry might go missing. When she had a concern, I checked her clothes and, if needed, checked with the staff.

For the first six months or so, she stayed in her room. She did not attend any activities. If she was urged to do so, she told the staff she did not feel up to it. She left her room only for meals and baths. She spent her time crocheting and watching TV. She did not make any friends. She said no one wanted to talk to her and the ones who did talk didn't know what they were talking about. She was not interested in joining in any family gatherings. She said it was too much trouble. No amount of convincing on our part seemed to help. Seeing her alone and unhappy and not doing anything to change it made me feel defeated and punished.

Mom became ill several times in the first few months. This did not help, as she felt the reason she was ill was because she was there. Fortunately she was able to have her own doctor looking after her.

She often told me she would like to come live with me. When she said this, my heart felt like it was melting. I reminded her that I worked all day and no one would be there to help her for hours at a time.

After about six months, she began to feel more comfortable. She started to enjoy being with the staff and began to talk to them herself if she had any concerns. She became more interested in what was going on around her. She started making some friends and going out into the hall to be with people. She began having her hair done more frequently. She started to feel like part of the group. I started to feel I could visit a little less, as she now felt better about her surroundings.

After eight or ten months, she was more like herself. She was friendly and made a couple of close friends. She felt comfortable with the residents in the hallways. She was happy but was still anxious to move to the facility closer to her home.

One year after moving in, she was able to move to the care home of her choice. She regretted that she was going to leave the friends she had made but was excited and positive about the move. The second move was less traumatic than the first. She was able to keep all of her things and was now closer to family and old friends. She knew what to expect and was comfortable in her new surroundings. She has been reacquainted with some of her old friends, who also live in the new place. She has already joined the cribbage league again. In less than two weeks, she feels at home. She is interested in her surroundings and is willing to venture out to acquaint herself with her new home. She is happy knowing that family and friends are close.

I feel that it is all right to visit when I can, but if I can't, it won't be such a disaster. She is comfortable and well cared for. I feel I can go on a trip and thoroughly enjoy it because I don't have to worry about her. I can again have time to enjoy the rest of my family as well as my mother, and have time for myself.

CHAPTER 8

Nursing Home and Assisted Living Systems

A major difference between assisted living and nursing homes, as noted earlier, is that the former are based on a social model and the latter on a medical model, at least historically. This means that assisted living residences often feel much more homelike than do nursing homes. They are often built to different building code specifications so that they look less institutional. They also perform fewer regulated and medical tasks, so they function less as a medical system. Many of them are newer than nursing homes, so they are built according to modern ideas to be like something other than an institution. Finally, because residents are supposedly (and generally are) less sick, more cognitively aware, or have fewer disabilities, they are able to be more independent in their decision making.

No matter how "homey" nursing homes try to be, usually they still function to some extent as institutions. They are a group living situation; they work on a schedule; people have to wait for things. There is a lack of personal space and an increase in the amount of time one spends in public places. Individuality, so valued in our society, is not easily fostered in nursing homes, so residents may easily feel devalued and "not special."

Nursing homes, and to a lesser extent assisted living, tend to take away many of the individual choices that we have in our lives. The result is that residents can have a feeling of loss of control over themselves. Often, it is in little things. For instance, in some areas residents are not allowed to self-medicate, or even to take an aspirin on their own, without a doctor's order. They may not be allowed a refrigerator or kettle in their rooms, so they must ask for a cold drink or snack or coffee. Even though they've had a glass of wine every night before dinner, they may have to wait for the nurse to serve them that glass or wait for the doctor to order it. At dinner there may be a choice of entrees, but still they are not deciding when to eat, what to eat, where to eat, or with whom to eat. At least in assisted living, residents often have their own cooking or food preparation possibilities, even if they do not have a full stove. Whether they use them is not the question—the question is who is making the decisions.

A residence must balance the needs and dignity of their residents with the safety and health of the residents and staff. They have occupational health and safety concerns they have to address. For example, nursing homes often have a high rate of injury to nurse's aides because of all the lifting they do. To counter that, they will often use a mechanical lift to help residents in and out of bed or on and off the toilet, often now ones that are installed on ceilings. There may be less "dignity" involved in moving someone in a sling on a lift, but how fair is it to ask aides to risk back injuries? Wearing masks and gowns may be necessary when a resident has an antibiotic-resistant infection, but it gives a hospital-like message. On the other hand, there are benefits—some research is showing that where lifts are used, a resident may be gotten out of bed more often and therefore be able to have more social interaction than in a facility where lifts are not used.

The focus in nursing homes (when it isn't on profits) is often more on nursing and less on home. For instance, monitoring bowel function is common in a home; every day a nurse's aide may ask your husband if he has had a bowel movement even if he has not had problems with bowel function in the past. It can be embarrassing. The nursing focus is partly because nursing is the largest department. This is true even though many functions performed through the nursing department do not require any kind of medical training. Being the constant recipient of care can symbolize dependence for someone.

You can easily become caught up in the way a home takes away your husband's individuality and independence. For instance, instead of asking your husband what he wants or talking to him first about his condition or behavior, the staff may phone you to ask what you think. If there is a problem, rather than talk to him, they may ask you to handle it. Whereas this may be appropriate if your husband has dementia, a lot of times it is not. Reminding the staff to ask him what he thinks or what he sees as the problem will help train them to treat him like a person, not like a patient. In turn, this will lower the burden on you and help you to keep treating him like a person. In assisted living, the reverse may be true. The residence may put more onus on him than he is able to handle, and you will have to step in to negotiate these decisions.

You can also try to help your husband maintain as much independence and responsibility as he can. Have him continue to handle his checking account, organize his taxes, and buy birthday presents for the grandchildren. If you feel he cannot do it, you may want to "consult" with him. Encourage him to take as much control as he can by making decisions for himself. Sometimes these are small decisions. If he is coming home to visit, what does he want for dinner? If he needs new clothes, take him shopping with you or ask what colors he wants. Life is made up of lots of small decisions, not just the large ones.

The younger or the more mentally able someone is, the more important it is that he maintain input into not only what happens in the care facility but also what happens at home. If there are young children or a financial portfolio, for example, your husband should be involved. These decisions and input keep him anchored to the family so that he doesn't feel isolated, rejected, or useless.

How the System Works

It is important that you understand how a nursing home system works (or sometimes doesn't). There are two aspects of which to be aware. First, a nursing home has several departments: nursing, maintenance, housekeeping, laundry, dietary, etc. One director may head several departments, but those departments tend to have separate staffs with separate job descriptions. Even though the staffs may cooperate, they function on their own. This departmental separation is one of the causes of gaps in communication and policy. Second, a nursing home runs on three shifts a day for seven days a week. That is twenty-one shifts per week. Over those twenty-one shifts, you can easily have six or seven different nurses and twice as many nurse's aides. You can have fourteen shifts of dietary personnel. When you include laundry, maintenance, recreation, casual or agency staff, and so on, there can easily be thirty people who will deal with one resident over the course of one week and more over the course of a month. If you think of the nursing home as a machine, think of all the shifts, all the departments, and all the staff members having to work together like the cogs in the gears.

If this were a perfect world, all the cogs would mesh together smoothly. Unfortunately, it's not, and they don't. Information is one of the first victims of the gap. If you think of information as going into a machine at one point and having to flow along a path to others, you can see that the more complicated the machine, the more possibilities there are for the information to get lost or changed along the way. Remember what used to happen when we played telephone when we were little? A sentence that started out as "Johnny has new shoes" ended up as "Mary got locked in the bathroom." The communication gaps, losses, and mistakes often lead to the lack of continuity in care and glitches that you will experience.

A Typical Day

It may help you to understand how a typical day in a nursing home runs. Starting about six in the morning, the night nurse will begin to give out morning medications and perform treatments. At the same time, the kitchen staff has arrived to start making breakfast. About seven or eight, the day shift will arrive. The nursing and care staff will learn what happened in the previous shift. The day nurse continues medications. The nurse's aides will begin to help residents get ready for the day. They will help them wash and dress. They will help them to the bathroom, or change them if they are incontinent. They may help with some treatments. They will begin to bring people to the dining room. Meanwhile, other support staff members, such as kitchen and laundry workers and housekeepers, arrive and begin to do their jobs. At breakfast, more medications are given out and the care staff members help to feed people. Some people eat and are ready to go back to their rooms in ten minutes; others need an hour. After breakfast, people are brought back to their rooms. Nurse's aides and nurses will help them use the bathroom, be bathed, and handle other tasks. Nurses will perform treatments, call physicians, do assessments, return phone calls from family members, and so on. During the rest of the morning, nurse's aides will give baths and help people to the bathroom. They will change people who have soiled themselves. They will answer call bells. During the morning, the recreation staff arrive and start programming, which continues until the evening.

At lunchtime, nurses and nurse's aides help bring people to the dining room, medications are given out, people are helped to eat. A routine similar to the morning happens after lunch until shift change. Also in the afternoon, caregivers help people to bed for a nap and then get them up again. Sometimes they have to get them up and down two or three times in the afternoon to use the toilet, or because they want to get into bed, then decide that they want to get out of bed, and then change their mind and want to go to bed again. The afternoon shift repeats the meal, medication, toileting tasks, and so on. Nighttime is the reverse, when people are toileted, changed, given medication, undressed, and helped to bed.

Besides making for a busy routine, many of the tasks take a lot of time, especially when they are done with the resident's dignity and comfort in mind. For instance, helping a resident dress entails choosing clothes and helping her feel right about how she looks. If she has arthritis, putting on the clothes means taking care not to hurt her. If a nurse's aide has many people to help dress, you can see what the workload entails. Another example is recreation. It can take almost as much time for the recreation staff to bring residents to a program as they spend on the program itself. Sometimes by the time they have brought the last resident, the first ones have forgotten why they were there and have left.

In the middle of the daily routine are medical emergencies, phone calls to and from physicians, and care conferences. Everybody is answering questions from residents and families. Sometimes there is a new admission or a room change. A tremendous amount of time is taken up in meetings and documentation related to governmental standards and requirements such as developing treatment plans. For example, in some areas if a resident has had an accident, such as a fall, the staff has to fill out a form that describes what happened and how it was handled. In all three shifts the care staff have to record in resident charts if there is a change in health status or some other issue.

While the nurse's aides and nurses are doing their jobs, the recreation staff may come to your husband's room to bring him to a program. A social worker may drop in for a visit. The housekeeper may come in to clean. There may be a volunteer who comes in. Your husband may choose to go down to the lounge, out for a walk in the garden, or try to go back to bed. He may have physical therapy or go to chapel for hymn sing.

In between all of the above, the staff have breaks, go for lunch, etc. When one person is on a break, this can mean that there will be only one staff member on the floor or unit. If one or two people are helping someone get out of bed or wash, it can easily mean that if you go looking for a staff person, she is not going to be easy to find. If you can't find a staff person, it doesn't mean that she is not busy or that there is no one on the floor.

You may have some anxiety related to staff people not being around and wonder, "What if he had a fall? How long would it take someone to find him?" You can see from the schedule I described that there can be someone in a resident's room several times during the day. Also, if a resident does not come down for a meal, this is a signal for the staff to check on him. This is also true for assisted living; a resident not showing for a meal triggers a call to his or her apartment. However, it is true that there is not going to be someone around your husband as much as you have been. There will be many times when he will be alone for several hours. This is not one-to-one care and, as I said earlier, staffing is often minimal. You have to accept that and work with it somehow. If you cannot come to terms with this at some level, then you should not put yourself or your husband in a situation like this. It is not fair to him, to you, or to the staff at the home.

Cyrus

When the lapses in my husband's memory first became apparent, I dismissed it as "getting older." However, when Cy's orientation and directions started to become a problem, I began to doubt my assessment of the situation. I took him to the university medical center for an examination, and there a diagnosis of Alzheimer disease was confirmed.

I was stricken by the blunt prognosis—that he would continually decline over a period of time and that eventually I would have to put him in a nursing home. At first I rejected that idea. I wasn't willing to accept that I would eventually be unable to meet the challenges that would arise.

Over the course of time, I saw that I was wrong and he would go downhill. I had to resign myself to the inevitable deterioration of a once razor-sharp brain. I became more and more of a caregiver. I sought out activities that could spark the interest of an individual with low vision (legally blind) and almost no hearing (even with the most up-to-date hearing aids). With two of the five senses badly damaged, stimulation was almost totally lacking. There could be no reading, writing, tapes of music or voice, puzzles, newspapers, lectures, discussion, TV, or radio. With life so limited, he slept much of the time. Activities ceased. Weariness, boredom, and depression followed for us both.

Before his condition had deteriorated to the point that he could neither reason nor understand, we discussed our problems of health and of living arrangements in the future. In the meantime, we continued to live as fully as possible, seeing close friends, visiting family groups, celebrating special occasions, taking short outings, attending church, and enjoying our precious, intimate moments together.

We made a move to an apartment, all on one level, close to transportation, shopping, and service facilities such as banks, entertainment, and future care facilities. Best of all, it was close to loving family help.

Eventually, I investigated the nursing home nearby. I knew it was necessary for his future care. It was only a five-minute walk. I was delighted to discover a bright, inviting residence with pleasant lounges and activity areas and a friendly dining room. The residents' rooms were cheerful. They had their own private toilets and sinks and were adequately furnished, with room to spare for personal pieces.

Pictures and memorabilia from home were encouraged. The dining room served nutritious food that was well accepted by the residents and could be individually adjusted. Juices, fresh fruits, and grain snacks distributed daily were a welcome diversion. The busy, caring staff were cheerful and efficient. Residents were kept active in varying small groups of their own choice singing, exercising, working with their hands, even watching TV. Bus outings could include family. Special activities were planned monthly by the creative, energetic staff members. Visitors were always welcome, including children and pets.

When the call came that there was a room available, my head responded with a rational "Yes" but even with all that I knew about the home and Cy's condition, my heart screamed "No!" It felt so unfair. I didn't know how I could do this to him.

In the few minutes I was on the phone with the social worker, an emotional battle raged within me. I went through doubt, fear, frustration, anguish, disappointment, sadness, and guilt. The rising inner turmoil left me unable to reason. I finally requested permission to temporarily escape. I hung up the phone and escaped in the comfort of home, where I thought I could put things into perspective.

I turned down the room. Later I changed my mind. They let me put his name back on the waiting list close to the top. When they called me the next time, finally, with the support and help of my children, I decided to go through with it.

The emotional struggle raged on. I was afraid. I didn't know how he would react to the news of his change of lifestyle and residence. How would I manage the whole situation and my own emotions? I tried to concentrate on the benefits to my husband that the new and stimulating surroundings provided.

After Cy went in, I continued to feel anguish, disappointment in my-self, and sadness at being without him. I tried to educate and involve myself in the goals and routines of the home. But at times I continued to feel frustrated and inadequate in that I couldn't take care of him myself. I tried to be flexible and find alternative solutions to problems when they came up. I didn't know if I could acquire the adaptiveness I needed to deal with the changes.

Eventually I realized that dealing with all my feelings would involve self-inspection and my acceptance of the inevitable. I also realized that I could solve the anguish, disappointment, and sadness only by fashioning a new and interesting life for myself.

It wasn't easy and it didn't happen overnight. It took tremendous personal effort and determination. I sought out new interests and ac-tivities, both mental and physical. I found that they proved stimulating and enjoyable. Every step of the way I had with me, always, the caring support of family and friends. They reminded me that I had been getting exhausted from caregiving. They told me that I had made the right deci-sion when I was doubting myself. I kept on telling myself that I had to maintain my own faith in an improving future. I kept walking this road, and after many months, things did get better.

PART III

MOVING IN AND SETTLING IN

CHAPTER 9

Preparations for Moving Day

As I said earlier, the transition to a residence is often a process of grief and loss. At the very least it can be filled with anxiety, as someone is facing an unknown. If your wife is being discharged directly from a hospital to a nursing home, you will not have much time to do any preparation. If she is coming from home and you have the time, adequate preparation before the move will help you and your wife through the process. There is both emotional and practical preparation.

How to Prepare Your Relative

If your wife was not able to participate in the decision that she needs to move or to place her name on a waiting list, then a good preadmission process can help her feel a part of the choice. It will also help minimize the stress and anxiety that will arise. This, in turn, will make postadmission adjustment easier.

Try to bring your wife to the residence for several visits before admission. See if there is a resident who can act as a buddy to her before she comes in. Obtain a schedule of activities and slowly let her start to participate in them, maybe even on a weekly basis. Maybe you can arrange for her to have a meal at the home one day a week. At first you may want to stay with her during the activity or meal, but gradually you may want to pull back and let her be there on her own so that she is used to your not being there. For this to work, you may have to work out questions of responsibility for medications, toileting, and emergencies with the staff.

Assisted living facilities in the private sector often have guest suites or rooms that are furnished. This allows someone to come in for a few days, a week, or a month to see what it is like. During the admission, this also allows for you to spend the first little bit of time with your wife.

In the time before admission, talk to your wife in general about what is coming up. She may focus a lot of anger toward you. Partly this is because you are a convenient target, one that is safe and visible. Sometimes it is easier to be angry with someone real and present than with God or even with oneself.

Have several discussions over time with your wife about what things she wants to take with her. Even if she has dementia, she can often still make decisions about this. What pictures does she want to take, what pieces of furniture? Talking about concrete things helps people prepare psychologically for the future.

It can be heartbreaking to have to choose only one or two possessions out of the many you have collected over a lifetime. When I moved from Toronto to Vancouver, I sold my house and all my things. I had a garage sale and even sold extra light bulbs. I shipped out ten boxes containing the only remaining things I had, including my clothes. The last day, when my telephone was shut off, I burst into tears. With everything I owned gone, I felt as if I had no identity, as if there was nothing left of the me that I had built up over years, and this was something I had a choice in. If someone is breaking up her home in the last years of her life, where she may have lived for twenty, thirty, forty years or more, and she does not have a choice, that feeling of losing the self is overwhelming.

I sometimes suggest that children not dismantle a home or apartment for a little while after admission if they can afford it. This can give people an out, if they are not sure and they have a choice—it tells them the door swings both ways, and they can go home. If they cannot afford to wait, maybe the family can put their father's things in storage. It may be comforting for him to know that his home is still there or his things are still available. Later he may tell you when it is all right to sell. Doing this may be expensive, but the advantage is that your father will "only" have to deal with the move, and not the permanent loss of so much of what he has built over his lifetime. It also gives him more control over the pace of his loss and grief.

One way to approach the breakup of a parent's home is to ask your father to whom he would like to give specific pieces. As you go around the house or apartment, talk about the different things in it. Reminisce about where they came from and what they meant to both of you. Let your father know how you will treasure his things; it is a way of saying that you treasure him. This can be a sad thing to do, but it can be part of the healing and letting go. It may also help you when you have to clean out the apartment: your dad has given you permission to have his things.

When you are deciding what to bring, make sure you pay attention to the guidelines of the residence. Your wife may have a tendency to try to take "just one more little thing." It may be hard for you to say no. If this occurs, call the staff and have them talk to your wife, so you don't have to be the one to say no. Remember that, especially in a nursing home, the staff need to provide care; they must be able to maneuver around furniture. There may also be limitations on electrical appliances. In an emergency, they must be able to get a stretcher or resuscitation equipment into the room and to a bedside.

It may be that you are helping an only parent, and a home or apartment will have to be closed down. If you would like some help with dismantling, disposing, packing, and moving, you can hire a professional mover or downsizer. These are individuals or companies who specialize in this area. They know where furniture and clothing and other items can be brought and which secondhand stores are buying. A good one will work with your mother to help her "sort and throw." They often have arrangements with moving companies. They will pack, unpack, and hang up everything. If you decide to hire one of these companies, get an estimate and find out exactly what services they will actually provide. Look in the Yellow Pages or search the Internet for "downsizers," look on elderpost.com, or contact the National Association of Professional Organizers (www.napo.net) or Professional Organizers in Canada (www.organizersincanada.com).

If you think that your wife will not remember her visits or is so resistant to the idea that preadmission visits would make things worse, then you may have to let that go. It does not necessarily mean that she will not adjust well. I have known many people who were memory impaired and absolutely refused to come for a visit or even consider the idea that they needed care. Their families were beside themselves with worry about how to bring them in and what would happen once they were admitted. It turned out that they were fine. Two days later they had forgotten they had just come in. They thought they had been living in the home for years.

If the admission is the result of an emergency or will be an admission directly from the hospital, you will not be able to do this kind of preadmission planning. Unfortunately, this can make your wife's admission and adjustment more difficult. (On the other hand, it can make some practical tasks easier for you because you don't have to worry about how you are going to move her out of the house or what you are going to say to her.) You can still do an abbreviated version of the process; just do what you can. Talk about care. Bring in the brochure or information book from the residence. Take pictures and bring them in. You can discuss what to bring and what will have to be left at home: which pictures, which dresses, and which purse?

Get to Know the Home in Advance

Try to get to know some of the staff people before admission. If your wife is able to be present at these meetings, make sure you bring her. You may not know the floor or room your wife is going to, but you can meet the recreation staff, the director of care (director of nursing), the social worker, and the administrator. If your wife is needing care, try to have a meeting with the staff before admission to talk about the kinds of things you have been doing for your wife and how you have been doing them. Are there any tricks you have learned that make it easier for your wife to eat, to get to the bathroom? Is there one kind of incontinence pad that has worked and others that didn't? Is she prone to some skin breakdown or infections? How does she sleep; does she get up at night? Has she had any falls, and when do they occur? All of the things that you do in terms of providing care are important for the staff to know; write them down and discuss them beforehand if you can. Even if they don't remember the particulars, this will help them remember you—and that will help in obtaining good care.

Many times I have asked a family member, "What do you expect for your Dad in the care we provide here?" and "What can we do to make this easier for you?" People usually have been unable to tell me. Clarify for yourself and the staff your expectations for care. What would constitute good care, in your opinion? What would make you say to your friends, "This has been a good place for Dad?" Try to be more specific than "he is happy." What will make him happy? What will make you feel safe? What will help you to sleep at night?

If it is a nursing home admission, do you want to be called every time your wife has a fall? Do you want to know every time there is a change of medication or there has been a routine doctor's visit? Do you want to know when there has been some weight loss? Do you want to know when she has had or is having a particularly good day? See if the home can meet these expectations. Find out what they think is reasonable and what their policy is on family communication. Try to let the staff know what kind of person you are. If you are anxious and tend to worry, tell them. If you are having guilt, let them know. They will most likely figure that out for themselves, but telling them will help them learn how to help you.

As noted earlier, assisted living may provide much less in terms of care and subsequently much less in terms of family communication. Be clear with yourself as well about what you expect or want from the residence. This is another reason to be honest about what your wife's needs are. If you want more communication than the residence is staffed for, you may have to hire private help, a geriatric care manager, or be prepared to visit more often.

Often a home will ask for some written information about a person. It is helpful to write down not only the physical care information but also your wife's daily schedule and activities (see questionnaire 2 in appendix 2). Include in this when she snacks and sleeps, when meals are, what time is bedtime. What are the little things that make her feel secure and comfortable? Is she used to looking out the window at the park or talking to her grandchildren at five every afternoon? Try to find out which of these habits can be replicated by the home. The more of her routine your wife brings with her, the less anxiety, fear, and adjustment difficulty she will have. If the home where your wife is going is not so good, preadmission meetings can help to ensure that the staff knows you are involved and will be monitoring care.

It is helpful to write up a social history of your wife. A social history is a document that describes a person and her life (see questionnaire 3 in appendix 2). It can be important for the staff. It helps them to see your wife as a person: who she was before she became disabled, and what her strengths and weaknesses were. It also helps them to assess her adjustment. If after three months she is never coming out of her room, that would have a different meaning for someone who was always a loner and shy than for someone who was always the life of the party.

If she is able to, your wife should write the social history herself or help you write it. This is another way to reminisce and to prepare for the changes that are coming. It puts life in perspective as a path or series of events and changes. The transition to a nursing home is a continuation of that path and another change, albeit a huge one.

Equipment

In the last few years, there have been some spectacular advances in equipment for disabled and elderly persons. You should have a good understanding of what is currently available and also what you need to bring. If your wife is using a walker or wheelchair, will she have to bring her own or do they have them at the home? Even if they do, it is a good idea for your wife to have one that is specifically measured to suit her. A proper walker will help her balance and gait and can prevent falls. In assisted living, will they allow wheelchairs in the dining room? If she uses a wheelchair, the wheelchair needs to be comfortable and one that she can maneuver. Poorly fitting wheelchairs can cause back problems and can reduce someone's ability to be mobile. If she spends most of her time in a wheelchair, it is like her home—it must be comfortable. Will your wife need a commode? Can she put in a pole next to her bed to help her get up and down? What about specialized utensils and plates to help with eating? If she has trouble putting on her own stockings, what about an aid to help her do that, or to reach things that she has dropped? A telephone with large numbers? A clock that speaks the time? An electronic pill dispenser, medication reminder? Something that will remind her to go to the dining room? Many cities have stores that specialize in equipment for elderly and/or disabled persons. Visit them or look on the Internet, for example, under "adaptive equipment," for equipment that your wife might benefit from. Even if there is nothing that you think she needs, look anyway. You can find things that help in ways you might never have considered.

Valuables

I have worked in homes where almost nothing went missing and in others where valuables went missing all the time. There sometimes seems to be no correlation between this and the quality of care. If you bring in valuables, have them insured or find out if the home's insurance will cover them. Residents should not keep large sums of money in their possession, but make sure that there is at least a locking drawer where money can be kept. See if you can glue or screw small mementos down, perhaps on a board you bring in. Maybe you can bring in a small, locking glass case or shelving unit.

The basic rule is, "If you don't want to lose something, don't bring it in." Accidents can happen, things break, and so on. No matter how much you are financially compensated, it might not replace the sentimental value of a ring or other item. On the other hand, if your wife wants a cherished item with her, maybe the risk is worth it. What is the good of her possessions if she cannot have them? As I said earlier, they are part of who she is. If she understands the risk even only partially, let her make that decision. Even if something has been promised to a grandchild, its value to your wife should be considered first, even with the risk of losing it.

Nursing home residents can usually keep money in a comfort account or personal needs account, but assisted living residents must often be able to be responsible for their own funds. If their care is being funded by Medicaid, there has to be a certain amount available from their funding for their own use. These accounts function as small bank accounts and are usually accessible during business hours. You can authorize a home to charge certain items such as outings or hairdressing to the personal needs account. You will have to monitor the account through monthly or quarterly statements. It is easy for a home to make a mistake with charges to a resident's account. *Make sure your wife actually receives the services or items for which she is charged.* Larger homes sometimes have a bank come in on a regular basis; this is done as a community service by the bank.

Even if your wife has dementia, she may want to have her purse with her, and she may want to have some money in it. She may lose her purse continually, but to many women a purse is a part of them. I have seen women with advanced dementia still holding on to their purses and feeling lost and upset without them. Having two or five dollars makes a difference to some people, even if there is nowhere to spend it or they don't know what to do with it. It is a good idea to put some other things in the purse, maybe some lipstick or a plastic holder for pictures of the children when they were small. Always make sure her name is on the purse somewhere.

Clothing and Laundry

There can often be a subtle or overt pressure on people in a residence, especially assisted living, to be stylishly dressed. People dress up, sometimes more so than they would in their own homes. This may not be such a problem in assisted living, but you will have to take a look at the clothes your wife will be bringing. They should be fairly easy to care for. This means washable. A lot of elderly people do well with jogging suits because they are easily put on and taken off, and are loose and comfortable. There are many companies that specialize in clothing for elderly and disabled persons. They have beautiful and stylish pieces and may make your wife's life easier. They may have Velcro instead of zippers, fasten in the front instead of the back, or be of material that is stain resistant. Make sure they are well labeled. Also, make sure you bring enough, in case the laundry isn't done often or clothes become soiled or lost.

Keep a list of all the clothes that your wife is bringing. After she is admitted, give a copy to the home, and if they wish to check it off with you, have them do so. Update it regularly when you bring new items.

This may also be a good time for you to review the shoes your wife is wearing. Are they appropriate to what her needs and abilities are? Many women especially wear some kind of heeled shoe for a long time past the time when they are at risk for falling. Do not take them away without careful thinking and maybe discussion, but they often present a danger. You might want to suggest running shoes or better support shoes she can try or use "for everyday use." Consider if she needs orthotics, or wider shoes. Would it be easier if she had shoes with Velcro instead of ties?

If the care in a home is good, laundry is often the most frustrating problem. Clothing can go missing (how many socks have you lost in the dryer at home?) or people find themselves wondering why ten pieces of underwear are not enough and how come your wife is always running out.

Sometimes a home may use more laundry than you do. A resident is changed more often because she is helped to the toilet less often. The result is that she goes through more clothes.

Also, sometimes they do not do laundry on weekends. Sometimes labels fall off in the commercial-strength machines or fade so that they can't be read. It is possible that the person in the laundry can't read. Usually a home does all the residents' laundry together in batches. It is easy to mix up laundry when you are doing many people's together.

Laundry is one of the services that may have to be negotiated in assisted living. Often the facility will provide linens and towels, and washing them is included in the price; personal laundry may not be. They will have either coin-operated or free laundry services. Pay attention to how far the laundry may be from your wife's suite if she is in assisted living. If it is too far or too hard to access for some reason, she may not use it and not do her clothes.

Many residences have some kind of arrangement with a dry cleaner; most will not dry clean in the facility. In a nursing home, dry-clean-only clothing is often put in the regular laundry and ruined. No matter how hard you try to avoid that it can happen. If there are special occasions for which you would like your wife dressed in better clothes, you can keep those at home, or bring them in in a plastic laundry bag that says "do not use," or "use on special occasions only."

In any residence, find out how the laundry works, how often it is done and delivered, and what the procedure is for lost laundry and dry cleaning. If all the residents' clothes are washed together, bring a mesh laundry bag so that all of your wife's laundry can be kept together. You may want to do the laundry yourself. If you do, bring in a hamper and mark on the top "Family Does Laundry." Some nursing homes also have a resident laundry for residents to do their own small things.

Plan Ahead for Moving Day

As mentioned earlier, fear, anxiety, and confusion are often mixed in with guilt when people are dealing with nursing homes or assisted living. About the time of admission, the former feelings are often stronger than the guilt. If you are well prepared, it might help, but no matter how well prepared you are, you feel them. First, remember that there are a lot of practical things to do in a somewhat short time. These include the logistics of carrying out the move itself. It may mean having to take time off work, find child care, or fly to another city. Several tasks to accomplish within a limited timeframe means there is pressure on you. Second, most people do not know what happens in a care facility. The unknown can be frightening. It can also be frightening to know that you are leaving your wife in the care of strangers, people in whom you have not yet placed very much, if any, trust. How will they know to do things the way you do? How will they know when she is upset? Will they get to her on time? These are natural concerns and in some ways can be answered only when they are answered.

Fear, anxiety, and confusion put people physiologically in a heightened state of arousal—somewhat like the fight/flight idea. There is a theory that talks about how people react in times like this, it is called crisis theory. Crisis theory says that when people are in a heightened state of arousal, it is hard for them to make decisions and process information. What this tells you is why it is hard to do some of the tasks and be organized around the time of admission. This is also why you organize your wedding in advance, plan your vacation in advance, and pack the suitcase two weeks before the baby is due.

Remember the confusion of doing those things at the last minute? It follows, then, that your goal before admission is to make as many decisions and plans in advance as you can.

Find out ahead of time what happens at the residence on the first day. What are some of the forms to be filled out (and can you fill out any in advance)? Obtain a copy of the admission agreement and read it ahead of time. Will you have to pay rent right away? How much, and to whom?

Try to do as much beforehand as you can. This means practical tasks such as filling out government forms and change-of-address cards. It may mean talking to the bank, the lawyer, the accountant. Anything that you bring should be marked with your wife's name. This includes dentures and glasses. Make a list of everyone who is involved in your wife's life and figure out who needs to be contacted. Do you have to call the cable company and the power company? Do you need to hire a moving company?

Of utmost importance is contacting the insurance company to preauthorize payment if private insurance will be used. Find out from the insurance company what they need to know and when they need to know it. If you do not do this, you can risk losing thousands of dollars in benefits.

If you have children, do you recall packing the suitcase a few days before the baby was due so that when your wife said, "Um, honey," all you had to do was remember to take it with you? This is like having a baby.

Well, okay, not exactly, but it will be especially helpful to make a written plan for what you will do when you are informed that a room is available and what you will do on moving day itself. Once you have a list, go back and number it from the first task you will do to the last one before you get into the car to leave. This will mean that when the call comes, and on moving day, you will not have to make decisions. Your list tells you what to do and bring; all you have to do is pack.

If you are bringing many things, plan to have one suitcase with essentials and comforts. This would be the most important items that your wife will want in the first day or two as well as the things that will make her most comfortable and secure. For instance, she may be attached to a doll; she may like certain candies or wear a certain perfume. There may be one piece of jewelry or one dress that is a favorite. It may be a picture of both of you on your wedding day or of your first grandchild—anything that would help to offset the strangeness and bring memories of home and family.

Have a plan for how your wife is going to be told that a room is available for her and that she will be moving soon. If she is alert and oriented, arrange for the home to call her and speak to her. If your wife is resistant or has some memory loss, it might be best if the doctor tells her. Maybe one of your children should tell her.

Decide how the move will take place. How will your wife get there? Who will go with her? Will someone meet her there? Will the rest of the family be involved? Are you going to be able to bring some of her things in first?

Plan to Take Care of Yourself

As you are preparing your wife, you are also preparing yourself. When she is saying good-bye to her home and to your relationship as it was, you are saying good-bye to her and the relationship as it has been. If she can handle it and respond, talk to your wife about what you are feeling. If not, talk to other family members or friends. Remember, however, that just because she is going into a home does not mean that she will not come back for a visit, that you cannot go on vacations together, or that you will never make love again. Your life, her life, and your relationship aren't ending; they are changing.

Once you have made all the plans for moving, make some plans for yourself. It might help you to have a buddy there to help when the day arrives. They can help "fill in the gaps" for you until you gain some equilibrium and do some of the practical, rational things that you are finding difficult. This is why it is good for there to be more than one family member around during the move. Plan for who these people might be; ask them if they will be there for you.

The time for placement will be a crisis for you, too. Those first few days after your wife has moved may be hard. You can feel lost, lonely, and confused in this time. Be aware that, after the fear and confusion settle down, the feelings of guilt and shame may intensify. During times of crisis, emotions are often magnified. Remember, the brain functions in a way that makes it harder to be rational in a heightened emotional state. This is a physiological fact. It means that you have fewer psychological resources to handle the intensified emotions.

You may feel at first relieved and not until a week or two later begin to feel the loneliness; or you may feel them both at once, wanting to change your mind and knowing that you cannot. Ambivalence is normal and sorts itself out over time.

Try to figure out what you will be feeling and make some plans to help you cope with that. Maybe you want to make sure you have dinner with your children or some friends. Maybe you want to have someone come and stay with you for the first week or so. Maybe you will want someone to meet you at your house when you come back by yourself that first day. Or maybe you will want to be by yourself. Whatever you think you may need, make sure you will have it. It is easier to cancel plans you have made than to make them at the last minute.

Don't be afraid to ask for support. This is not a time for heroism or stoicism. People want to help you. Let them. You will not fall apart because you have let someone help you. You may break down and cry, but your tears will stop, and you will be stronger for having shed them.

Betty

On a rainy morning in April, my sister and I moved Mother to Mountain Ridge Home. She was ninety years old and had lived in Elm Manor, a congregate care seniors' residence, for five years.

A couple of years after she went to Elm Manor, we began to get concerned because she was going downhill. We phoned the health department, who did an assessment. They sent us to Dr. _____, who diagnosed Mother with Alzheimer disease.

But now she was having increasing paranoia and hallucinations. She was hearing things that weren't there. She was missing meals and needing help with medication for glaucoma. Elm Manor couldn't deal with these things. Mother would have to move.

After touring a number of facilities over a year, my sister and I liked Mountain Ridge the best and put her name on the waiting list. We toured it twice, the second time with Mother. She did not really comprehend what it was all about, but it made us feel better that she was involved in the decision in some way.

Her name came to the top of the list once and we declined because we felt she wasn't ready to move. The second time her name came up, we felt the move had to be made.

I organized things by phone with my sister. I do not recall a meeting about the move or about Mother with anyone at Mountain Ridge. We moved a desk and chair into her room and put pictures and a bookshelf on the wall to make it welcoming for her.

The admission itself was confusing and chaotic, and it appeared no one was prepared for her. Reception did not know she was coming. I staggered in with boxes of clothes and had not been told I could park in the back, much closer than the side street where I had parked. No one helped me. The bed in Mother's room had not been made.

We had understood we would be meeting with the senior nurse and administration, but this did not happen. The recreation therapist and dietitian came into the room. They were friendly and welcoming and asked Mother questions about her likes and dislikes. The timing was not appropriate. She was too confused and was incapable of answering the questions.

That day was difficult for all three of us. It did seem that not much effort had been made in preparation for a new resident. Mother's comment was, "Can I go home now?" It was heartbreaking for us, as you can imagine. However, we were invited for lunch, which helped us get a sense of the procedure for meals. Also it gave us a way to be supportive to Mother.

The first few days at Mountain Ridge were confusing and frustrating for my sister and me, as well as for Mother. We did not know who to talk to with our questions. We needed to know who the staff were. What were their roles? What was the daily procedure? How much care and attention was available for Mother? We needed to know what to expect from the home. Perhaps our expectations were high, but we didn't know because we had nothing to compare it to and no one to talk to about it.

From my experience, I would recommend that family members clarify expectations, such as: What can you expect the home to do? Who are the staff, and what do they do? Whom can you contact with your questions?

CHAPTER 10

Moving Day

Stay Calm

Moving day can be as traumatic for you as it will be for your wife—and maybe even more so. The call will come to tell you a room is available. You will find out the day and the time of admission. You will hang up the phone. Then you may have a sense of panic, "Oh, oh, what do I do now?" You might forget everything that you were just told on the phone.

Sit down. Have a cup of coffee. (Or maybe a drink if it's after lunch. Well, okay it is a special occasion. Have it anytime, as long as you have gotten out of bed first.) Let yourself think for a minute. Allow for the fight/flight reaction to dissipate a bit. Let the feelings pass through you; you may have panic, fear, anger, sadness. Take some deep breaths. Give yourself some time to do nothing but regain some equilibrium. Call the person who is going to help you with the move. This will give you someone to lean on as you go through the immediate crisis.

Reread your plan and list of things to do that you wrote earlier. The plan will make the task easier because it is something concrete. Reread the home's information materials that you received on the tour. Although you may have read them once, you may have forgotten much of the information because you didn't need to act on it right then. Now you do.

If Your Relative Refuses to Go

It may happen that your wife starts to hesitate. If she does, and she is able to reason, remind her that she can try it for a month or two and then decide if it is the right place for her. The home is not a prison; the door swings both ways. I have had people move in gradually to a nursing home. For the first while, they may go back to their own home to sleep several times during the week. Little by little, they end up spending more time sleeping in their room at the home. People adjust and grieve at different speeds and in different ways. Some people hold their noses and dive in, and some put in their little toe to test the water first.

If your wife has dementia, it may be difficult to enlist her cooperation. She may refuse to go into care and insist that she doesn't need it. She may honestly not know that she has deficits and not understand what is wrong. It is part of the tragedy of dementia that one's ability to make decisions and judgments is impaired. Often however, at some level, people do know and are so frightened that they deny it. Sometimes, at some level, people want someone else to make the decision because they cannot. Mum may rail at you, refuse to speak to you, but also know that you did what she wanted you to do but could not admit to needing. Many people with dementia do accept it when their family member tells them they are no longer safe living in their own home. Some accept it when a spouse or child tells them they can't provide the support anymore. But there are many people who will refuse to understand or go.

There are a number of ways to approach someone with dementia about the move to care. You may say that it is for only a short time while you have a rest or while you go out of town. You may say that the doctor wants her there for some tests; she will stay until the doctor says she can go home. Some people have said that it is for financial reasons. With a parent, you may say that the apartment building has been sold. Think of what or who might make sense to her in her world, and use that as an explanation. Sometimes it is better if the doctor tells her. When it is the fault of someone or something else, she is not fighting you directly. If she is going to have a private room, you might see if you can spend the first night or two with her. Ask if the home can put an extra bed or cot in the room. That way, your wife has someone with her.

It is beyond the scope of this book to discuss ethics, coercion, and individual rights. Clearly, there is often an element of coercion when someone has to enter a residence, especially a nursing home. When an individual has dementia, the coercive factor can be even more pronounced because of the individual's impaired ability to make decisions. You may have to tell your wife that she is going. You may bring her for lunch or an activity and tell her then that she is going to stay for a while. You might tell her you are going for a drive.

A friend of mine is also a geriatric care manager. When his mother, who had advanced Alzheimer disease, could no longer live at home, he arranged for his mother to go for a spa day with his wife. While they were out at the spa, he and his brother moved her things into the residence. Then when it was done he called his wife on the cell phone, and she then turned to the mother and said, "Oh, Mum, that was Danny. A terrible thing has happened. There was a flood in your house and the fire department was there and said it is too dangerous for you to go home. But luckily he has found a place for you to stay until everything is fixed." Mum said, "Oh, that is terrible." But she went with Danny's wife to the residence and agreed to stay. She never went home.

I have seen some elderly people who were living on their own deteriorate to the point that they were hospitalized for health reasons and from there were transferred to a nursing home. As I discussed earlier, be aware that, in most areas, people have the right to make their own decisions until they are deemed incapable by law—whether or not they are obviously and significantly mentally impaired. If your wife refuses to stay, it may be that legally you cannot make her stay, nor can the nursing home keep her. It could happen that the facility will tell you after a while that she has to try again at home. Find out what the policy and laws are in your area and with the home where your wife will be going.

Walking through the Door

Sometimes when I am looking for housing for a client, I go to see a residence where I have never been. Walking through the door is like going through the looking glass—into a strange world that is full of sounds, and colors, and objects, and directions that somehow look different from other places and times I have encountered them. I don't know which way to turn, I don't know to whom I should talk. If it is a nursing home, I see rows of wheelchairs. If I am in an assisted living residence, I may see no one and I walk around as though in a large empty, beautifully furnished morgue, the silence screaming of loneliness.

And I am just there to visit. I know I will leave, I know I have truly chosen to walk through that door.

Many of my clients, and maybe your wife, do not have that luxury.

What is it like to wonder about what your meals will be? Who will you talk to, who will take care of you? Will you find gentleness and compassion, or will you have to be on your guard? What will it be like to have to find your way around when your memory is no longer what it was, and what will happen if you are a bit incontinent? Will you make friends? Will you have the right clothes? The ability to be on your own after being married for sixty years?

Sometimes I think about how much courage it must take to walk through that door, how much strength it takes to put one foot in front of the other (or roll in a wheelchair, or push a walker) when you are dragging fear, and sadness, and anger, and resentment, and confusion, and maybe some hope with you too.

For those of us who work in nursing homes, this is what we need to pay attention to, and this is what we should be responding to, when we see your wife, and you, walking through that door. It may look to you like we don't. Sometimes we forget. Sometimes we say we understand but act as though we don't. Sometimes we feel pressure or time constraints and want to take your blood pressure instead of offering you tea and time to talk. You can remind us; remind us of what it is like to be you in that moment.

When You First Arrive

What happens on moving day depends somewhat on the level of services provided at the residence you are moving to and on the requirements for the provision of service. At an assisted living residence providing fewer services, the arrival may feel more like a move to a new home with an added business arrangement. At the time of arrival in a nursing home or assisted living with a high level of care, there is usually an initial interview with a nurse, who will take vital signs (such as pulse and blood pressure readings). He may also conduct a more in-depth interview and ask about physical health, emotional issues, and practical abilities such as going to the toilet, feeding, dressing, and washing. Your wife will probably be assigned a seat in the dining room and tablemates. Other staff members will probably try to meet her at least to say hello. If too many staff interviews are taking place, ask if some of them can be spread out over the next few days. It is easy to be overwhelmed by staff members who think they need information right away. Someone will probably give you and your wife a tour. If they don't, ask for one. Although you may have been there before, things will look different this time.

During that first day, there are usually several administrative tasks that you have to complete. These can include signing preadmission agreements, reviewing payment options and plans, and receiving information that federal and state law requires you be given. The forms can be somewhat confusing. The details can take a bit of time. If your stress level is high, these things can feel onerous and you may feel pressured. That is why it is a good idea to know in advance what you will have to do that first day and to see if any of these tasks can be done beforehand, especially obtaining a copy of the admission agreement.

See if you can stay for the first meal with your wife or at least sit with her in the dining room and have coffee during the meal. Stay as long as you can that first day, or stay for a while and come back.

Even if you have written down and presubmitted care issues that you think are important, talk to the admitting nurse again about them. Unfortunately, you cannot assume that the nurse and nurse's aides who are on duty that day have had time to read what you wrote or, if they did, that they will remember. If you refresh their memories, there is a better chance that the important things will be done in the way in which your wife is accustomed.

In the United States a nursing home must inform residents of certain rights if their care is being covered by Medicare or Medicaid.

Many state regulations require the same for assisted living. These include what items and services the programs will pay for, what they may not charge for, and how much they do charge for additional services. They also include a resident's legal rights concerning a personal-needs (comfort) account and information about state agencies, advocacy groups, and advance directives. If these are not provided, ask about them.

Joan

My mother's condition had been deteriorating for several years when we took her to the doctor. He gave us a diagnosis of Alzheimer disease and confirmation that she should not be living on her own. This finally made it clear that something had to be done. She was only seventy-two years old. We put her name on a waiting list for a nursing home and were told she would have to wait a year. The last few months of that year were by far the worst. Her memory was fading rapidly, and her inability to handle the basic needs of daily living had put her in physical danger.

As moving day grew closer, Mom would talk about how happy she was living in her own apartment. She had no idea she was on a waiting list for a care facility, but she knew something was up. Whenever we tried to broach the subject of moving, we were met with fierce opposition and a long history of how she had raised four boys and always been in control of her own destiny. "How dare you even suggest you know what's best for me?" she said. "I love where I am."

With less than a month to go, we received a call from the social worker. She said that our mother's name was getting to the top of the list and that a move could happen at any time. And when that time came, she said, we had twenty-four hours to accept the spot and another twenty-four hours to move her in—forty-eight hours for the entire move. We had a plan and were prepared for the move, but, still, forty-eight hours seemed almost impossible. We had full-time jobs, small children, and no idea if we could pull it off.

"Are we talking about her name coming up in a week, a month, or several months from now?" I asked the social worker.

"We're not sure," she replied. A pending nurses' strike had made the uncertainty worse. It became a nervous waiting game.

On the eve of the July 4th weekend, we were told that a bed was ready and that we should be moved in on the following Tuesday. Fortunately, we had a long weekend working in our favor, but the task still seemed beyond reach. My brothers and I had dreaded this day since we first put our mother's name on the waiting list.

We brought our mother to her new home, carrying only her most precious possessions, her family photos. Later we could bring a chair, a TV, and her piano keyboard. She had been a concert pianist, and her music was close to her heart.

"I don't belong here. I wish I was a thousand miles away. It's like being in jail." Her words hit me deep inside. "It's a nightmare," she continued. "You can't make me stay. I'm going to run away."

My mother's condition in the days after the move deteriorated faster than we could have imagined. There was almost total confusion and disorientation about her surroundings and her whole existence as a person. She could not understand why she was there at a time when she had been so happy at her old place. Just one week earlier she would go for walks to the local coffee shop and return home safely. Now she couldn't find her way back from the elevator, just thirty feet away from her new room. I was told that this was typical and that within a week or so she would regain her sense of orientation. But after several months she has not returned to the level she was at before moving into the home.

Eight weeks after she moved in, the staff at the home scheduled a care conference with my brother and me to discuss our mother's progress. The staff at this meeting consisted of the head of each department. Each gave a report from her own perspective. The general thinking was that my mother had settled in well and that the staff found it a pleasure to work with her. She got along well with the other residents, they reported. This was great news to me and my brother, and we felt compelled to tell the staff how grateful we were for all their help and support.

But for the family members of persons with Alzheimer disease, nothing is ever certain. Things are always changing as the disease progresses. You never know what is around that next corner.

I started receiving reports from the staff that our mother was exhibiting "unusual behaviors" and that a doctor from the mental health agency was being brought in to examine her. I couldn't believe she had changed so fast.

The staff at the home would be the first to agree that my mother is one of the most passive, loving, and honest residents at the facility. This was evident from the reports at the team meeting. Clearly, she would not intentionally harm or even inconvenience anyone living at the home. Knowing this just made me have more questions than answers.

I received a call from the director of nursing, who informed me that the decision had been made to move my mother to another ward, the "Special Care Unit," for people unable to cope in the regular part of the facility. I had heard about this ward during my initial tour of the home, but few people had talked about it. The doors to the ward were locked and the people inside were isolated from the outside world. That's where Mom would live. It didn't seem like we had a say in the matter.

When I heard the news, I thought, "Not again. She was just getting settled." My brothers and I went to visit our mother that weekend. When we got there, she was looking better than she had in months. She was visiting a friend on her floor who was playing the harmonica. She was more oriented to her environment than she had been, and she even recognized someone sitting outside her window.

After personally touring the Special Care Unit that weekend, it was clear that the residents were at stages far beyond that of my mother. I thought that the staff at the home were rushing it. She may not have many years left before she reaches that point, but I didn't see any reason to cut those years short.

With the hope of delaying the move to this ward, I set up a meeting with the social worker and the head nurse for her floor. The staff at the home had been open and accommodating in the few months she had been there. Perhaps a meeting is what we needed. I wondered if I had been too demanding on the staff time. But then the nature of this disease requires as much participation from the family members as possible. I wasn't sure how the meeting would turn out or what my options would be, but I was sure it wouldn't be the last intervention I would have to make in my mother's care, or the final crisis left to solve.

In the meeting, we explained to the social worker and head nurse why we were concerned. They told us what they saw as problems. They agreed to try to do some other things. When they heard what my brother and I had to say, they reevaluated what they thought. They agreed to wait.

It is now several months after that meeting. My mother is still in the same room and she is doing well. I am just glad that we were able to ask for a meeting and didn't take what the staff told us as the only course. We had to have the courage to speak up and believe in what we saw and knew about my mother. But they also didn't act like they were the experts and we were "just the family." They listened and I think they learned something too.

When we deal with the home, the only consistent thread holding things together, it seems, is clear and open communication between us as the family and the staff. This open communication and the sincere efforts of the staff to keep us informed give us comfort in knowing that our mother is getting the best treatment possible.

CHAPTER 11

Settling In

Resident Adjustment

A move for any elderly and/or ill person is disconcerting and can be confusing. As I mentioned, in times of high stress, people's coping abilities are often impaired.

For people who have memory loss, a new situation is particularly difficult because they have trouble learning. In their own home with familiar surroundings, they can use old habits to guide them in their daily life. In a new situation, such as a nursing home, they cannot use those old habits. The familiar cues are gone. Remember, people with dementia retain long-term memory, but it is short-term memory that people need first in new situations.

For any new resident, whether or not he has some memory loss, adjustment to a residence can easily take three to six months. I cannot emphasize this enough. After your husband has been there for four months, it may feel like a long time, but it isn't. Some of the complaints, behaviors, and emotions that you continue to hear about from your husband or the staff will be the result of trying to adjust, even though they may seem completely unconnected or may occur months after the move.

In some ways, coming into nursing care or assisted living is like moving to another town. There are new customs and new neighbors, new ways of having needs met and getting things done. Especially for someone who is memory impaired, finding the way around is like learning the streets in a new neighborhood. If you've ever moved, think about how many times you might have driven around looking for the turn into your new street or even driven right by your house. Remember too, what it felt like when you realized you had done this.

Changes and Differences in Behavior

You may be surprised to find that your husband is acting differently in the residence than he did in your own home. It may look to you like he has suddenly gone downhill and his confusion has increased. In fact, what you may be seeing is

1. The extent of his memory loss without the cues in your house that helped him hide it
2. An increase in confusion due to the new situation
3. An anxiety or fear reaction
4. The effect of medications being taken as prescribed, which may not have been the case at home
5. An unrelated medical condition that coincidentally started around moving time, such as a urinary tract infection or pain.

Unfortunately, depending on the residence he is moving into, your husband can go into a decline because the care is not very good, because he is being overmedicated or mismedicated, or because his needs are not being attended to. In a home that you don't know (say, for instance, it has been a fast or unsought transfer from the hospital) or one in which you do not have confidence, you will have to be there often to monitor what is going on and try to figure out why it is happening. If the care and caring are not good, you will not be able to depend on the staff to rectify the problem or help you figure out what it is.

It is possible that after a while, your husband's functioning will return to normal or improve. He may even start walking better, communicating more, or doing more on his own than he did at home. People's functioning sometimes improves when their personal attendant (you) is not around. If it is a parent who has moved into a residence after living alone, he may improve because he is receiving adequate nutrition, proper medication, social stimulation, or effective therapies. There are several reactions that may occur on admission.

DEPRESSION

Your husband may adjust easily or, for several reasons, he may go into a depression. Causes can include feeling abandoned, acknowledging the reality of his condition, and reaction to all of his other losses. The crisis of the move can activate a preexisting low-level depression. Even though this is a normal reaction to change, it still can be painful for you to watch and may cause you additional feelings of grief and guilt. It may make you think you have made the wrong decision.

It is difficult to be a family member of someone who is depressed. It can make you feel particularly helpless or angry. Your response may be to try to cheer up your husband. The problem with that approach alone is that, to a point, it denies what he is going through. Keep open communication and talk about what he is feeling. Tell him what you are feeling. Remind him and yourself that it will get better. After you have acknowledged and talked, then you might want to find things to do or talk about that distract him. Come back to the subject when you feel or he feels it would help to talk.

WITHDRAWAL

Your husband may adjust to the move to a residence by withdrawing. This looks like depression, but it isn't. It is simply his way of coping with an onslaught of new people, routines, and so on. He will probably gradually come out of it, sometimes starting in a week, sometimes starting in a couple of months. If after several months of withdrawal your husband has not started to come out a bit, and if he was a gregarious person previous to admission, then it is time to consider whether he has become depressed or something else is occurring.

If your husband withdraws, he may withdraw from you too. You may have a tendency to try to draw him out because you feel abandoned or rejected. That may even be how he wants you to feel, because that is how he is feeling. You can try to draw him out, but at the same time try to respect his way of coping by allowing him the emotional space to withdraw. If you feel your own anger rising, talk to the social worker or another staff member, a support group, or a family member.

At some point you may want to try to tell your husband to "snap out of it" or "stop feeling sorry for yourself." Sometimes this can be therapeutic. Just be careful about how and when you do it. I once told a resident who was not doing well, "You know, Mrs. Martin, you are here to live, not to die." For her, it helped her realize that she could still have a life.

AGITATION

Your husband may go through a period of agitation on admission. This is especially true of people with some kind of dementia who do not have the skills to deal with a change in environment. They do not understand what is happening and they may not believe you when you tell them why it is happening. They may not like where they are and feel imprisoned. Often they are not able to express what it is they are feeling directly—the agitation is that feeling.

Sometimes a resident's agitation, anger, complaining, or aggression is part of the grief reaction and fear. Talk about the feelings that you suspect may be under the behavior, not about the behavior itself. If he is unable or unwilling to express the underlying feelings, you may want to respond by trying to change the subject, or even not responding. When he sees that his behavior is not eliciting a response from you, it may change. He may also talk more to someone else, such as the social worker, than to you. My experience is that staff are often extra nice and gentle when a resident first moves in. However, agitation can be the result of interaction with the staff. You will have to be aware of this too. It may not be abuse, it may just be discomfort, fear, or embarrassment as someone they don't know tries to help them bathe, dress, or use the toilet.

Usually, someone who has become agitated due to the move will settle down. It may take some investigation to see how his environment can be adjusted. You may have to figure out if there is anything in particular to which he is reacting. This is where you need to work with the staff, because you know your husband much better than they do. You may even have to take some leadership in requesting that they do all the investigation possible.

If your husband is a younger man, his anger may be greater and more intense than that of an older person. It also may take him a lot longer to deal with his admission. Not only will he be dealing with the loss and grief, but also he is probably surrounded by people much older than he who have lived their lives much more completely. It will emphasize to him his situation, the unfairness of it, and what he hasn't had and most likely never will.

In turn, your guilt, anger, and distress may also be greater. As unfair as it is to him, it is also unfair to you. Even though you don't mean to, you may notice yourself directing your anger toward him and not the situation. This is clearly a case in which a competent therapist would be helpful for you and for him. At some point, he and you both will learn to turn the anger where it should go and then move to come to terms with it.

A decline in functioning, changes in behavior, depressed mood, or withdrawal can be much more intense and take longer for someone who has come directly from the hospital or who enters the home in an emergency than for someone who has been adequately prepared. It can be a shock and a crisis. The feeling of loss of control is exaggerated. This is not to say that adjustment doesn't happen in this situation. It does. But the person is more fragile, both emotionally and physically.

DELAYED REACTION

Some people have a kind of delayed reaction to moving. They seem almost unaffected at first and manage to get to the dining room, go to some activities, and talk to people. Their true reaction may not come until several days, weeks, or months after the admission. This can be because of some level of denial; in the beginning they cannot even admit to themselves how hard it is or how they feel about their loss. It may be because only when they feel safe in their new surroundings are they able to allow themselves to feel what they need to. It may also be because they start out in a type of shock, a common first reaction to a crisis or grief.

MEDICATION AND ADJUSTMENT

Whether your husband exhibits depression or agitation, the staff may suggest some kind of medication to help with the transition. A word of caution. Medication is not necessarily a bad course of action if it helps the staff provide care. If they absolutely cannot get him changed or bathed or dressed or to sleep, then medication may be a win-win situation. Medication can also help your husband settle down if he is overwhelmed by fear, agitation, and panic. People suffer with those feelings. I have seen medication make a world of positive difference for a resident; at times it might have been cruel not to use it.

There can be a thin line between using medication to help someone settle in and using it as a form of restraint. Under the U.S. Nursing Home Reform Law, medication can be used only to treat a person's medical conditions, not to control behavior. Keep your eyes open. Make sure you understand what the side effects of the medication are. Watch to make sure that your husband doesn't become overly tired or at risk for falls. Make sure that all options have been tried and all potential causes of the agitation have been investigated. For instance, if he is struggling when they try to help him change for bed, maybe he can just sleep in his clothes and change in the morning.

If medication is used, make sure that it is reviewed regularly so that it can be stopped when he doesn't need it any more. Find out for whose benefit the medication is being prescribed. Is it to help your husband or is it to make it easier for the staff, or both? (For more on this, see the sections on medications and on restraints in chapter 12.)

A resident's adjustment may seem different to family than it does to the staff. Often a resident will talk and behave differently with his family than with the staff. It is not uncommon for a resident to complain bitterly to her daughter but never open her mouth to the staff. Your husband may eat only if you feed him, or he may not be able to move without his wheelchair when you are there. Yet when you are not around, he may be feeding himself and walking independently with a walker.

Your husband may complain to you but be reluctant to complain to the staff because he does not want to be a "troublemaker." He may be concerned about maintaining an image of "a nice person" and will not want the staff to think ill of him. He may be afraid of retaliation. It is hard to complain when you are feeling vulnerable and the people you wish to complain about are the ones who are taking care of you. Also, many elderly people are not used to being advocates for themselves in the medical system. If your husband thinks medical personnel are the authorities, he will question, ask for, and complain less.

The reason for the differences between what you hear from your husband and what the staff sees can sometimes be found in your relationship. If he lets you know that he is unhappy with the situation, that is a way of retaliating for being abandoned by you. It may be a sort of angry gesture. Sometimes complaining can be a way of keeping you as his champion and involved in your relationship—if you are not there, something is going to happen to him; if you worry about him, you will be around more. All of these can be unconscious processes and not something that he is willfully planning. This is also not to say that his unhappiness or problems are not real. They are, but you need to look at some of the dynamics that occur between the two of you and their meaning as they relate to the three-way relationship (your husband, you, and the nursing home) in which you now find yourself.

You may have to stop responding to some of your husband's complaints. This can be difficult, as it will feel like you are further abandoning him. Explain what you are doing by saying something like, "Honey, I know you are a little frightened and don't like being here, but you need to get used to it and I need to help you. So when I come to visit or when we talk on the phone, I want to hear the good things that are going on. I don't want to hear complaints from you unless they are serious. I want you to try to solve them yourself by talking with _____." Then set up a system with the social worker or another staff member who will check in frequently with your husband. When he sees that the complaints are no longer eliciting from you the effect that he wishes, he may start to acclimate to the new situation. If you do this, you first need to be absolutely sure that there is no abuse or neglect occurring and that you have thoroughly investigated his complaints. If you are not satisfied, keep checking, digging, and monitoring. As mentioned earlier, agitation or withdrawal can also indicate abuse.

The second hardest experience you will have in the process of having your husband settle into a residence may be when you want to leave and he wants to go with you or doesn't understand why he is being left there. This can be heartbreaking. Until he gets used to it, he may repeatedly feel abandoned and angry. For you to continually go through this can be like picking a scab. I talk about how to handle this in chapter 14, "Visiting." Here, I want to emphasize that it will get better. Also, be aware that it is possible that fifteen minutes after you have left, he may have forgotten that you were there, what he is upset about, or even that he is upset. Unfortunately, you are not around to see that part. The staff can tell you what he is like after you leave and how long it takes him to settle down.

One of the most troubling things that can happen is that your husband will call you constantly to tell you that he wants to go home. You can talk to him, he will forget that you have done so, and he will call you again in five minutes. Usually that stops after a while, but it can lead your guilt machine to kick on at high speed: you were right—you were a terrible person to do this to him. You may have to buy some kind of call-monitoring device, a specialized answering machine, or even a second line. You might want to ask the staff to limit his calls. You might want to put another message on your service temporarily, saying something like, "If this is Jack, I love you and am thinking about you. I will call you as soon as I can." You may have to stop answering the phone or turn off the ringer for a while. You can make him a DVD of yourself and the family reassuring him, talking to him.

Keep reminding yourself that your husband is adjusting. That can be difficult to do when he is calling, complaining, depressed, and agitated. The emotions that keep you involved are the same ones that make it difficult for you to step back and view the whole picture analytically. One way to help maintain this perspective is to make an adjustment calendar. To do this, take at least twelve sheets of paper and mark them Week 1, Week 2, Week 3, etc. When he enters the home, jot down during each week what he and you have been going through—complaints, emotions, and so on. At the end of each week, write up a short summary. Just the fact that it is a time-limited calendar will help to tell you this is a temporary situation. Most people are surprised at the end of twelve weeks to see what they have been through and how the process has been resolving. If things are not resolving, the calendar is data you may need later. This is another area where it is also important to have support of other people, especially other people who have been through what you are going through. See if there are family members available at the residence to whom you can talk.

Dementia and Behavior

It is not my intention or ability to educate you in geriatric medicine or psychiatry. That would be presumptuous. However, there are a few essential things that anyone who is a caregiver for an older person needs to know about aging, dementia, and memory loss. I have said some of them above, but they bear repeating.

First, remember that "old age" is a description, not a diagnosis. If someone tells you that a change in your husband is due to old age, they are not telling you anything. Dig deeper. Ask for a more precise reason. If no one can tell you, then ask what they need to do to find out. This is one of the reasons that you want a physician who has a knowledge and interest in geriatric medicine. She will go the distance for you. To find out why a change has occurred or is occurring may take some invasive procedures that you or your husband do not wish. It is also possible that even if you find out what is happening, there may not be anything you can or wish to do about it (for example, chemotherapy for cancer). But that should be your choice, made with appropriate information.

Dementia is a syndrome (a cluster of symptoms) that is chronic, usually not reversible, and progressive. It is characterized by memory loss, personality changes, behavioral symptoms, and/or other cognitive changes, such as loss of what we call executive function: the ability to plan, reason, and make judgments. It affects about 5 percent of people over sixty-five years of age and 20 percent of people over eighty.

There are several kinds of dementia. Alzheimer disease is one of the most common. So if the doctor tells you that your husband has Alzheimer disease, she is also telling you that he has dementia. But if she tells you that your husband has dementia, it doesn't necessarily mean that he has Alzheimer disease. As of this writing, it is difficult to make a definitive diagnosis as to whether someone has Alzheimer disease or another kind of dementia.

Strokes can also cause dementia. This type of dementia is often called *vascular dementia* or *multi-infarct dementia*. It can occur from major strokes or it can be caused by many small, sometimes imperceptible strokes called *transient ischemic attacks (TIAs)*.

Dementia can also be caused by Parkinson disease, Pick disease, chronic alcohol abuse, and many other diseases. You may hear the terms *Lewy body dementia, Korsakoff syndrome,* or *AIDS-related dementia.* As of this writing there is no cure for most dementia, but there are a few medications that can sometimes slow its progression.

Often what looks like dementia is something called *delirium.* Delirium is a syndrome characterized by a sudden or fast onset of symptoms such as memory loss and confusion, with fluctuating levels of alertness and impairment. There are also behavioral symptoms, including falls, restlessness, agitation, listlessness, and aggressive behavior. Delirium is common in the elderly. As you can see from the causes below, delirium is often the result of a condition or illness that has different symptoms in younger people. Delirium is usually reversible. That means that the confusion and behavioral changes will be resolved when the underlying cause is treated.

Some of the causes of delirium include

1. Urinary tract infection, or UTI (this is extremely common and recurs often in elderly persons)
2. Pneumonia and other chest infection
3. Electrolyte, thyroid, or potassium imbalance
4. Medication overdose and medication reactions
5. Chronic pain
6. Bowel impaction/constipation
7. Sleep deprivation or sleep disorder
8. Malnutrition and dehydration.

Dementialike symptoms can also be caused by depression. It is estimated that 25-50 percent of the population in a nursing home has some level of depression. Delusions can also cause dementialike behaviors. Delusions are a set of false beliefs based on an incorrect perception of reality. They are maintained despite all evidence to the contrary. You cannot talk someone out of delusions. Delusions can be a symptom of delirium or can exist on their own. Depression and delusion are usually reversible and treatable.

Reduced hearing and eyesight can contribute to an older person's behavioral presentation. He may withdraw because of an inability to interact. He may try to mask cognitive losses and end up answering questions or interacting in a way that seems to indicate that he has not understood. Once someone withdraws because he is unable to participate in the world, he can become isolated, which can lead to depression.

If your husband begins to exhibit any of the signs of dementia or if his behavior or condition deteriorates, it is essential that he be investigated to see if any of the above reversible conditions are occurring. Do not permit a continuing medication order that modifies behavior without investigating the causes of the behavior first. You do not know if something can be done until the tests have been completed. All of the causes of delirium can be tested for fairly simply with minimal discomfort. A physician who is knowledgeable about geriatrics and who cares enough to pay attention will automatically screen for reversible causes of problems before prescribing medication.

Having given this warning, I want to emphasize that the causes of dementia are not reversible. You need to be willing to accept that. If your husband has Parkinson or Alzheimer disease, he will continue to decline. These are progressive diseases. People die from complications that arise from them. Many family members end up in denial because it is so painful to acknowledge this. But the pain and pressure of denial weigh more heavily in the end than the process of acceptance.

Numerous Web sites deal with dementias. Try the Alzheimer's Association Web site, www.alz.org. They have an excellent interactive piece about what happens in the brain when someone has Alzheimer disease. There is also the Canadian site, www.alzheimer.ca. Another excellent site is the National Library of Medicine / National Institutes of Health site, www.nlm.nih.gov/medlineplus/alzheimersdisease.html. There are many links to other sites there.

Sex and Relationships in Nursing Homes and Assisted Living

Many years ago I was on the staff in the geriatric psychiatry unit of a large hospital. We had recently admitted an eighty-four-year-old woman who had severe depression. She was from out of town, and her husband was not with her, so I called him on the phone. I was asking him about her and about their relationship. At one point I asked him how their sex life was. There was a long pause, and I thought, "Oops, shouldn't have asked that." But then he said, his voice shaky, "Thank you so much for asking. No one has talked to me about that before."

Much of our society associates sex with young people. The implicit message is that older people are not sexual, or they should not be. They are and they should be. Our skin is a sense organ. Touch, whether sexual or not, is one of the most important means of communication. It is important to our mental and physical health. This is true if you are twenty or if you are ninety. Long after someone's memory has gone, touch and intimacy are still valuable. When you talk with older people, it is clear that people never lose our need for touch, intimacy, and desire for some kind of sexuality.

Seniors residences, nursing homes especially with their multiperson rooms, set things up so that intimacy is harder to come by. This is compounded by staff members either not knocking at doors or knocking and then entering without waiting for an answer. In one facility, a staff member told me about finding a resident and family member having sex in a closet.

Staff attitudes toward residents' sexuality are at times problematic. There is often no sensitivity training regarding this population. I remember in one facility where I did some consulting, one of the staff members recorded in a chart that she had discovered a resident involved in a sexual act. There was no problem—except for the staff member. There was no reason to note this kind of thing in a chart.

For gay men and lesbians, the issues of relationships and intimacy can be even more difficult in residential care. Often you will find people going back "into the closet" after living an openly gay lifestyle for most of their lives. In the close to thirty years that I have worked in nursing homes, I have met only about two or three openly gay residents. I know there were others, they just weren't open about it. For sure, as of this writing, many older people come from a time when being gay was not acceptable, and they do not welcome gay people. It can be difficult for a gay or lesbian couple to try to live openly in assisted living as a couple. There are a few residences that are open, and more coming, that are oriented to this population. Staff attitudes about gay men and lesbians may be even more rigid or conservative than their attitudes toward sexuality in general. Many of them are from cultures where being gay/lesbian is not acceptable. They may not be comfortable with it for religious reasons or their own fears. It is hard to be open about oneself when the people on whom you depend are not comfortable and seem not to like you or to be judging you.

Residents do become involved in a range of types of relationships, everything from kissing and hugging, to intercourse, to moving in together, to marriage. Ask whoever is giving you a tour about how they handle resident relationships and sexuality. Often, the person who has the most difficulty with residents having sexual relationships may be you. It can be difficult for you to see your parent involved with someone.

Where relationships become problematic is when there is a discrepancy between the parties involved and their ability to give consent. If one or both have a dementia, that may impair their judgment at some point. There are times when one resident can become predatory with others. The question to consider is whether your mother knows what she is doing. Would she have done this if she were truly cognitively aware? Is this harmful or beneficial? Is the problem more you or your siblings than her? I have many times seen residents with fairly advanced dementia find each other and become sweethearts.

It may happen that your husband with dementia will become involved with another resident. This may be because he thinks the woman he is involved with is you, his wife, or he may have forgotten he is married, or other reasons. Marriage is a concept, an idea about two people. As people lose their reasoning ability, they lose the ability to formulate or hold onto concepts, so the idea of marriage is not something they are *able* to understand. This may feel like a betrayal to you. It can feel like this is one more step in the slow disintegration of your marriage. You may know that this is not what your husband would have wanted to do, or how he would have wanted to be acting, if he were able to hold on to himself. You may want to prevent the relationship and will have to talk to the staff and see what they can do. It may take you some soul searching to let go of the pain. But it is not about your marriage or your relationship; it is about illness and the toll it takes.

On Staying Healthy

There are four elements to maintaining good health in old age: good nutrition (including fluid intake), exercise, social interaction, and mental/cognitive stimulation. They are essential for all of us, but with elderly persons, deficits in any of these areas can mean a much shorter route to ill health or even death. Whether your husband is at home or in a residence, pay attention to all four.

Malnutrition and dehydration are common in elderly persons. Similar to many single persons living on their own, they do not eat as well. Women who used to cook for a husband or family may just "pick" at making food. A man on his own may not ever have cooked for himself regularly, so he lets himself eat poorly. A medication can make food taste bad or funny. Elderly people often have reduced sensations of smell and taste, so food tastes bland. When food tastes bland or funny, people tend not to eat as much or as well. People with dementia may forget to eat even if a meal is placed in front of them, or they may forget how to eat. Someone may not be able to shop for food, so reduce consumption. Older people may not take fluids for the same reasons that they don't eat well. Plus, if someone has problems with incontinence, especially nighttime incontinence, he may reduce fluid intake so he doesn't have an accident.

Both malnourishment and dehydration occur in nursing home or assisted living residents. This can happen because a resident is not getting sufficient help with eating, he does not have enough time to eat, he has developed swallowing disorders, or for the same reasons that he may not eat or drink at home. It may be necessary to closely monitor intake. Do not assume that the nursing home staff is doing this, even though it is their job. Assisted living may have even fewer people monitoring eating, and certainly fluid intake. As noted, they may call if someone does not come to a meal, but they may not.

Exercise is one of the most important parts of care for elderly persons. Older people lose muscle mass and strength relatively quickly when they are inactive for even a short period of time. Activity has all kinds of physical benefit for elderly persons (as it does for the rest of us). It has a positive impact on bowel function, heart and blood pressure, and diabetes. With increased physical ability, people feel better about themselves. When they maintain their physical abilities, they maintain their independence and social life. If someone cannot get around, the ability to interact with others can be impaired. Lack of mobility or impairment in the ability to transfer (get out of bed, on/ off the toilet, for example) may be one of the triggering factors in an assisted living facility saying they can no longer provide care.

Social interaction decreases for many people as they age. As they lose a spouse, their friends, and the ability to drive, their worlds shrink. They can become shut-ins. A couple of years ago, I was hired by a nursing home to do a study of people on the home's waiting list. Issues concerning social interaction were one of the major reasons for which people were going into care.

Social interaction is nourishing for most people, although not all. I am convinced that many of the behaviors that we see in nursing home residents are the result of loneliness, isolation, and despair. Unfortunately, they are often diagnosed as depression. When this happens, they treat the victim and not the situation—by which I mean they treat the resident, not the residence.

Social interaction is not assured in a residence simply because there are activities. Your husband may not wish to make new friends, or there may not be appropriate activities. He may not have the competence to develop relationships. He may not want to come out of his room, even if the staff encourages him. If he is not independently mobile, he will have to depend on the staff to be taken to activities or to be somewhere that encourages interaction. You cannot assume that he will even be gotten up and out of bed, never mind be brought to activities or helped to relate to others.

Be aware that social interaction means relationships, not activities. Relationships give people their sense of self and satisfy the need for intimacy. Relationships can develop and be nurtured through activities, but people can go to a residence's activities without being involved in relationships. Relationships also develop outside activities in homes. For instance, people come to know their tablemates in the dining room and other residents in their rooms or hallways.

Stimulation at the cognitive level means a variety of things. For sure it includes social interaction, but it also includes learning and challenge. It can be crosswords, painting, and board games. Several different "brain fitness" programs have been developed to help with cognitive stimulation. This stimulation aids in *neuroplasticity,* which refers to the brain's ability to change and develop throughout life. Cognitive stimulation is tied to emotional well-being and vice versa. Your husband will not be able or willing to participate if he is isolated, anxious, or depressed.

Your Emotional Adjustment

Your first impression of a residence, especially a nursing home, may be that a bunch of old people are just sitting around; you may perceive a sea of wheelchairs. This can be upsetting, but it will change. Over time, you will begin to know the people and become friendly with them and their families. You also may react with a feeling of "my husband is not as bad as they are." This may be true, but it also may be that you know him, and he is at his best with you. You don't see him as "an old person sitting around in a wheelchair" because you see the person he is. Other people are saying the same thing about their husbands.

When you come back to visit the first few times, you may be overwhelmed to see your husband sitting in a wheelchair like the other residents or wandering with a blank look on his face. You may experience him differently from how you did when he was in your home. You may have a feeling that this is a different person. This may be more of the feeling you have already had: "My husband is gone." In a sense, it is true; he is not the person who was able to talk to you the way he did or to function the way he used to. That doesn't mean that you are not important to him anymore or that he needs you any less. What's changed is the give and take. It is you who are doing the giving for the most part. Remind yourself that you are experiencing grief and that it will get easier.

A family member's adjustment often parallels the path of the one who is in a residence. Partly that comes about because you will not feel comfortable until you have the sense that your husband is feeling comfortable, that he is safe, or that he is getting adequate care. So, your initial adjustment may also take three to six months.

Your husband may adjust better than you do in the beginning. Many people have told me that after the initial move occurred, their relative did fine—they were the ones who went through the crisis. People who were afraid to say anything to their spouse about the move to a home found that he accepted it well. I know some family members who called the home every evening, after having been to visit every day. Their husband was fine; they were the ones who couldn't sleep.

The Gap in Your Life

Even if the move to a residence is a relief, and you are confident that you have made the right decision, it is still a major lifestyle change for you and everyone else who has been involved in the caregiving process. You will have to adjust not only to the home and to the change in your relationship but also to having a different life on your own in which you are not primarily a caregiver.

Many caregivers have given up part of their lives as they became more and more involved in caregiving. Sometimes they stopped going to a bridge club or bowling league, sometimes they let go of friendships. When your husband goes into a residence, you may suddenly realize how much you have given up and who is no longer around because you have let them slip out of your life.

Now there is a big gap in your daily life. You are no longer wondering "what is he doing?" when you are not around. You are no longer organizing medications, toileting, and monitoring for the majority of your day. Whether or not you feel relieved, you may also feel a loss.

This can lead you to feel envious and be critical of the people who are doing the tasks you used to do.

You may also feel in some ways at a loss about what to do with your time and your thoughts and your energy. It will feel strange at first, like something is missing. To fill this gap, you may have a tendency to grasp onto visiting or becoming involved in the home.

A couple of years ago, I admitted a ninety-three-year-old woman to a facility. Her son and daughter-in-law had been caring for her in their home for ten years. They had renovated the home and had arranged their lives around taking care of this woman who had advanced dementia. When they had finally exhausted their resources and those of the system, they admitted her to care. The daughter-in-law had been the primary caregiver—she had become an expert in Alzheimer disease, medications, heart disease, and local support systems. When the woman was admitted, her daughter-in-law had a terrible time. She continually called, asking about problems, medications, and so on. She told us that she wanted to ensure that her mother-in-law got the best care possible. But underneath that was an inability to let go. She had been on the caregiving train so long that she didn't know how to get off. She had an important role on which she could focus a lot of her energy. At some level, she was also getting what is called secondary gain—a lot of attention and admiration from people in her church and community because she was such a selfless, giving daughter-in-law. On admission, she lost that. Caregiving also diverted her attention from an unsatisfactory marriage. Not until she was able to look at some of these underlying issues directly and honestly was she able to shift her caregiving role.

Begin to think about how you want to fill the gap. Slowly start to plan things that are healthy, enjoyable, and functional for you. Make a schedule for yourself and put into it some activities you want to pursue or people you want to see even if at first it is only one activity or person per week. When you are feeling stronger, take a piece of paper and write down some goals for a year from now. Write down how to reach those goals.

Then start to do what you wrote, even though you may not feel like it at first. Activities can lift your feelings or change your emotional state. Once you are doing them, you will be glad you did. At first it may be hard for you to believe that you can feel better. It is like setting sail for another continent—you have to believe that it is there even though you can't see it and you have to get there before you can feel it. Activities and people will help contain your feelings and distract you from them. They will help you balance and regain your life.

There are a number of books written about loss, though there are fewer about the process of moving on. You might want to look through *How to Survive the Loss of a Love*, by Melba Colgrove, Harold Bloomfield, and Peter McWilliams, or *To Begin Again: The Journey toward Comfort, Strength, and Faith in Difficult Times*, by Naomi Levy.

Phases of Adjustment

It may be helpful to think of your adjustment as happening in phases. These can be more intense for family members of nursing home residents than for family members of someone moving to assisted living, but it is situational. The first phase is the crisis. It occurs from the time when your husband is offered a bed through about the first week. This is when you first encounter the new system and experience the change. It is the time of highest stress and when your emotions are running high. During this period, you may feel abandoned, angry, and helpless. You may feel alone in having to deal with the institution. You may want to ask some questions and may not know where to turn. This is the time when your support needs can be highest, but you will be focusing your attention on your husband.

The second phase comes in about the second to fourth week. By then the initial crisis is over, and you begin to figure out some of the more practical things, such as to whom to talk, what times particular things happens, or where to find something. It is when you are doing your initial problem solving. You may begin to feel like you are able to come up for air. At the same time, you may feel that one day everything is fine and the next day nothing is right. Expect that this is a time of ups and downs for both you and your husband. This is also the time when you may begin to feel sharply your own loss and separation. As the initial crisis settles, you realize what "this" is going to feel like.

During the second phase, you begin to establish relationships with the staff. You both are figuring out what the others are about. It is also when the staff begins to develop a feel for what your needs are and how to assist you. Look for the people you feel could be helpful to you.

Establishing relationships with the staff and the home is the development of trust. Developing trust takes time, and in some ways you will need proof that your trust is justified. This happens through a series of small events and interactions over the initial period. It would not be normal for you to have that trust from the first day.

After having been a caregiver for so long, you may find it hard to let someone else take over. Partly this relates back to guilt, and partly it relates to the grief process. But partly it is fear—fear that no one can take care of your husband the way you have, fear of what is going to happen if you are not around to take care of him. If this comes up for you, ask yourself what you are afraid of. Write it down and then look at each item you have written. Ask yourself if the fear is realistic or not. If it is, talk to the nurse or social worker about your concern.

The care your husband receives in a residence will not be the same as the care you gave him. But that doesn't mean he will not receive good care. There are often glitches in the first few weeks, but even that does not mean that the care will not be good or that you have done the wrong thing. It means that the system is learning and routines are not established yet. In fact, it may turn out that his needs might be met better in the residence.

The third phase goes from about the second to the fourth, fifth, or even sixth month. It is when you start to figure out some of the subtle but important details about the home and the care, such as what to do when your husband has an outside appointment and when the podiatrist comes. During this phase, you are learning what your role as a family member is. You learn what your expectations are and what others expect of you. You learn what the home really does, as opposed to what they say they do.

In the third phase of adjustment, your trust in the staff should grow as you see that they are competent. This will happen as you see your husband settle in. That is why your adjustment parallels his. If you do not ever feel that you can trust the staff or the home, and it is honestly because of the quality of care, then it is time to move your husband or become an active partner in a process of change. (See chapters 12, 13, and 16.)

Although the beginning of this phase may be marked by the continuing pain of your loss and separation, it is often during this period when you may begin to let go. You start to face living without your husband and without caregiving as the central role in your life.

The final stage is when you and your husband have developed a routine for living. You have a routine for visiting. You have at least begun to reestablish your life outside, with some new habits and daily patterns.

The fourth stage does not mean that you're smoking a cigar with your feet up on the desk. It means that you have surfaced with a feeling of equilibrium in your life. You may still feel some guilt and depression. You may still feel some emptiness or anger.

As I suggested earlier, you might want to see if there is a family member of another resident who has been in the home for a while who can act as a "buddy" or mentor for you during adjustment. Or try to get to know some of the other relatives who are visiting at the same time you are. These people can become a type of informal support system. They know how the home works and have learned to get things done. They know what you are going through. I have always found that family members are willing to help other family members.

You should also go to the family council or the family information nights. There may also be a family support group, often run by the social worker. These can give you an opportunity and a forum to figure out the system. Even if you feel you do not need the emotional support, you may benefit from the practical information that these meetings provide.

Acceptance

Some people have told me that, in fact, they never fully come to peace with having their relative in a nursing home. They always have a feeling of sadness when they walk out the door. What they have been able to do is accept it. They say that the feelings of guilt and loss become more manageable, and they have been able to move on. They have to keep working at letting go and accepting their feelings in order to come to whatever stage of adjustment they are able to manage. It is easier for them when they see their relative happy, and this is why families of people in assisted living often find it easier— their loved one often feels that they are in a new home and not in an institution.

You may have to work at acceptance. You can do this in the same ways you worked at the resolution of guilt. Talk with your husband about what the two of you are experiencing. Write down your feelings in a diary. Write letters to your husband about what you feel and are going through. Post a note on your mirror that tells you what you need to hear.

The staff understand what you are going through as you adjust. They may not understand it the way someone who has been there would understand it, but they do know. In a good home you can talk about it with the social worker or one of the nurses. It is their job to take care of you also.

If the care and home are acceptable or better, then what you must learn to do in that first year is to come to emotional terms with the situation as it is. Know that it may change. Know that there will be ups and downs. Take and give what you can, and let go of your expectations. In some ways, this is an attitude of "one day at a time." Acknowledge your anger and your grief and acknowledge how and when they are coming out. Try not to be ashamed of your feelings or to hide them. Let them be a signal to you that you need to work on acceptance and take care of yourself.

New Relationships

There may come a point after your husband has been in the residence for a while when you have made a new life for yourself in the community. For some people, this means developing romantic and intimate relationships. Especially for people whose spouse has dementia, this becomes a possibility because you have truly lost not only physical intimacy but also emotional intimacy. Becoming romantically involved with someone else can bring up tremendous conflict and guilt. It goes against your marital vows. Your children may be extremely upset. You may feel your community is judging you.

A new relationship does not mean that you are abandoning your husband or that you love him any less. It means that you have adjusted in a way that is right for you. You are the only one who can decide this. It is not uncommon. Let me tell you that many people who have walked in your shoes will not judge you.

Bill

We came together in midlife from vastly different worlds. "Soulmates at last," we said. Our joy was indescribable.

We lived the good life for a few years, my Bill and I. We had each devoted a great deal of time and energy to our respective careers, and it had paid off well. We enjoyed meaningful work and an enviable lifestyle with exotic travel, interesting social events, and, most of all, each other. We had waited a long time for this and thought we deserved all we had.

But our dream was cruelly interrupted a few short years later. Slowly but surely, this proud man of dignity and intelligence was thrown into the neverland of dementia and disability, and I became his caregiver.

I began to pray and bargain with the cruel God, who, I decided, was responsible for this devastating turn of events. I begged for a nice predictable stroke, something that people don't survive. I forced my confused husband to visit every quack up and down the coast, drink unpalatable potions, and swallow pills that made him choke.

Although I kept a journal for most of the four years of my husband's illness, there is a painful void in the record once placement had become imminent. My last entry for almost a year was: "This all seems so hopeless, I can only watch him deteriorate further, but I want him with me anyway. My intellect tells me I am deranged for wanting to continue living this way, but it seems to be the only thing that has any meaning."

Etched in my consciousness forever is the dark, rainy day I sat sobbing in the parking lot after viewing the chosen facility. In hindsight, I can see that this was the point of acceptance: acceptance that I could no longer cope and that I had to release my love to the care of others and to a simpler world.

It was so painful to know I would be placing Bill in care. I felt bound by promises: ones I had made to him and to myself, and ones he had made to me. It made me wonder about who I was, about how I had formed and shaped my life to this point. I felt I was being untrue to our relationship and to the things we had built together. When I made the decision to put Bill into care, I was filled with feelings of guilt, loss, failure, and self-doubt. I thought that maybe I was not loving enough, that I was being cruel and heartless. I was sure that there was a way to avoid doing this if only I kept searching and trying.

The day Bill was admitted to the nursing home was both the worst and the best day of my life. It wrenched me away from the destructive path we were on and signified the end of my life as it was. Despite all my feelings, or maybe among them, I knew it was also a relief to turn him over to people who were trained and equipped to care for him. Although Bill couldn't speak, I think he was able to cope better in this new world of routine and simplicity.

Several months later, when I was offered a job, I wrote in my journal, "My love, I am leaving you behind, and that makes me so sad." Then a few passages later I wrote, "I can't handle it. What used to be most important to me is now insignificant. Bill, I am lost in the same neverland as you are."

Eventually when Bill's physical condition began to deteriorate, I decided I wanted him to die at home. Because he was not able to get up and down stairs, I began the process of modifying our two-story home to accommodate him on the main floor. When my plan became known at the nursing home, the head Nurse cautioned me about the time and energy it would take, and what that would take away from Bill. She pointed out that I would be too exhausted to give him the same attention I now could when the staff was bathing him, preparing his special food, changing and dressing him, toileting him, etc. I hated her for her honesty, but I was thankful someone had helped me see the folly of what I was trying to do.

Now as time has softened my wounds, I can see that placement is sometimes a predictable and practical step as we near the end of life. Current lifestyles do not accommodate home care in the way that they did in my mother's generation. I know that although medical advances have extended life, people are older and sicker than they were then too.

During the years Bill spent in the facility, I had a ringside seat from which to observe others and myself. I heard people complain about the most trivial oversights as though they were life threatening. I saw healthy seniors spend their remaining years focusing on a relative who no longer knew them. I noted the ones who dealt with their loss by staying away. I came to understand that if I let caregiving become the focus of my attention, then giving it up and moving on would be extremely difficult.

For me, letting go was a gradual process. Eventually, Bill's placement provided me with the space to grow and move back into the mainstream of life. What I perceived as the worst day of my life was actually the first day of moving toward a new and interesting segment—one of appreciation and thankfulness for the experiences I had, and of greater understanding about the passages I would have to go through in life.

PART IV

BEING THE FAMILY MEMBER OF SOMEONE IN CARE

CHAPTER 12

Care and
Care Planning

Basic Standards of Care

Care should be about enabling and allowing people to have their individuality, dignity, and respect. I think certain basic standards and rights should never be violated. When I started out as a geriatric care manager, I wrote the following list as a response to how I saw elderly people being treated, and allowing themselves to be treated, as they went through the health care system. I would like to see people use this list of rights as a guide to obtain adequate care from their health professionals, whether or not they are in a residential facility. If any of these standards is violated as you work with the health care system and health care providers, it is a signal to demand a change.

1. You have a right to be valued as an individual.
2. You have a right to a physician who is knowledgeable about geriatric medicine.
3. You have a right to a diagnosis for a problem, if one can be identified, and to know what that diagnosis is.
4. You have a right to information about your treatments and medications.
5. You have a right to be spoken to, not about.
6. You have a right to be treated as an adult, not a child.
7. You have a right to live at risk if you have the capacity to make that decision.
8. You have a right to be consulted about decisions that affect you in any way and to make decisions about yourself for as long as you are able and competent to do so.

9. You have a right to determine who will make decisions for you and in what situations when you are unable to do so.
10. You have a right to make advance directives and have them carried out.
11. You have a right to say when you have had enough.
12. You are responsible to make sure your rights are respected and to use your rights appropriately.

As I have mentioned several times already, in the United States, the rights of nursing home residents are enshrined in the Nursing Home Reform Law of 1987, which covers a wide range of rights for residents and regulations for nursing homes. These include transfers, admissions and readmissions, payments, refusal for care, discharges, restraints, medications, and others. If you are told by a home that they cannot do something or you cannot do something, this law, as well as the laws on Medicare and Medicaid, are probably the ones you will need to find information on first. Canadians do not have a similar law, as health care is a provincial responsibility. However, all areas have standards of care and licensing bodies that look after nursing homes and assisted living facilities. Nursing homes are regulated and must follow guidelines of local health authorities.

How Care Is Organized

Usually, the provision of care is organized around what is called a care plan. In assisted living, it may be called an individual service plan (ISP). Note the difference in approach—care versus service. Medical model versus social model. A care plan is a document that identifies an individual resident's problems and strengths. For each problem a resident has, the staff will identify a goal or objective. The care plan then lists the actions to be taken to achieve those goals.

The basic components of a care plan identify a resident's level of independence in the areas of eating, dressing, washing, grooming, bathing, walking, and transferring (the ability to stand up, go from the toilet to a wheelchair, etc.). These are known as activities of daily living (ADL). The staff will determine through observation and, one would hope, through talking to you and your mother how much help your mother needs. Abilities such as dressing are categorized as, for example, "independent," "needs partial assist," or "needs total assist." With walking or transferring, the care plan will identify whether your mother uses a walker, wheelchair, and so on. If she needs help to transfer, it will say whether she needs one or two people to help. Sometimes a chart will be posted in your mother's room identifying what kind of help she needs. It is almost always kept at the nursing station as well.

A care plan also addresses more complicated needs, such as medical, social, nutritional, recreational, psychological, and spiritual needs. This is the part where special diets (such as diabetic or low salt) will be identified. The plan may note skin integrity (meaning whether the skin is intact or there are ulcers, wounds, etc.), tendency toward depression, and behavioral issues. It may also identify family needs or issues such as caregiver stress or if there are conflicts in the family that could affect the resident's care or decision making.

An individual service plan may identify some or all of the above, or it may not, depending on the level of assistance that the facility provides. If there are concerns that they are not addressing, you need to talk to them about it to see if they can and at what cost.

The goals in an individual service plan describe an optimal level of desired functioning and list the actions to be taken to attain those goals. These are based on a realistic view of what is possible for each resident. For persons with diabetes, a goal may be simply to maintain appropriate blood sugar levels; the actions would be appropriate diet and exercise. For depression, the goal may be that your mother express contentment. There may be several suggested courses of action, such as a mental health assessment, medication, appropriate activities, pet therapy, and bus outings. For walking, the goal may be that she is able to walk fifteen feet safely with her walker. Courses of action may include physical therapy and new shoes.

In nursing homes with Medicaid-funded beds, an initial assessment must be done within fourteen days of admission. A care plan must be developed by seven days after that. The facility must use what is called the Minimum Data Set and a Resident Assessment Protocol. These are fairly complicated instruments that create a problem-solving path for the staff as they examine all areas of a resident's functioning. If used well, these instruments are an excellent guide for the provision of good care and for problem solving when something is amiss. Assisted living residences that accept Medicaid are also usually required to develop an individual service plan, but even facilities that do not take Medicaid should have one. It is an industry standard.

The care plan is one of the areas in which the social history that you wrote will be important. It tells the staff what your mother was like before all this started, so they have a basis for determining what success will look like and what is normal for her. For example, if she was always somewhat underweight, her care plan would probably not have as a goal that she reach her ideal body weight.

Unfortunately, sometimes staff members do not read care plans, write down changes, read the changes that have been noted, or pay attention to them if they do read them. First of all, some staff members are illiterate. Second, a nurse's aide with fifteen people to take care of every day might not have the time to be aware of all the changes. For casual staff or agency staff members, remembering the care plans for all these people they've just met is hard. These problems should be addressed, but remember that the setup of the system can mean communication and continuity problems among departments, staff members, and shifts.

You should try to involve yourself in the development and monitoring of your mother's care plan, and you may want a copy of it. (For more about care plans, see "Nursing Homes: Getting Good Care There," from NCCNHR [formerly the National Citizens' Coalition for Nursing Home Reform], www.nccnhr.org.) The best way to involve yourself is through a care conference.

Care Conferences

A nursing home care conference is the occasion during which you, your mother (if she is capable), and representatives from all disciplines meet to talk about your mother's care. Usually it is attended by a nurse, nurse's aide, recreation worker, social worker, dietitian, and other therapists employed by the home. Ideally, a physician and pharmacist will be there as well. Often a housekeeper, dietary aide, and pastor will attend. During the conference, people from each discipline will discuss issues that they have identified and look at ways of meeting needs. Assisted living facilities may or may not have similar meetings. If they do, the staff attending may be more limited, reflecting the lesser variety of assistance provided in these residences. You are still welcome to call a meeting of the staff members the facility does have. At some facilities, this will not be something they are used to, and their reaction may be less than enthusiastic, partly because they do not see themselves as providing "care."

If your mother is unable to sit through a meeting or would feel too threatened or confused to handle one, you can talk to her beforehand and see what her views are. Ask the social worker to do the same. Some people who are nonverbal or who have dementia can make clear some of their needs or problems. Your mother is the "team leader" and you are the co-captain. Make sure her voice is heard.

Some family members feel intimidated in a care conference. The process is new to them, there can be many staff members there, and unfamiliar medical terms are used (see the list of abbreviations in appendix 3 for terms that may come up). Just think of the staff as people who happen to have knowledge in a specific area. You do too, in other areas. You are not stupid if you don't understand their terminology. They are rude for using terms that you might not understand without explaining them to you. Ask them to explain, speak up, slow down, and go over something again. Keep on asking until they get it. If you have a feeling about something, you can state it—your opinion is valid, and your feelings deserve to be heard. If you need to, you can bring someone with you, either another family member, a friend, or a professional such as a geriatric care manager.

The care conference is your chance to give and receive information. Your mother and you are the experts on your mother—you know how she has responded, what she used to be like, what was normal for her. You know her limits and the meaning of some of her behaviors. You know her psychological strengths and foibles. You have the right to ask questions about what is being done and why. You are the one who can give some insight into how and why the goals that the staff sets can or cannot be met. You should discuss the goals and hopes you have.

You also have the responsibility in a care conference to listen with some respect to what the staff says. They may see the picture differently from you. They may not feel that the goals you have are realistic. They should be able to tell you why they believe what they do and present data to support it. You may not like what they have to say, but that doesn't mean that they are wrong. It may be that the result of a care conference, in assisted living especially, is that you and the staff (or just the staff) make the decision that they cannot safely provide service for your mother. If that is the decision, you have a choice of accepting it, attempting to negotiate it, or going to the ombudsperson or another state or provincial official.

You may still believe that the goals you have for your mother are realistic. I have many times seen people achieve goals of rehabilitation or improvement after a stroke that no professionals thought were possible. The people did it through willpower and perseverance. If you disagree with the staff and believe that your goals are realistic, you may have to find the evidence yourself. You also may have to work with the staff to find ways to try to achieve what you hope. There may be limitations on the staff and budget that will interfere, and you may have to accept that and find another way around it. The Nursing Home Reform Law says that nursing homes have to help residents achieve their *practicable* potential. That is where the dispute may arise.

You may also have to look at your goals and ask yourself if you are hanging on because of the grief of seeing your mother deteriorate. If that is what you are doing, then you need to take a look at your grief, anger, and other feelings. Dealing with them by denial is not helpful to you and can be difficult for your mother. I have seen people hang on long after there was no realistic hope of improvement and long after even their parent wanted it to stop.

This is not to say that substandard care or practices are acceptable. It is saying that you must be honest with yourself about what is going on. It is not easy to do. Letting go of some of your goals may mean facing that your mother's condition is progressive and that she will die. This means that you will have to accept that you will lose her; that you will have to go on with your life without her. I wish I could say something that would make this easier for you, but I don't know what that would be, except perhaps to remember that, in the end, the best thing you can do for your mother is to help her find peace and a peaceful and easy exit from life.

At the end of the care conference, you should feel that you are working with the staff and your mother in a team. You should understand what the staff feel they are doing for your mother and what they need to do. You should also have confidence that they understand both you and your mother and that they know how she is experiencing her life in the home. Even if your mother is deteriorating, you still can look for the quality and comfort of life free from pain.

There should be an initial care conference about four weeks after admission and not later than eight weeks. It is good to check in with the staff informally before then, but it can often take four weeks for the staff to develop a clear idea of what your mother's care needs and abilities are. There should be a care conference yearly after that.

It is also a good idea to have a care conference when there is a marked change in your mother's condition, either for the better or for worse. This gives everyone the opportunity to sit down and revise plans. It also gives you a chance to talk over how you and she would like to handle this phase of her care. Maybe you would like to be more involved. Maybe you would like more aggressive tests to be undertaken, or maybe you don't want anything more to be done.

Charts

In a nursing home, a chart and records are kept for every resident. Assisted living residences will keep a file, with at least the individual service plan, as well as some contact data, but it may not be anywhere near as complete as in a nursing home. In the nursing home chart should be the care plan, medical history and medical examination notes, as well as results of blood work, X-rays, and so on. Usually, each discipline will do an assessment, which will be written up in the chart as well. The form of the main body of the chart varies, but usually it is a historical narrative that highlights problems and actions taken by the staff. It includes discussions with the physician and will document different incidents: for example, if your mother has had a fall, if she has had some behavioral problems, if there was a particular family interaction. The doctor also writes in the chart.

Sometimes the staff will also keep records similar to flow charts that document a resident's pattern in regard to a specific problem, such as sleep, pain, or behavioral disturbance. These are particularly effective in determining what the cause or specifics of a problem may be. For instance, if your mother is agitated, the staff can look for a disturbance in her environment and see if it corresponds to a certain time of day. They can then look for clues as to what may be happening at that time. Maybe her pain medication has worn off and she needs a higher or more regular dose, or maybe she is tired or hungry.

You have the right to read your mother's chart (if she has given you permission). If you do so, it may be helpful to sit down with someone who can go through it with you rather than to examine it yourself. The staff may insist that they be present, but you can also ask your own physician or other consultant. If you do want to read it yourself, don't jump to conclusions about what is said in the chart. Although charts should be written with the idea that they will be read by the family or resident, often they are not. It is easy to misinterpret what is in a chart. I heard of one family member who got upset when reading that her husband was SOB. She thought the staff was saying he was a son of a bitch. Actually, he was short of breath.

In both Canada and the United States, there are laws restricting access to information to protect privacy, and these are often used to deny family members or residents access to charts and files. In the United States the relevant privacy law is HIPAA (Health Insurance Portability and Accountability Act). In Canada there are provincial laws called freedom of information legislation or a similar name. You may be able to sit down with someone in the residence to negotiate you reviewing the files. However, you may have to fight if the residence uses these laws to limit your access, and this fight can be difficult. You can go to your state ombudsperson, licensing agency, or a lawyer.

Medication and Care Planning

You should pay particular attention to the issue of medications. Older people react differently to medications than do younger people. Their bodies do not eliminate or metabolize medications as easily or in the same way as a younger person's, so it is especially important that your mother be on the minimal medication possible.

It may be that medications have been gradually added to your mother's routine over a couple of years as different illnesses or conditions have arisen. All of the medications may make medical sense individually, but they may have interactive effects that can cause problems. Or they may help one problem but cause another. If they were added slowly, she may not ever have had a comprehensive medication review.

It is also possible that medications that were appropriately prescribed and taken have built up in your mother's system. This can happen slowly, and when it begins to have some adverse effects, the medications might not be diagnosed as the cause because they have been stable and effective for so long. It may happen that they need to be cut back or stopped or another drug prescribed in their place. People who needed certain medications at home may not need them now. If your mother needed medication to help settle in to a residence the first month, she may not need it in the third month. A medical condition may have changed, and the medication may need to be adjusted. Sometimes at home people weren't taking their medication as prescribed. When they come to a nursing home and have it dispensed properly by a nurse, the medication can start to affect them differently. Medications need to be reviewed regularly and discontinued when they are no longer needed.

I have frequently seen medications prescribed in nursing homes without residents' families being informed. The residents may or may not be told that they have a new pill to take, and/or why they have it. It is common for a change in dosage to occur without family members being informed. Partly this happens because one nurse can have many medication changes to deal with over the course of a day. For her to call each family, discuss it, and so on would take an extraordinary amount of time. Ideally, there should be a minimal list of specific medications that trigger a call. Without question families should be called when a medication is prescribed for behavioral or emotional reasons (which can be in contravention of the law anyway).

You should know not only what medications your mother is taking but also how they are prescribed, especially those prescribed for behavioral concerns and for pain. Medications can be prescribed on a regular basis (for instance, twice a day, or two tablets once a day in the morning). Or they can be prescribed on a PRN (as necessary) regime. "As necessary" can mean it is up to the discretion of either the resident or the nurse. If a medication is prescribed PRN, find out how often it is in fact being given.

Sometimes medications have lifestyle effects. For instance, if your mother is on a diuretic (water pill), she will have to use the bathroom more often. If she is slow on her feet with a walker, she may be afraid that she will have an accident before she can get to the bathroom. This will cause her to stay in her room and decrease her social interaction, which can lead to depression. Or she may be on some medications that affect her sense of taste. This will have an impact on her eating, so her nutritional status can be affected. Some medications can increase the risk of falls. Some medications or combinations can cause delirium or other changes in behavior.

The above are the reasons why it is so important to have access to a good pharmacist. Drug interactions and effects are their area of expertise. A good pharmacist will be able to say whether medications and dosages are appropriate for your mother's diagnoses. He should also be able to advise you if behavior you are seeing could be related to medications. If you suspect that medications are inappropriate and/or are having an adverse effect on your mother, try to find a good pharmacist or ask for another medical consultation. To find a pharmacist, go to your local drugstore or call the professional body in your state or province.

Several Web sites offer information on medications and medication interactions.

Medication and Pain Control

Some studies have indicated that up to two-thirds of all nursing home residents are undertreated for chronic pain. Other studies have shown that people with dementia receive less pain medication for the same conditions than do people who do not have dementia. There is no need for either of these situations to occur.

Sometimes staff do not even ask if someone is having pain. Twice lately I have had clients who told me their pain is between six and eight on a scale of ten. The staff did not think they were having pain at all, or thought that if they were, it was not very bad. A pain assessment should be part of the admission process in a nursing home. You need to ask your mother about her pain and then tell the staff. Levels of pain should be reviewed regularly, and certainly when a resident has an incident or illness known to potentially cause pain.

Pain management has changed and improved greatly over the past decade. The staff in a nursing home or assisted living facility may not be trained in pain management, or not to a high degree. However, there are professionals of several disciplines who specialize in pain control. These include doctors, nurses, occupational therapists, acupuncturists, and psychologists. You may have to ask the residence to call in a pain control specialist, or seek one out for yourself.

The approach to pain control today is to give medication so that the pain does not "break through," as opposed to giving it only when the pain becomes too great. When a medication has been prescribed for pain PRN, the result may be that your mother is not getting it often enough, especially if she has dementia and is unable to tell someone when she is having pain. One result can be behavioral disturbance: she will "act out" her pain.

Many residents don't want to bother the nurse or believe that they should be able to stand a little bit of pain. They will ask for something only when it becomes unbearable. By then it is harder to control. Also, if a nurse is busy, she may not be able to respond to a request for medication. If it is prescribed on a regular basis, there is a greater likelihood your mother will receive what she needs when she needs it. If your mother is reluctant to ask for pain medication or tell the nurse when she is experiencing discomfort, you might want to ask the doctor to prescribe it regularly throughout the day. If your mother is reluctant to take it that way, it should be her decision, but perhaps she would be willing to try it for a month and then reevaluate.

As I alluded to above, people with advanced dementia or impaired verbal skills are often unable to directly state whether they have pain. They may act it out behaviorally, which may lead to results different from appropriate treatment for pain. You may have to be the one who identifies for the staff the meaning of your mother's behavior.

Different types of pain medication are administered in different ways. For example, some are delivered gradually and continuously by wearing a patch. If one kind of pain medication isn't working, find out what options are available. You may have to do your own research and suggest something.

A word of caution: most medications have some side effects on some persons. Don't read a physician's desk guide to medications, have a panic attack when you read about all the potential side effects, then insist that all your mother's medications be stopped. The point is to be aware of the potential for problems and to be able to discern if a condition or a change in condition is caused by medication.

Restraints

I remember the smell of urine being the first thing that hit me when I walked into the nursing home where my grandmother was living in about 1972. It was before people understood Alzheimer disease or dementia care. In the lounge the people were lined up in rows as though they were at a theater performance. They were sitting quietly, staring straight ahead. Some were slumped over the side of their chairs or wheelchairs. My grandmother was in the front row, secured to her chair by a restraint that immobilized her whole upper body. This was how they stopped her from running out of the home into the street. When she saw me, her face shattered like a mirror and she started to cry.

Restraints are still in use today. A restraint can be chemical—medication that alters a person's personality or mood or slows her down to the point where she is immobile. Physical restraints restrict someone's mobility or movement; for example, she may be tied into a wheelchair or confined to bed through bed rails.

The reason a home usually gives for restraining a resident is that it is for the resident's own protection or to protect the other residents or staff members. Research shows that restraints do not generally prevent injuries such as falls; in fact, they may increase the likelihood of injury. Restraints end up being used sometimes because there has been an inadequate problem-solving process. It takes time and effort to figure out why some behaviors are occurring. Once figured out, it can take considerable staff time to meet the needs that cause the behavior.

Ideally the staff will go through the steps necessary to understand and intervene in a problem. Don't fool yourself. The reality is that limitations on the staff and resources may prevent them from doing so. The reality is that they may not have the education to figure it out. The reality is that they may see your mother every day and not recognize when her behavior is abnormal or has changed. Even if they do try to do all the problem solving, they still might not figure out what is wrong or why a behavior is occurring.

In the United States the law specifically addresses restraints under resident rights: "The right to be free from . . . any physical or chemical restraints imposed for purposes of discipline or convenience, and not required to treat the resident's medical symptoms." The law also says when restraints may be used. There are regulations to document and monitor the use of both chemical and physical restraints. Although Canada does not have a similar law, many homes have a no-restraint policy and will apply restraints only following a physician's order. Usually, however, this only applies to physical restraints. Medication is frequently used to modify behavior. Despite the laws and the policies, you still need to keep on top of this issue.

There is often a fine line between the use of medication for responding to a resident who is anxious, irritable, or difficult to manage and using it as a restraint. When does it become restraint? The difference may be in underlying purpose—is it for the resident, or for the home? Is it about safety, or is it about time management? Again, the reality is that sometimes, in a group living situation with limited resources, the ideal is not going to occur.

There is no excuse for basic problem solving not to be done. You may have to be the detective. If the home tells you that your mother needs some help with her behavior, you may have to step in and prepare a checklist of everything that should be tried and all the tests that need to be done. You may be able to tell the staff what the problem is because you know your mother—you may understand what she wants, what is bothering her, or what she is missing.

It may make you uncomfortable to see your mother at risk for falls if she is trying to walk instead of using a wheelchair. You may wish for her to be restrained. But she may prefer taking that risk. If she is not mentally aware at present, you need to ask yourself what she would have done. Your mother has the right to live at risk if she chooses, or if this is something that she might have wanted. The fact that you are her caregiver does not give you the right to make decisions that go against what she would want because of your own needs or fears. If she makes a choice that leads to injury, you need to accept that it was not your fault.

The NCCNHR (www.nccnhr.org, formerly National Citizens' Coalition for Nursing Home Reform) has two excellent guides that discuss restraints: "Avoiding Physical Restraint Use" and "Avoiding Drugs Used as Chemical Restraints," by Sarah Greene Burger.

Toileting and Incontinence

Many older people have some kind of incontinence problem that leads to the wearing of pads or diapers. If you think about it, one of the first symbols we have of being "grown up" is when we are toilet trained. To lose control over bladder or bowels brings us back to being a child. It is a shame-inducing problem. It can also cause someone to limit social involvement for fear of smelling bad or having an accident. You almost never hear it discussed; it is one of those "closeted" kinds of problems. Yet, the use of incontinence products in care facilities is common; up to 80 percent of residents wear some form.

Bladder incontinence is a complicated problem and often misunderstood, even by well-trained staff members. For example, your mother may constantly feel that she has to urinate, but when she is on the toilet be unable to do so. When she asks to go to the toilet often and the nurse's aides see that she has not voided, they may think your mother is malingering or trying to be difficult. Some people also have continued dribbling. Your mother may have a bladder that doesn't empty completely, so she has to urinate frequently. The staff may think, "She couldn't possibly have to go so often; she is just wanting attention."

If your mother starts to have problems with incontinence of either bowel or bladder, pay particular attention to how the home is handling this. A resident who becomes incontinent may do so because of neglect. The staff may not respond to her needs to use the bathroom and may find it is easier to put her in diapers. Incontinence can be indicative of a urinary tract infection, changes in medications, side effects of medications, or other medical problems. See if the staff or doctor can diagnose the cause of the incontinence. There is often something that can be done. This includes bladder retraining and exercises, surgery, and medications. Once again, however, to be able to use some of these solutions can take staff time and money. Often the staff does not have the training or time to be able to implement some of the behavioral solutions. Also, your mother may not be able to do the necessary exercises. (For more information on urinary incontinence, see www.agenet.com.)

If there is an ongoing problem, see if your mother is on a toileting schedule and an appropriate bowel protocol. Maybe she needs to be reminded to use the bathroom more frequently. Maybe she needs more help in getting there. Sometimes confused residents simply cannot find the toilet or need more directional cues to go to it. If they are helped with this, the incontinence will clear up or decrease.

If your mother is incontinent of bowel, this may take additional investigation. Has something changed in her food or medications? Is there an actual problem in the bowel? Is the home using an appropriate bowel protocol, which guides them on what to do when there is some kind of irregularity? Bowel incontinence can often be managed, or better managed, when the appropriate routine is followed. Bowel incontinence, like urinary incontinence, can sometimes respond to exercise or other interventions, if the resident has the cognitive ability to respond.

Toileting routine should include nighttime. It is generally not appropriate to have someone sleep through the night if he is wet or soiled. This leads to skin breakdown and infections. It is also a loss of dignity. Many times residents have told me the nursing assistant said to them something along the lines of "go in your diaper, that's why you are wearing it." Diapers or pads are not an excuse for the staff to ignore a resident who needs to be changed. Having said that, some diapers are incredibly absorbent and can hold urine safely until someone is changed.

If your mother was wearing pads or diapers and managing on her own at home, make sure that she is able to manage by herself with the ones she is wearing at the facility. A change of system can make it difficult for her, hence decreasing her independence as well as making her incontinent.

Be aware that the staff can be excellent about changing your mother on time and you will still come in and find her wet or soiled. Sometimes someone is put on a toilet, then fifteen minutes later she has an accident. Caregiving is not one-to-one, the way it might have been when your mother lived in your home or when she had someone with her all the time. It can be upsetting to come in and see your mother soiled or wet, with the accompanying loss of dignity. Your first reaction may be, once again, guilt and then some anger and frustration with the home. Investigate the circumstances, but you must understand that there may be times when she will be soiled or wet.

Falls

Falls happen for a number of reasons, some preventable and some not. Some of these reasons are

- malnourishment or dehydration
- osteoporosis
- arthritis
- cognitive impairment
- general weakness
- a problem with balance or gait
- dizziness when going from sitting to standing
- medication problems
- large or small strokes (TIAs) or seizures
- illness
- improperly fitting shoes
- being pushed or abused
- visual impairment
- equipment that is inappropriate or in poor condition
- variations or changes in flooring
- placement of furniture or equipment
- unsecured carpets or floor mats.

If your mother is falling, find out why. This may entail the staff's keeping a record of when and how she falls, which will illustrate a pattern and may help to find a means to prevent it. It can also pinpoint a staff member if it is a case of individual abuse.

Have a physical therapist do an assessment, even if you have to hire one from outside. Try to find one who is knowledgeable about geriatrics. Once she assesses the problem, she may be able to develop a strategy to prevent or lessen the incidents occurring. If your mother is getting some rehabilitation or strength training to improve walking and prevent falls, make sure that strength training is included for her upper body as well.

Sometimes people fall from weakness, because their condition is deteriorating. There is no abuse. There is nothing that could have been done. They may have to start using a cane, walker, or wheelchair. This is another transition, one that people often fight against, especially the wheelchair. That explains why people refuse; it is not about "being stubborn," it is about loss. How it is introduced and the understanding that it is something that someone has to get used to will have a huge impact on acceptance, as well as sense of dignity and self.

Pressure Sores

Pressure sores (bedsores or decubitus ulcers) occur when the skin has been rubbing against something like bedsheets or the seat of a wheelchair for too long without being able to breathe. They also occur from contact with irritating liquids, such as urine. After a while the skin turns white, then red, and eventually breaks down, opens up, and festers. The sore can be so deep that it goes right to the bone. Gangrene can set in, eventually leading to amputation and possibly death. Pressure sores generally should not occur. If they do, a good home with a good nursing staff will catch them early, and under most circumstances can resolve the problem. There are creams, lotions, and medications to help prevent them, and there is equipment such as special mattresses and coverings to protect the skin. Information on the incidence of pressure sores at a facility should be available from inspection reports.

An older person's skin may be fragile and can bruise easily. Problems such as dehydration and poor nutrition can make it even more fragile. Medications such as blood thinners can lead to skin being more easily bruised. A bruise does not necessarily mean that your mother was abused or that the care is bad. If she is in bed or uses a wheelchair or is otherwise stationary for long periods of time, she is at risk unless she is turned or moved regularly. You may want to check her skin frequently. If you find that your mother's skin is bruising easily, speak to the nurse, physician, or dietitian to see if there might be measures you can take to improve it.

Depression

As I mentioned earlier, it has been estimated that the incidence of depression in nursing homes is up to 50 percent. This number is for people who have the number and types of symptoms that make up an *actual* diagnosis of depression according to standards of the American Psychiatric Association's *Diagnostic and Statistical Manual of Mental Disorders* (DSM). The number of people having *some* of the symptoms and behaviors of depression would be much higher.

Dr. William Thomas, the originator of the Eden Alternative philosophy and care model, said he once started putting on death certificates "died of loneliness" and similar causes. After seeing these kinds of deaths, he started talking about the plagues of loneliness, helplessness, and boredom in nursing homes. Yes, there is depression, but often it is because of these three plagues and the loss of purpose and meaning accompanying them. Medication is often the treatment given in nursing homes. The real treatment should be fighting the plagues.

You as a family member can also suffer from these plagues. Fight them with more than medication. If you feel helpless, find other people with whom you can work for change. Exercise, go on vacation, see a therapist, make friends, play bridge again. See chapter 16, "Making a Home Better."

Alcohol, Drugs, and Other Addictions

An often-overlooked issue in seniors housing is addictions—usually to alcohol, sometimes to illegal drugs, and sometimes to prescription drugs. With the arrival of the Internet, addictions to online gambling, games, and sexual material have become a problem as well.

Addiction can "take hold" when an individual is lonely, depressed, or angry or has a lot of free or unstructured time. There is a lot of loneliness and depression in seniors housing, and, despite the presence of activities and recreation workers, there is isolation. Certainly people have unstructured time—time with no obligations, appointments, or things they "have to do." Thus, there is the potential for abuse of alcohol and drugs and for other compulsive behaviors to take hold.

Some residents in assisted living and in nursing homes have an addiction when they come in. Some residents develop an addiction or an alcohol abuse problem while they are there. It is easy for some residents in assisted living, and sometimes for those in nursing homes, to go to the local store and purchase alcohol and then hide it and drink it in their rooms. It is simple to telephone the local store to have it delivered. Often, well-meaning friends (or drinking buddies) will bring alcohol or drugs for a resident. Online addictions are sometimes the easiest to develop, because people do not have to go out or order; it is right there for them. The easier it is to access the focus of addiction, the easier it is to become addicted to something.

A residence may or may not notice that someone has an alcohol or drug problem. You may have to be the one who identifies it. Or the residence may identify it, and you may dismiss it as "not a big deal." It is important to recognize the problem, because alcohol and "recreational" drugs can interact with medication and increase the risk of falls and of behavior that becomes irritating and unacceptable. Their use also can isolate your mother from other residents or lead her to isolate herself.

If you know that your mother has an alcohol or drug abuse problem, check on alcohol and medication administration policies before you choose a residence. Find out if there is a happy hour and, if so, how it is structured. Find out the policy regarding alcohol at meals and, in the case of nursing homes, in rooms. (Assisted living residences usually have fewer guidelines, as residents are supposed to be, and often are, more independent.) Whether you tell the residence or not is tricky. On the one hand, they may choose not to admit her.

On the other hand, if they are going to take care of her, they should know, especially if they are giving her medication. If you do not tell them, their liability may be limited if an incident occurs.

If you do tell the residence, you can discuss the extent of the problem and how it is handled. It may not be an issue once she goes into the residence, and it may be something that the residence has had experience dealing with. You may just tell them that your mother drinks sometimes during the day—that she always has, that you are aware of it, and that it has never caused a problem. Or you can say that she has had a prescription for a certain pain medication and has self-medicated for a long time. Remember, if you do not say something, you may be setting your mother up for failure.

Alcohol or drug abuse may be a signal that your mother is not able to handle loneliness or depression. If you or the residence finds your mother is abusing alcohol, you may have to work with the staff to involve her in activities and review her care or service plan. You may want to bring it up to your mother. You may wish to refer her to a counselor. There are agencies and counselors who focus on addictions among seniors.

Sometimes an older person will admit to drinking too much or using too much medication, or to drinking when she feels sad or lonely. It may not be necessary to identify your mother as an abuser of alcohol; it may be enough to identify that she is trying to cope with something. You can be supportive in helping her find solutions and involve her in staying away from alcohol. She may be able to do it by herself, or she may need some counseling or other support.

If she is not able to recognize a drinking or drug problem or is unable to deal with it because of a cognitive deficit, the residence may have to intervene structurally. They can prohibit alcohol. They can insist that they administer all medications. Sometimes they will end up regularly searching a resident's room (although that brings up privacy and legal issues). Sometimes a doctor can forbid a resident to drink alcohol because of "medical" issues or tell her he is discontinuing a prescription. You may have to contact friends and ask them not to bring alcohol or drugs, or even have certain people banned from visiting in a room. Work with the residence; it is in their best interest to help.

In some cases, if the behavior that is the result of drinking or drug abuse becomes a problem, a facility may have cause to evict someone. You can fight it, but they may have the legal right to do so, especially if you misled them about the issue or withheld information before admission. It is to be hoped that, before this happens, you and they will have been working together. If not, you may want to talk to the local ombudsman or, in Canada, the representative from the health authority.

Other compulsive behaviors, including online gambling, games, and viewing of sexually oriented websites, while not causing the physical risks, are still a concern. This is especially true for younger residents for whom computers and the Internet are already a part of life. For anyone, however, online addictions can pose a threat and can end up costing thousands of dollars. Whereas the Internet can provide a diversion for people who are isolated due to lack of mobility or other restrictions, its online activities can also lead to isolation, depression, and shame. People can give out personal information and be conned into trusting someone online who will take financial advantage of them. If your mother is cognitively impaired and has access to the Internet (and this will be the case for more people over the next few years), she may be at risk. You may not realize this is happening until you see a credit card invoice. As with alcohol or drug use, you and the residence may have to confront your mother, you may have to put some kind of controls on the computer, put a limit on a credit card, or even remove a computer. If you suspect some kind of Internet fraud or abuse, tell the residence and then the police.

Roommates

I don't know about you, but when I think of the word *roommate*, I think of summer camp, college dormitories, or maybe my first apartment. I do not think of the situation I would like to be in when I am eighty or ninety. Yet more than likely your mother will have to have a roommate at some point if she goes into a nursing home. More often than not, assisted living situations provide one unit to each person, although there are some that also have shared accommodations of some kind.

The good news is that some people like to have a roommate. If they are immobile, if they are lonely, or if they are frightened, it can be comforting to have someone in the room with them. If it is someone with whom they get along, a bond can develop. They can watch out for each other, or one can watch for the other. If one or the other at least has a certain level of awareness, it will cut down the opportunity for abuse or neglect because it is not going to happen so easily while someone else is watching. Roommates may share family visits. The other family and you may help each other monitor the care and condition of each other's relative.

The bad news is that a roommate can be horrendous. If your mother's roommate is cognitively impaired, she may go into your mother's belongings and take them, wear them, or even try to eat them. Certainly she may lose them. She may have different sleeping patterns, she may be incontinent, she may be loud. She may be deaf and turn up the television so loud that your mother can't sleep, or may demand that your mother turn off her television so that she can sleep.

Whichever of the above situations occurs, if your mother has one or more roommates, she will have minimal privacy and no place for intimacy. She will have no place to entertain you and no place to call her own.

You may want to try to be creative in establishing some private space by the way you arrange furniture. Maybe you can bring in a nice room divider, or if there are curtains between the beds, make some nice new curtains yourself. Can you put up shelves or hang things from the ceiling (like a bead curtain)? When I read these suggestions, they almost seem pathetic, but something is better than nothing, and what they do give is meaning to your mother—that you are and have been there for her.

If she can't entertain you in her room, see if there is somewhere else she can be your hostess. Is there a kitchen where she can get or make you coffee or tea? Is there an out-of-the-way corner where she can take you to sit and talk?

Find out what the policy is on switching rooms and roommates if there are problems. If there is a waiting list for a private room, make sure you understand how it is made up and how people move up it.

Is it by need or by date of request or by funds available? Also find out what the home's procedure is for resolving roommate problems. If you are looking at homes, see if you can wait for a single room to become available and enter directly into that.

If your mother is having trouble with her roommate, make sure you hear all sides of the story and look for all the possible reasons for it. Is it to keep you involved? Is she jealous because her roommate's family visits more than you do? Is she jealous that you spend time with the roommate when you are supposed to be visiting her? Is she being a difficult person to get along with? As with any other problem, you must be a detective and keep your mind open.

How your mother accepts her situation is similar to so many other aspects of nursing home care: it is influenced by how you deal with it. If she is upset, acknowledge her feelings. Make sure, however, that you are not projecting your own feelings and upset onto her or encouraging her to feel upset because you are. Stay aware of your own feelings. Guilt can be worse for you if your mother is in a multiple-person room because it may emphasize to you how much she has lost.

In the end, your mother may accept the situation better than you do. Often, older people are good at being stoically accepting, especially if they know that, in time, the situation can change.

Louise

My mother had multi-infarct dementia, the result of frequent small strokes that affected her memory and reasoning abilities. We realized that there was something wrong when she began having memory lapses and time became a problem. During a summer vacation we went on a boat trip one morning, returned to our cabin for lunch, and then set off in the other direction down the lake in the afternoon. Mum remarked that we had gone the other way yesterday. She didn't remember it had been just that morning. We said nothing to Mum but at least, with some humor, we saw the positive when Dad remarked that Mum would have a longer holiday than the rest of us.

We knew we could not change her perception of time. We could easily adapt and, of course, we hoped that this was all that Mum would confuse. It was not. It soon became apparent that she was unable to remember things that had taken place just a few minutes or hours before. When we traveled, she forgot where she was all the time. At the end of a trip, Mum would have no recall of it. However, she loved all kinds of things in the moment.

As time went on, Mum lost more functioning. Her walking became unsteady and she could no longer sign her name. Gradually, she was not able to manage daily tasks that had been part of her repertoire all her life. She needed help with food preparation, bathing, dressing, going to the bathroom, and other things. Someone had to be with her always. At first, my father cared for Mum largely on his own with some help from my sister and me. But we soon found ourselves overwhelmed. We added services like adult day care and home help.

The amount of care Mum required was gradually going beyond our ability to cope. We began talking about a nursing home as opposed to supporting Mum at home. Despite realizing that we were beyond our ability to cope, we gave it the old college try. We set up an elaborate system that involved Dad and homemakers in the day.

My sister and I juggled full-time work, families, and all-nighters with Mum. Sometimes, it was truly exhausting but sometimes it was truly funny as well. We compared notes about how many times we got up each night. It was frequently at fifteen-minute intervals. Mum, of course, had no idea that she had just been in to see us and was perfectly cheerful throughout. It was impossible to be angry with her because she was either happy to see us or as fearful as a young child might be in the night.

When we made the decision to look for care for Mum, she had to be further assessed. That was when we discovered that she had added Alzheimer disease to her multi-infarct dementia. After the assessment was completed, it was clear that Mum needed to be in a locked area of a nursing home because she had no idea where she was and she was wandering outside. As it happened, there was a placement available in the secure unit of the Royal Care Center almost immediately. Had Mum been more alert, she would probably have had to wait as long as two years. The bed's being available was a godsend because we were all getting tired. I don't know how much longer we could have kept on. But it was also hard that we had to make a decision so quickly and live with it. We had no time to prepare ourselves emotionally.

When we come to see Mum, she always knows us and is thrilled with our visits. She searches for my father when he is not there. She constantly asks to come home. We can explain where she is and why and she is accepting in the moment, but then the question is repeated over and over. It is immensely sad not to be able to help Mum when she becomes upset and confused about a situation that she cannot explain and that cannot be explained to her.

Living with Mum's being in a nursing home has probably been the most difficult thing we have had to do as a family. We know that it was the right decision, but having Mum separated from the family unit is hard. Our parents had been married for over fifty-five years. They fully expected that death would part them at some point, but they did not think that something like Alzheimer disease would.

In many ways, Mum's dementia is like death. She is not the person we once knew. But at the same time, aspects of her character and personality continue to shine through. We can't walk off and leave her behind as if she had died, but we don't have her with us anymore either.

Many staff members at Royal Care Center, where Mum lives, have helped us in this difficult situation. They are used to seeing residents and their families learning to live in this new world. However, they don't seem to gloss over the feelings, but take time to listen, to reassure, and to make suggestions that might help.

I cannot say enough for the support of other families at Royal who have shared this journey too. Once a month we attend a support group and in between we often see other relatives on the ward. It is helpful to be with others who are experiencing similar problems. This gives us a variety of solutions or at least ways of tolerating the issue. You begin to see families as whole units with a history that didn't always include Alzheimer disease. Now they are learning to include this disease and their relative in their continued functioning. Somehow, that continuing becomes the focus instead of the disease.

In some ways, my family has been strengthened by what we have been through. We clearly see the love between our parents. As daughters, we have been given the opportunity to be useful and caring to both our parents. Our husbands have demonstrated their respect and commitment to the family they joined through marriage. The grandchildren, who range in age from teens to adults, have not shied away and are much more prepared for helping their own children through tough times as well as us as we age. They have helped both their grandparents at home, have visited Royal Care Center often, and have attended support group meetings. Even the first great-grandchild in this clan has come halfway across the world to be the best hug therapy that Mum (and the rest of us) could have had.

I don't want to minimize the pain that we all feel in this situation. There are times when it is unbelievably sad to see our mother in her separate existence. It is hard when she cannot understand and we cannot make it better. Not to be able to take her home when she asks or, worse, cries is dreadful. However, Alzheimer disease does not mean that we stop being a loving family or that we cannot laugh. It does mean that we have to find new ways to do things together and to support one another.

CHAPTER 13

Communication and Problem Solving

Working the System

Most family members experience a sense of confusion when they are first dealing with a residence. They can be complicated systems, so it will take some time for you to learn how to navigate them. You probably learned to do this with the hospital system or home care system before your mother was admitted. Although there are ways to speed up your "learning curve," it will take time, just as it took you time to learn to be a caregiver or to learn how to maneuver in other systems. There are several reasons for this:

1. Before you can ask a question, you have to figure out what it is you don't know.
2. Even if you have read all the books and literature, you will have individual questions that will arise as you go through the process, and each residence is different.
3. Doing it is different from reading about it.
4. You will have to be involved in the system to learn its gaps.

Until you have figured out the system, you may experience a good deal of frustration with both it and yourself. Be prepared for needing the time to learn. Try to be patient with yourself and remind yourself that it takes time.

As mentioned earlier, it is helpful to sit down with the staff before admission to talk about expectations, both yours and theirs. This may be especially important when dealing with assisted living, where often staffing any services are limited. Make sure your expectations can be met, and at the price level you are paying. However, it may not be until your mother is actually living in a residence that you realize you had some expectations and they are not being met. You may expect the physician to call you or come in when she hasn't. You may expect the home will be using the same kind of incontinence pads that you did. You may expect them to provide shampoo and soap, and so on. Some of these issues can be discussed at a care conference. You can also discuss them with the director of nursing, the social worker, or the nurse on the floor.

Communication

I remember when I was on the staff at a nursing home and admitted a particular woman with a hearing difficulty. After a couple of days, the daughter told me that her mother had two hearing aids, and they weren't being put on. Her mother, ninety-six and forgetful, was unable to do it for herself. First I had to find the hearing aids, which her mother had misplaced. Then I went to one of the nurse's aides and asked her what happened. She said the woman dressed herself and didn't need help in the morning. I explained that she did. I wrote it down in the communication book and told the nurse. The next day, the woman still wasn't wearing her hearing aids. I went back to the nurse's aides. A different nurse was on duty that day. This happened on three days before the information got into the system where all staff working with the woman knew her care needs, abilities, and habits. Two weeks later I again saw the woman without her hearing aids. I asked a third nurse's aide where they were. She told me that the woman must have forgotten them and that she dressed herself. This aide hadn't worked with this resident before. I just had to keep working and tracking this until the information became part of the system.

Communication in a complicated system is difficult. You need to learn how to make your communication effective so that the system works for you. You may tell a nurse that your mother hates orange juice, and three weeks later she is still getting orange juice in the dining room. After you have said it five times, you may feel like tearing your hair out. Most likely you will feel like tearing out someone else's hair.

Monitor care and services especially closely in the first few weeks after admission. This can be particularly important in assisted living, where there may be fewer staff members and where there is a greater onus on the resident or the family to be able to direct care for themselves. There is a lot for the staff to learn about a new resident. This is the time when you are passing the torch to the staff. You may want to make sure that they have grasped it firmly before you let go. Don't let yourself feel bad if you feel like you are "checking up" on the staff. In a good residence, that isn't what you are doing. What you are doing is tracking the system. (If the residence is not so good, checking up is exactly what you are doing, and you will have to continue to do it carefully as long as your mother is there.) There will always be gaps in a system's functioning. That is often where problems occur.

There are tricks to make information flow more easily. The first is to ask the staff how they make sure information is communicated through the system. For example: "How do I make sure my mother is signed up for a bus trip?" "How do I make sure the staff knows my mother just got a hearing aid?" "What do you do to make sure the aide knows my mother has a new treatment for her dry skin?" Different residences have different systems. You need to learn what works in the residence where your mother is. When you want the staff to have some information, write it down. Keep a copy for yourself and date it so that you have some notes to refer to. If it is information that affects more than one department, such as nursing and dietary, give a copy of the note to each department. You may also want to give a copy to the director of the department. Let them know that you are doing all this simply because you know it is easy for information to be lost.

Even after you have written down what you want the staff to know, don't assume that what you wish to happen is going to get done. Track things for a few days and follow it through a few shifts. In the dining room, for example, check to see that the weekend and weekday staff members have received your concerns and followed through on them. In one assisted living facility I have a client in, I told the staff that she now has a new foot cream. When I saw her a week later, I made sure to look at the tube. It was clear that they had not been using it every day.

When you are giving information, make sure you give it to someone who is there on a regular basis, not a casual staff member or someone from an agency. Ask the person to write it down in the communication book. This is a book for the staff that documents information about residents' changes or needs. They may or may not go into the resident's chart. It is kind of like a documentation of highlights of what happened on a shift, similar to an overview or snapshot.

If your concern needs an active response, don't wait for the staff person to call you back. Let the person know that you will visit again or call her back, then wait a few days and do so. If she hasn't gotten the answer, tell her you will call back in a few days. If you keep calling back, it puts you at the top of the list.

There is a good time and a bad time to talk to the staff. Bad times tend to be at change of shifts. This is when people are going home and trying to finish up their day. They usually are trying to communicate to the next shift staff what has happened during the day. You will not get their full attention. (On the other hand, it might be a good time to schedule a brief meeting—maximum five minutes—if you do so in advance. That gives you the advantage of being able to talk to two shifts at once. The key is to make it brief and focused on information. It is not a time to problem solve.)

It is also not a good time just before, during, or just after meals. These tend to be labor-intensive times when the staff are focused on helping residents into or out of the dining room, dispensing medications, or helping people to eat. Other labor-intensive times are when residents are being made ready for the day: nurse's aides are toileting, dressing, washing, grooming, and so on.

Ask the staff when a good time to talk to them is. Usually they want to help. If you communicate when you have people's attention, there is a better chance that what you say will go into the system.

Be clear about who is to be the spokesperson in your family. If there is a spouse and three children, it is not reasonable to expect that the residence will send everybody notices of conferences or call everybody when your mother has a fall. I remember a frustrated daughter calling me to complain because the family had not gotten notices of conferences or meetings. When we investigated, we found they had originally told us that the mother was aware enough to be given notices directly. She had not been passing on information to her daughter. When we discovered this, we started sending notices to both the resident and her daughter.

If there is some conflict in your family about how decisions are to be made, see if you can work that out, or at least let the home know, so that they are not contacting one person and asking for a decision or giving information, only to face a backlash from other family members because they weren't included. If one person, usually a son or daughter, lives out of town, try to keep that person in the information loop.

Gaps in the System

Communication problems also exist and occur between systems, for example, between a nursing home and a hospital or the assisted living facility. People are often transferred between various systems, and their medical or psychosocial information does not always come with them. They can wind up taking new medications, having medications stopped, or having newly identified medical problems, without these things "following" them beyond the point at which they were identified. I once worked with a resident who was transferred from hospital to a nursing home. It took us three days to find out she was diabetic, because the hospital had not included that on the transfer documentation. A facility cannot be held responsible for information it was not given. Therefore, it is up to you or your mother to be alert enough to make sure that all of the information is transferred between systems, especially if your mother goes from a residence to hospital and back again, or if she is discharged to a residence directly from a hospital. You may want to consider a care conference after discharge from the hospital, even if your mother is going back to a residence where she was already living.

When Things Go Missing

It is amazing what goes missing in a nursing home! Beyond valuables, people lose glasses, toothbrushes, dentures, and telephones.

Sometimes things are stolen. Sometimes a staff member will accidentally break something and be afraid of the family reaction, so he will clean it up and not say anything. Sometimes possessions are misplaced. Sometimes the resident will throw them out. It is common for a confused person to take out dentures, wrap them in toilet paper, and throw them in the toilet or into the garbage—or drop them into an unfinished bowl of soup, which then is collected and thrown down the sink by the dishwasher, who doesn't notice something at the bottom of the bowl. It is also common for a confused resident to walk into someone else's room and put in that person's dentures, sit in his chair, or sleep in his bed.

It is true that things are stolen. That is why you want to have a list of the possessions and clothes that you brought in, and you want them clearly marked. But don't jump to the conclusion that something was stolen. Investigate. Learn the lost-and-found policy of the home. Search for things that are missing. Ask the staff if they have seen it somewhere else or with another resident. Go look in the laundry.

Your Role

As I indicated earlier, the most important aspect of your role as a family member is to provide your mother with the love and attention that make her feel valued and important as an individual. No one else can do that the way family and friends can. It is your history, trust, acceptance, and intimacy that make your relationship irreplaceable. You are the only one who can "anchor" her—give her a sense of her place, history, and importance: in short, an identity.

Sometimes family members describe themselves as advocates. I prefer to think of them as partners, because the word "advocate" can take on an adversarial tone. You want to work with the staff, not against them. Even when you do not like what is going on, I think that when you are changing things for the better, you are still being a partner in care. The result may be conflict, but the goal is the partnership and supporting the staff to do their jobs as they should be done.

As a partner in your mother's care, you need to continually monitor how the residence is affecting her. Continually does not necessarily mean frequently. Your trust level in the residence will affect how vigilant you are, as will your mother's ability to take care of herself and her willingness to speak her mind. If she is receiving minimal help in an assisted living residence, it will be less, if she is cognitively impaired, it will be more. If she is the kind of person who will not speak up, then you may not have to monitor the residence, you may have to probe with her. Is your mother getting back her laundry? Was she missed when the podiatrist came to see the other residents? Is she signing herself up/being signed up for outings on the bus or dinners out with the supper club? Has she had falls or bruises? Is there a subtle change in her behavior? Does she need all the medications she is getting? How is she eating and drinking? Is she participating?

Being the family member of someone in a residence, especially a nursing home, puts you in a dual role: you are both partner and client. This is not often discussed, but can make things difficult. For example, you are going through your own reactions and feelings about her being in care, and yet the staff may call you because your mother is anxious and want you to help settle her. It can be hard to manage both at the same time.

Remember that systems and people change. What was working at one time may stop if there is a new nurse or nurse's aide who wasn't privy to the conversations you had with the one who was there for the two years previously. A new administrator or director of care can change whole systems. With so many different staff members providing care over the course of a week or month, they may not have the consistency to pick up on the things you would. Casual staff members especially will be less aware because they are on site less frequently.

Keep things in perspective when you notice that something hasn't been done—if toenails haven't been cut, they can be next week. If you cannot take this stance, you will never sleep. You will feel that you are continually at war with the home and will never be satisfied. You need to trust that the major issues and most of the care is being done properly. As I said, if you can't, then think about finding a place where you can.

On the other hand, there are many homes where you will have to be constantly on top of things, where the care does not meet high standards, and where some of the staff, the management, or the corporation is either incompetent or uncaring. Then your role can go from a partner to a police officer.

If your mother is in a home where you have to be more police officer than partner, you will need to learn how to do this effectively so that you don't burn out. (Reread the section on abuse in chapter 5, see below on "Making Complaints" and "Throwing Bouquets," and see chapter 16, "Making Homes Better.") Here are a few things to remember:

- Pay attention to your feelings and what you sense. If you think something is wrong and the answer is unsatisfactory, keep looking.
- It is your right to read the chart. Do so if you are suspicious.
- Rely on outside experts if you must—pharmacists, physical therapists, and specialists in gerontology.
- Not all the staff will be incompetent or uncaring. Search for the ones you can trust; rely on them, and ally yourself with them.
- Visit at varying times during the day and at care times so that you can develop a total picture of what is happening and how care is done by different staff members.
- When you find the staff members who are competent, see if there is any way you can make sure they are providing care to your mother, or at least are in the same unit or area as your mother.
- Build bonds with other family members and work together to monitor care.
- Talk to residents whom you feel are competent and able to stand up for themselves and listen to what they have to say.

Making Complaints

After your mother has moved into the residence, you may find yourself criticizing how care or service are given or continually feeling that they are not up to standards. Sometimes you will be accurate in your criticisms, sometimes maybe not.

As I mentioned above, during the first phase of the time in which your mother is in the home, it is important that you keep focused on your feelings and what you are going through. This is especially important with regard to complaints or problems.

I recently was referred a man whose mother was placed in one of the city's best nursing homes. She had been transferred there because, ultimately, the man had burned out the first home with his anger and hostility. He was rapidly doing the same in the new home. He was a big man who yelled at the staff, intimidating them. Underneath his anger was his grief about his mother's decline and his guilt that he was unable to help, along with his anger that he had had to look after his mother since he was about fifteen years old. He was unaware and unable to acknowledge any of these underlying issues, so he had no idea that he had a problem or that he was being inappropriate. Despite several meetings and different approaches, he was unable to understand it.

When you have a complaint, take a minute to look inside yourself and ask what else is going on for you. Often people find that their anger or distress about an occurrence in the home is really tied to feelings of guilt or sadness about their mother's being in a residence. It can be less painful to criticize someone than to accept your own feelings. Have the courage to ask yourself if your criticisms or concerns are really about the care or if they are the result of your trouble accepting or even acknowledging some of your feelings. Sometimes it is both. Solve the problem, but don't let the system or staff become the whipping post for your guilt. It is easy to let this happen, but it is not fair to the staff nor, in the end, to yourself.

You may need to be able to talk about your criticisms with someone. If there is a social worker, that is her job; if not, it is often the director of care's responsibility. You might also talk to a caring nurse, recreation director, or pastoral counselor. Verbalizing your criticisms to someone can help you take another look at them and see them differently. It doesn't mean that you are a bad person because you are critical. Nor does it mean that the care is not good care because you are critical. It may be that you are right about the care or the incident, but the way you have approached trying to solve a problem is inappropriate because of your feelings about the situation. When you can separate the two, you will find that it is easier for you to communicate, and you become a better partner in your mother's care because you are more able to listen.

If you have a complaint, make sure that you have gathered all of the information and you know exactly what the problem is. If it is something your mother has complained about, remember that you are getting only one side of the story. Try to find out from the staff, preferably more than one staff member, what they know about the incident or issue. It can look a lot different when you have all the information. For instance, you might think that the recreation staff is not bringing your mother to baking. When you talk to them, you may find that she wanders away before the activity is over. But because you have come in at the end of the activity, you think that she has never been.

Sometimes people feel confused about what they can "legitimately" complain about. I had a client once whose mother was in a nursing home. They had told him he was not allowed to stay with her while she was in the dining room because it would upset the other residents. In fact, they did this because they considered him a "difficult" family member. He was confused about this policy, but it sounded somewhat reasonable to him. As in this man's case, you may be told that something is policy, or that it can't be done, or that "we don't have the staff." You may be intimidated at first by such a response. If it sounds reasonable to you, or if you are feeling already burned out, you may let it go. You don't have to.

If you are unsure about what is "legitimate" to complain about, know your legal rights. In the United States, that means knowing what the federal Nursing Home Reform Law says are your rights, and what a facility can and cannot do. The law says that a nursing home must provide care that a resident needs to reach the highest practicable level of functioning. It also specifies under what conditions therapy can and cannot be terminated, under what circumstances a resident can be discharged and when they cannot, and other issues. Unfortunately, there are no similar requirements for assisted living at a national level, although individual states, as mentioned, do have regulations. For more information, see the National Senior Citizens

Law Center's "Twenty Common Nursing Home Problems—and How to Avoid Them" (available on their Web site at www.nsclc.org).

Canada unfortunately does not have a similar law, even at the provincial levels. However, there are standards of care and regulations protecting residents of nursing homes and, according to the province, varying degrees of protection in assisted living. You can speak with someone at your local Health Authority if you have questions about what a nursing home or assisted living residence must provide and can or cannot do. The effectiveness of the Health Authorities and their willingness to be involved varies from province to province.

I want to warn you that sometimes family members become labeled as difficult, as in the situation with the two sons in the example earlier, for different reasons. This is why it is important that you be able to

- look inside yourself and see where your anger or disappointment is coming from
- understand that care is not one on one and will not be as you did it at home
- understand what is realistic
- understand the disease, and the system

When problems are honestly about care, services, and standards, then you need to put aside your concerns about how you might be labeled or whether the staff like you or not. You will have to keep firmly in mind that your number one priority is your mother. This can be hard to do—most of us want to be liked.

Sometimes your mother may honestly have problems with the residence or staff. Yet even though you encourage her to say something to them directly, she may not be willing to do so. Form a good picture of why not. Make sure it isn't because she is intimidated by the staff, has been threatened or abused, or has seen other residents abused.

You may have to teach your mother that it is all right to voice what she wants or doesn't want. One good way of doing this is to have a small meeting with the appropriate staff member and your mother. When you meet together, you can support your mother and model for her that it is all right to say something. If she has the experience of voicing her concerns a couple of times, she may be more willing to do it for herself.

In recent years people have started to use video cameras and other systems through the Internet to monitor their relative's care. Some systems (for example, see www.eldervision.info) allow voice and video interaction, so you and your mother or her caregivers can see and talk to each other. If you do this, remember that it can be an invasion of your mother's privacy. Video monitoring can also cause some resentment from the staff, even those who are doing their work (and who theoretically have nothing to hide). How would you feel about being video monitored throughout your working day?

On the other hand, some homes allow video cameras in residents' rooms because they can protect the staff from false claims of abuse or neglect. Staff people who are confident about the care that they provide may have little objection to being on film and might even welcome the occasion to show that they are doing a good job. I suspect that cameras reduce the incidence of abuse just because people know they are being watched. If you do wish to use a video camera, it may help if you present it in a positive light, saying, for example, "My mother has been complaining and I am worried. I know you have a good staff in a difficult situation with a lot of residents and limited funding, so I would like to use a video camera to help you show that her care is good."

In the end, if something is bothering you or your mother and it is not solved by talking it out with the staff, you may have to gear up for a harder time. Going "higher up" can be intimidating for some people. You may fear that the result will be worse care for your mother. You may feel that you don't have the skills to address the problem. If you are tired from caregiving or are pulled from your work or your home life, you may feel you don't have the time or the energy to take on what needs to be taken on. You may feel confused about where to turn and become more confused by a system that seems unresponsive. The longer the problem goes on and the further you have to go, the more helpless and unsure of yourself you may feel.

I want you to know that you do have what it takes. You can learn to advocate using the same skills you learned to be a caregiver. Talk to other people, find another family member who feels as you do, be part of a support group. Join a group that advocates on behalf of elderly people or the Alzheimer or Parkinson association. Use the Internet to communicate with other caregivers who have done what you have to do. Hire a geriatric care manager (www.caremanager.org) who has the skills and experience to advocate for you. I have often coached people on how to advocate. Do whatever you can to make sure you have the support that you will need so you don't burn out as you take your complaints higher in the system and government. Use your anger and your sense of justice to keep your goals clear and your end in sight. You will find yourself with strength and resolve that you did not know you had.

Keep on forgiving yourself. You did not choose the situation, and you would not have chosen a poor home if you had the option or the knowledge. It is not your fault that problems are occurring. Don't feel guilty about shaking things up if you must. Reread chapter 4 on guilt and do those exercises once again. Remind yourself that the energy you expend on guilt will take away from the energy and purpose you need to obtain the best care possible for your family member.

Your first step beyond the floor staff, social worker, or director of care will be the administrator. Be clear about what the problem is, what you expect, and what you have tried to do. Come up with some possible solutions. When you are making a complaint, present it calmly and rationally. Tell whomever you are talking to that you are angry and frustrated instead of blasting her. Be specific if you can, giving dates, times, and staff involved. If you think you are too angry, practice at home, saying out loud what you want to say. Say it in front of a mirror, and record yourself, so you can hear what you sound like. You may want to write a letter and then put it aside for a day or two and reread it before sending it. The goal is to solve the problem. Set up the conditions under which that can be done.

In the United States every facility must have a formal procedure under which someone can make a complaint. There should be a staff person designated to hear complaints. The home must respond to your complaints within a reasonable length of time.

If the home is owned by a chain or larger company, find out whom you can talk to in that company. Let the administrator know that you will be doing that. You may also be able to become a shareholder in the company. This will permit you to attend the annual general meeting. If all the families in the home and many in other homes become shareholders, this can have an impact on the company.

If, after going through the home's formal complaint procedure, you feel that you have not received an adequate response or that the issue is still not being dealt with, seek out the health department; licensing agency, or area agency on aging, or, in the United States, the state ombudsperson for aging issues or adult protective services. The ombudsperson will help you negotiate with the system. This office also reports to the licensing office. You have the right to go to those people or agencies. You can find them through the Eldercare Locator (800-677-1116) or online at www.eldercare.gov/eldercare.net/public/home.aspx. They will have the most up-to-date names, addresses, and telephone numbers. In Canada, problems with assisted living may be dealt with through a different system than the nursing home system. Call your local Health Authority to find out who is responsible.

If the situation is one that you feel constitutes abuse, you can go to the police or adult protective services or other agency that is responsible for seniors. The police may tell you that this is not an appropriate issue for them; however, abuse may constitute assault, and that is certainly a matter for the police. Better that you should go to them when you are concerned about assault than when you have to report a death from abuse or neglect.

You can also go to the local media, picket the residence, or talk with a lawyer. These may be necessary, but they do carry consequences. If you are going one of these routes, take one more look inside to try to ask yourself how much is attributable to your own feelings or other issues. You owe that to yourself and the residence. Ask other family members or go to the nursing home's family council to learn what they think. Listen carefully to the ones who disagree with you, because they are giving you information that you might not want to hear, and this makes it more valuable. Remember, you can destroy people's lives if you go after them by mistake.

If you do go outside of the residence to address your grievance, make sure you have documented everything that has happened concerning the issue and the efforts you have made in trying to solve it within the home.

Throwing Bouquets

Working in a nursing home is physically and emotionally draining for several reasons. Staff members become attached to residents and families; at a death they experience grief. Having few staff members to provide care means they often work overtime, often unpaid. It also means that sometimes they are not able to provide care as they would like or as they should, and they know it but cannot do anything about it. They often do not get breaks because of emergencies and paperwork requirements. Lifting residents in and out of bed, on and off the toilet, and so on, is tiring and can easily lead to back and other injuries. The staff receives the brunt of the family's emotional turmoil in the form of anger and criticism. The pay is minimal.

Nurse's aides, laundry assistants, and dietary aides are often seen by residents (and sometimes family members) as servants. They are often treated that way. If they are of a different racial or ethnic background, they are often the recipient of covert or overt racism and prejudice.

I know some residents and families have had awful experiences. I know that some staff members of nursing homes have no business being in a position of responsibility anywhere near another human being. But there are many, many dedicated and caring people out there. Many of the staff people in the worst homes would desperately like to give better care. It is agony for them to see what is going on and to be part of it. It is wrenching for them to have to make decisions based on limited staffing and lack of support. It goes against their sense of humanity and against their professional integrity and code of ethics. There are many who are intimidated by their employers but who need a job. These people are as caught in the system as you and your mother are. Find them, and help them to be the staff they want to be and the caregivers you want.

Remember to throw some bouquets. Treat all staff people as professionals or as experts in their field. See if there is some area or action for which you can give them some respect. A simple "thank you" is extremely rewarding. It means that you have noticed what the staff are doing for your mother. It can give them the energy and impetus to keep on making an effort to provide good care despite the trying conditions of their work. Ask after their families or activities. Get to know them as people. When you notice someone doing something positive, go up to her right away and reinforce that with a "thank you" or by saying, "I admire the way you handled that." This will increase the likelihood of the behavior happening again.

If I can make a completely unscientific statement with no research to back it up, I would say that, from what I have seen, the ratio of complaints to bouquets is about twenty to one. This may be because of genuine problems with care and funding, but think how you would react if, for every time your boss told you "good job," he made twenty complaints. If you are already feeling stressed and overwhelmed in your work, this does not make for good incentive.

Write a note to the staff and send a copy to the administrator. You don't have to wait for a significant event or for Christmas—just a note to say that the efforts are appreciated can go a long way with the staff. Send flowers or a fruit basket to a nursing station. You may not realize it, but often the complimentary notes are posted at the station or in a staff room. Send chocolate—staff like chocolate. Well, anyway, *I* like chocolate. Send me some.

It is appreciated if you ask if you can do anything to make it easier for the staff to help care for your mother or someone else. It may be something simple like including another resident in your visit. Usually it is appreciated if you help feed your mother if she needs assistance. The simple fact that you asked shows the staff that you care about them.

Remember, you are in a relationship with the staff, too. In some ways the relationship is separate from the one they have with your mother, but if it is a positive one, it can beneficially influence the relationship they have with her. Relationships are two-way streets. Care about the people you want to care about you and your mother, if you can.

Alvin (part 1)

When my husband, Alvin, became depressed over the murder of his son, over losing his vision, and other tragedies in a short period of time, he was placed in a convalescent home and given an antipsychotic drug that was not monitored. The effects of the drug, combined with his Parkinson disease, left him "frozen" stiff eighteen hours of each day for a month, winding up a virtual vegetable. To save his life, a G-tube was inserted to feed him and he was sent to another convalescent home as a full-care resident. He was unable to move, push a call button, scratch his nose, or turn on the TV. All he could do was talk, and he was so brain damaged from the drug that he often didn't know anyone or anything. I was told there was nothing they could do for him except keep him calm and as comfortable as possible. Because they also discovered inoperable lung cancer, no one, including the doctors, expected him to live six months.

I realized that if my husband was going to be anything more than a vegetable, it was up to me to find the solution. Thanks to our faith in God, and my insisting to the doctors that he have certain treatments, and surreptitiously sneaking some to him on a daily basis, there was a remarkable difference. Even the doctors and staff could not believe it. Gone was the depression; Alvin began recognizing people and talking, singing, whistling, playing his harmonica, telling jokes, beating the others at trivia—he became his old, happy self. It took several months, but it was worth being a bulldog. At the same time, he was off his Parkinson medication with no symptoms and his lung cancer started shrinking.

I became known as "the doctor" (they didn't want to call me what they really thought), but I did gain a reputation for being persistent and loving, not only to Alvin but also to the staff as long as they did a reasonable job. That was the problem: most of them wanted to do their jobs but they were so overwhelmed by the workload that it was impossible. Because I was nipping at their heels when I arrived in the afternoons or weekends, Alvin got better care, but still it was appalling much of the time. I found if I backed off, they did take advantage, so I didn't dare; however, I also made sure I helped whenever they needed it. Alvin and I entertained often, and I tried to be a "nice" person, if a bit dogmatic.

Alvin was musical, and we were fortunate to be in a facility that had many retired professionals performing for the residents. I had to insist that they get him up and out to activities. Because he was also blind at this point, it was all he had to look forward to. He enjoyed every minute, singing, whistling, smiling, and participating in all activities, and he made everyone else happy as well.

I was fortunate to have good health, which held up in spite of long hours and hard work after my daytime job and forty-mile commute to the home. I found that checking on Alvin en route to work at 5:00 a.m. and coming in unexpectedly caused panic, as well it should have. The staff's neglect almost caused Alvin's death several times and did cause numerous hospitalizations. I wanted to transfer him, but because of the entertainment and the convenience, I put this off. Also, it would have meant moving him out of town, as there was no other facility in this town that I wanted him in.

After a CNA taught me how to lift Alvin, I started to take him everywhere I could. Using a portable wheelchair that folded up like a stroller and with just a little help from Alvin, we would sing "Hold Me" and he would grab me around the neck while I lifted him into and out of places. We were able to again be a part of things on the outside. Had I not learned to help him and insist that he go out, he would have been left to vegetate in the facility.

During the next two years the facility became a "House of Horrors." We had life-and-death incidents constantly, primarily due to lack of staffing. The last year of his life included:

1. A tube feeder that never lay down flat, a large hiatal hernia, and a lot of congestion. Had I not taken off work that day, he would have drowned in his own vomit. As it was, he ended up in a hospital due to aspiration pneumonia and internal bleeding.

2. I checked him every night, but one morning I came in to find that his scrotum was totally burned, looking like a piece of raw meat. He had been fine the night before but had been allowed to sit in his feces for hours. He was on Vicodin for the pain for a week. You don't just visit your loved one; you'd better do body checks regularly.

3. My life was threatened at one point and, in the presence of Alvin, I was threatened with not being able to visit him if I visited anyone else in the facility. Not only was my life threatened, I was told it took only a minute to put a pillow over my helpless husband's face. Because of these threats, I had to watch a resident literally die of starvation and malnutrition across the hall without being able to do anything except report it.

I began the process of trying to move Alvin. I felt it was no longer safe. Even though the nurses and nurse's aides liked me (except for those few who were causing the problems), the power people felt I was a threat to them, as I knew and saw too much. So when I asked that he be transferred, the blackballing began. I learned that you do not request a transfer; you go to the facility where you want to move, make the arrangements, and let them send for the records. The old facility will still try to make the care seem much more than it is, but you have a better chance.

At this point, again due to lack of care, Alvin became very ill, but the facility refused to transfer him in spite of high temperatures for days, congestion, brown urine, etc. I finally had to insist they put him in my car (unhealed broken femur and all) and I took him to the hospital, where the hospital staff had some unmentionable things to say about a facility that would allow a car transfer and not know a person was so desperately ill. Alvin was hospitalized with tubes suctioning his lungs for ten days. When they felt he was stable enough to transfer, we could not find a bed within a fifteen-mile radius, thanks to the blackballing by the House of Horrors. I even visited facilities, taking his medication list and care list.

We were fortunate to have someone on staff on our side and were able to get the director of care of the best facility in the area to come to see him to see why he couldn't be placed. She couldn't believe it, stating he was such a sweet person and his care was no more than many others. So we got him into our first choice and the best facility in the area.

Alvin spent seven wonderful weeks in the new facility before he joined the angels. We were so thrilled finally to be where it did not stink, did not look like the typical facility (even had lounge chairs in the rooms and only two beds per room instead of three). It made us realize there are still some great facilities out there, even if you're on Medicare and Medicaid. But you have to look hard to find them.

The two main things I learned from my husband's time in care facilities are that you'd better visit regularly, if not daily at least a couple times a week, and at irregular hours, and do a body check or have someone do it for you whom you can trust. Pressure sores quickly get away from you and are killers. You must stick up for your loved one; there's no one else to do it. There are great places out there, but you have to be willing sometimes to go the extra miles to see that the person is happy and comfortable. Alvin told me shortly before he died that he couldn't believe he'd had such a nice day. He finally felt safe, cared for, and loved, and I was able to relax for the first time in three years. We felt we'd finally gone from Hell to Heaven, right here on earth.

CHAPTER 14

Visiting

How often to visit, what to do when you are visiting, how long to stay, and how to leave are important issues that may trouble you. They certainly bear some discussion as you try to balance your needs and those of your wife.

Visiting in an assisted living facility can be a different experience from visiting in a nursing home. Assisted living often feels more homelike; residents may have their own units that feel like small apartments. Compare this to a nursing home, where a resident may not even have their own room, let alone a place that feels like their own private home. Also, residents in assisted living may look and be healthier and more able. Things in assisted living can seem more "normal."

Some people do not want to visit a relative in a nursing home. For them, it is too upsetting to see "all those people in wheelchairs." Or it is upsetting to see their relative in her present condition. Sometimes friends are frightened; the thought in their minds is that "this is where I could end up pretty soon." You can move beyond those feelings if you are willing to confront them. They do subside. This is another situation in which you may wish to seek some professional help. If you avoid visiting, the guilt from doing so can be overwhelming. After the death of your relative, you could feel intense regret that will stay with you for a long time.

Just as in every other aspect of care, there is no one right way to do your visiting. Your situation, relationship, needs, and time schedule are different from those of the daughter of the lady whose room is next to your wife's. Unfortunately, your wife might not take those differences into account when she tells you that Mrs. Smith's daughter is here every day (implying, therefore, "Where the heck are you?").

Your tendency in the beginning may be to do what you think your wife needs; at some point, you will have to figure out what your limits are. If you don't, you might as well have kept her at home. What is it that you honestly feel you can and want to manage? Write down your limits. It can help you stick to them. It is kind of like writing a care plan for yourself. If you trust the home enough not to have to do surprise visits to monitor care, tell the staff how often you will be visiting. That way, they can tell your wife, when she starts to worry, that you will be in soon.

Remember that at the end of the adjustment phase—both yours and your wife's—the goal is for her to be integrated into the residence. So when you think about visiting issues, remember to ask yourself the question, is this going to help or interfere with her adjustment to the home?

How Often to Visit

It is fine to visit the home every day for the first couple of weeks or so, up to a month. There is a psychological assurance for both or all of you in that kind of pattern. It also helps you begin to see how the home works on a day-to-day basis and to know the staff. Because it is also the time when the staff is getting to know your wife, they may have questions for you, or they may be missing some part of her care that you wish to review with them.

It is good to vary the time of your visits so that you see different staff members and different routines, and so that your wife doesn't become dependent on "this is the time when he comes to see me." The more she depends on you for reassurance, social interaction, and so on, the less reason and willingness she may have to integrate herself into the home. Remember, you are fostering adjustment—for both of you.

You might also find that a shorter visit, done more often, is better for both of you than coming for a whole afternoon. Just dropping in for half an hour can be meaningful. If there are several family members, set up a schedule so that you are coming on different days. This will help you avoid burnout.

Sometimes shortly after admission, the staff may recommend that you stay away for a week or even longer. Usually when they do this, it is because your visiting is interfering with your wife's settling in. It is a little like when you leave a child at school or camp for the first time. Without you there to hang onto, she will get used to it more easily. The difference, of course, is that your wife is not a child. If you think you can trust the home, and they recommend this to you, you may wish to consider it.

There can be less agitation when families don't visit frequently in the beginning. I have seen many people who were calm throughout most of the day end up being upset after a relative's visit. It seems to bring up their feelings of being abandoned and alone and reminds them of their home. Their reaction can also be a bit of a manipulation so that you feel guilty or so that you change your mind. Is it better to visit and have your wife be agitated and upset when you leave, or is it better to stay away for a while? I think it varies with the individual and situation. Generally, however, I think it is better to come and pay the price of the agitation when you are leaving. You will have to discuss the situation with the staff, then try it and see.

Before you decide to stay away for a week, do some in-depth problem solving with the staff to see if there is anything else going on that is causing the agitation, or if there are any other ways of dealing with it. If you do decide to stay away, see if a friend can come to visit in your place. Often, a friend's visit will not stimulate anxiety the way a family member's visit does.

Generally, most professional people recommend that after two weeks to a month, you stop coming every day. This is done to protect you from burnout. It also says clearly to you—and you might not want to hear this—that you need a life outside of your relative in the facility. If you are unable or unwilling to do this, at least give yourself permission to take a day or two off every now and then, at least once a week. If you don't, you can burn out.

The first time that you skip a day may be hard; you may have to make yourself do it. It will be easier if you plan something to do rather than sit around at home and wonder how your wife is doing. Visit friends or other family members. Fix the roof or clean the house; do some of the things that you have put off doing. This is another situation in which a friend could visit in your place. A "no visitor" day could be a second step.

Some family members do come every day. Depending on the home, you may feel that it is the only way you can monitor for abuse or neglect. Or maybe visiting every day is how you want to express your commitment to your wife. Just because she is in a home does not mean that she cannot provide you with love, affection, and companionship. You might enjoy coming in and just sitting and reading or watching television with her. Even in a good residence, you might want to help her eat dinner or walk. Your marriage does not have to be over because she is in a home. You need to do what is best for you in your situation. The trick is figuring out what is best as opposed to what you want. Sometimes the two are different. Take some time and ask yourself what you are hanging onto and why. Ask yourself if there is anything you are avoiding because you don't want to face it. If you do visit every day, remember there may come a day when your wife dies. Then you will have a gap in your life. Make sure that you do not give up friends, activities, and interests. You need a balance in your life.

Visiting a resident in a nursing home can be difficult for practical reasons. There is little private space in a nursing home, especially if your wife has a roommate. This is difficult to get used to because close relationships are not lived solely in public. If your wife liked to entertain, in a home she may not have a place to do so, and even if she does, it is not hers. If you think about it, the act of "visiting" is symbolic for both of you of a power difference—she is in an institution and governed by its rules—and of a change in your relationship.

Visiting Someone Who Has Dementia

Even if your wife has advanced dementia and, two minutes after you leave, she phones to ask when you are coming, your visit has been worthwhile. People who have dementia can experience the moment, and they may be living only in the moment. If your wife is nonverbal, she may understand a whole lot more than she is able to respond to. Speech, hearing, and comprehension are different functions in the brain. Also, the fifteen minutes you spend holding her hand is important even if there is nothing said or she is unable to respond.

You might want to leave a guest book in your wife's room and sign it when you and other family members come in. This gives your wife a visible reminder of who has been to visit. If you have worked out a visiting schedule with more than one relative or friend, this lets you know if it is working. You might also want to write down what you did together and to whom, including staff members, you spoke.

If you live out of town, or even if you live in town, sending a letter or postcard is nice because your wife can look at it when you are not there, and the staff can read it to her over and over.

American culture tends to view social interaction as primarily conversation. This idea can make visiting difficult because conversation with persons with dementia is often limited and frustrating. Family members often say they don't know what to do when they are visiting.

Your visiting may be more satisfying if it is activity based. Activity can be something as simple as holding hands while watching television or listening to music. Do a simple woodworking project together. I sometimes walk up and down a hall with a client holding hands and singing songs with her, and, believe me, you do not want to hear me singing. But I don't care, my clients enjoy it. You may want to bring in some old photographs and make albums, or review the albums. If the home has a residents' kitchen, maybe you can make some cookies together. See if you can find some games that are within your wife's ability range, such as a simple jigsaw puzzle. Do her nails, or do a craft. See if the home has any activity boxes that they can lend you. Maybe there is a book of old photographs of the city where she grew up. Take old family photographs and make them into videotapes you can play and watch together. Bring in a book of songs and sing together. Sit together in a chair and watch the people go by in the main hallway. See if the kitchen staff will let you set some tables for dinner. Clean the room together. Schedule your visits with other families, so you can all visit together. Remember, there are many ways for people to be together; talking is just one of them.

Going Out and Going Home

Older people living on their own often experience a withdrawal from the larger community due to physical limitations or losing their driver's license. When they move into a residence, especially a care facility, this interaction decreases even more. Everything is there and done for them. Your wife doesn't have to shop, or go to the post office, or out to the doctor; the food is there, the staff will mail her letters, and the doctor may come to the residence. Think about how you would feel if you never, ever, left your house, or got out only one day a week? It's called cabin fever.

Your wife is still a member of the community. Think about ways in which she can continue to be part of it. Maybe bring her to church on Sunday for at least part of the service. If she had a bridge club, see if she can continue to go, or see if the bridge club can meet in the home. You can take her with you when you do your grocery shopping or when you have an appointment with your doctor. Your visits don't have to be in the home; take her out for coffee, lunch, or a walk.

Younger people particularly need to see themselves as part of the larger community. The more connected they are, the more normal they feel. This connection validates their worth and identity as persons, and it counteracts the feeling of uselessness that people with disabilities can experience.

If your wife has dementia and you do take her out, it might be wise to limit the stimulation she will encounter. People with dementia often do not do well in situations with many people, multiple conversations, or a lot of noise (which is why sometimes a well-run dementia unit is a good idea). So even though you want to bring her to a family wedding or dinner or to the club, it might not work out well. Try it and see, but be prepared to bring her back early.

If you are wondering if you should bring your wife back home for a visit, try it after a few weeks. This can be especially important if she was discharged directly from a hospital into a nursing home. She never had a chance to say good-bye to her home, possessions, or pet. See what happens while she is there, and then ask the staff to monitor what happens after she comes back. It is not necessarily a bad thing if she is upset on returning; it is part of the grief. You and she will have to judge whether taking her home is like "picking a scab."

If you do decide to make a clean break rather than the slow transition that visiting your home would entail, wait a significant amount of time, even two to three months, before taking your wife back home. A good guideline indicating that someone has settled is when the person begins to talk about "my room" or being "at home" and means the residence.

Remember, too, that you can bring your wife out for vacations, even if it is just a weekend or overnight. Many hotels and resorts are built so that they are able to accommodate people with disabilities. I have known people who have gone on cruises to Alaska with their families and to Las Vegas with other residents they met in a nursing home and their families. Some have hired a companion to go somewhere. Everyone needs a vacation.

Ending a Visit

Ending a visit can be harder than the visit itself. Your wife might not let you go. She might be angry with you and tell you never to come back. Even if she is not agitated, the look on her face may intensify your guilt. Especially in the beginning, you may feel each time you leave that you are abandoning her, and you may experience a twinge of pain knowing you are going home to an empty house. It will get better, and you both will get used to it. It just takes some time. That is hard to remember when you are in the middle of it, but just take one day at a time.

If your wife has dementia, you might have to experiment with what works and what doesn't. For some people, it is helpful to say, "I have to go to work now," or "I have to go have my hair done/go grocery shopping/go to the doctor's" rather than to say that you are going home. You may just be able to say, "I have to go to the men's room" and she may not remember that you have gone. Sometimes it is helpful to say right at the beginning, "Honey, I can stay for only an hour today," and then remind her after forty-five minutes that you will have to leave soon. If there is a hairdresser, bring her there, and you can leave while her hair is being done. Take her to an activity and sit with her for a while. When she is involved in the activity, you can leave. Maybe you will want to visit just before a meal so you can get her seated in the dining room and then say good-bye. Or ask the staff to take over and distract her for a minute.

Monitor your stress level if visiting and leaving are hard on you. Try to have people in your life with whom you can debrief when you come home, especially at first when you are adjusting to the changes. It can be helpful just to be able to say to someone, "That was a hard visit."

Companions

Family members often hire a paid companion for their relative. There are both advantages and disadvantages to this. The advantage is that a companion gives extra, individual time to your wife. This helps provide the one-on-one relationships that can be lacking in a care facility. It gives added stimulation and encouragement. A companion can help you monitor the care your wife is receiving. Sometimes a companion can help with exercises or other rehabilitation if she is trained and/or monitored by a physical therapist. She may be able to give an extra bath. However, a companion can prevent your wife from integrating into the residence if she doesn't take her to activities or if she prevents her (either intentionally or not) from interacting with other residents. Companions can also create a dysfunctional dependency. Sometimes they do this because they are afraid they will work themselves out of a job. If your wife has a companion before admission, this person should maintain involvement for at least a little while after.

If your wife is able to participate in the decision, ask her if she would like to try a companion. She may want someone to alleviate the boredom. You may have to explain that you will not be visiting any less, that you need a break but you will still be coming, or whatever is true for you and reassures her. You can also discuss it as an experiment: "Let's see if you enjoy having someone else come to visit."

If you do decide to hire a companion, the decision can be part of the overall care or service plan. Consult with the staff or have a care conference to discuss the goals and objectives of the companion. What do you expect the person to do? What would the staff recommend in terms of hours per day or week and time of day? Find out what the rules of the residence are concerning companions. Rules can include signing in and signing out, not taking work from union personnel, and issues of insurance and liability. Although the home will not supervise the companion, someone, perhaps the nurse on the floor, the social worker, or a recreation worker, should be able to give you feedback on how the relationship is functioning. The home will also have a good idea of the pay scale for a companion in your area.

You can hire a companion privately or through an agency. I would not generally use a staff member from the home, even if the person has some extra time. It is a conflict of interest for the staff member and seriously divides her loyalty to you. If you want to hire a private companion, ask other family members whom they use or ask the home if there is someone whom they would recommend. Some people have success through notices in community newspapers. Or you might see if there is a local school that trains nurse's aides or LPNs and ask if they can recommend someone. If you hire privately, look into your responsibilities concerning paying taxes and benefits. Screen the person carefully, ask for a police check, and call references. If the person says she has worked for someone else in this capacity previously, call the home where this other client lived as well as the family who was involved.

If you hire a companion through an agency, the agency will take care of screening, payment, and insurance. Agencies do not always make the best choice of whom they send—if they don't have someone who meets what you need, they may try to send someone whom they think might work. That is why you should interview the person beforehand—to see if you think the fit will be good. The agency may charge you for the time because they may have to pay the person to come to an interview. Ask the agency about the companion's training. Make sure the agency will send the same person consistently, not a different person each time. You should meet with the companion or call the agency supervisor regularly, at least once a month.

Whether you hire privately or through an agency, follow specific procedures. Have the companion sign in and sign out of the residence. You might want the person to keep a notebook in your wife's room of what she has done each period. There may be a staff member in the home who is willing to countersign the companion's sign-in book in your wife's room. Specify to the companion (and the agency) what you want the companion to do and the job description, and write it down. Make sure that the companion is helping your wife take advantage of activities and that she is assisting your wife to adjust to and integrate with the community. You may want to start by having the companion be there when you are visiting. This helps your wife become accustomed to her and can teach the companion some of the ways in which you interact with your wife.

A Few More Words about Sex

Just because your wife is in a residence does not mean that you have to stop having sex. It can just make things more challenging. There is also no reason for you to stop holding hands, cuddling, or having your arms around each other. Younger and/or disabled people can also still have sex, but they may have to learn to work with or around their disability. A physical therapist can be extremely helpful in this area, as can your local organization for people with disabilities. Your wife may also need to know that you still want to have sex with her.

If you wife has her own room, you can lie down on the bed together and watch television. You can cuddle up and listen to music. You can make love, and you can nap together. A good facility will try to accommodate you in that way. If they are unable to because there is a roommate, then allow yourself to have as much intimacy as you wish within what is available. To have more, you may have to go home. You can also go to a motel or a nice resort that is equipped for people with disabilities. Many people do this, although they may not talk about it. Some higher-end residences have guest suites that are available to family members.

If you are using your wife's room for sex or other intimacy, tell the staff that when you are visiting you want some privacy. Sometimes they use a passkey and enter a room with only a cursory knock, or simply knock on a door and enter. This happens because often a resident is unable to respond or cannot hear (or because the staff member is rude or in a hurry). Emphasize to the staff that when the door is closed, they are to knock. Put a "Do Not Disturb" sign on the door.

Jane

My father cared for my mother in their apartment for several years. During these years, Mom traveled down that terrible path we all hope and pray won't happen to a loved one. Even now, writing this is so painful, tears stream down my face as I recall the heartache and the decisions we had to make.

As the only child and a nurse, I think I expected more of myself than I ever expected of client families. I've worked in the long-term care setting for over twenty years. Distressed, loving families were people I saw on a daily basis. My heart went out to them as I tried to ease their guilt and anxiety. All the objectivity is gone when you have to deal with your own situation.

My father, dear stubborn man that he was, decided that he and Mom would be better off in the country. Against all advice, he bought a house in a small town an hour's drive from any medical services. Of course, it wasn't long before it was clear that without family and friends they were alone and isolated. My father's workload as a caregiver increased dramatically with no support.

Many frantic trips followed, and I admit I was resentful at having a six-hour return trip to see them. By this time, I had been suddenly widowed and was feeling ticked off at everyone, especially at my father for having taken Mom so far away when she needed a lot of care.

The decision to move Mom to a care facility wasn't difficult to make when Dad became ill. It became obvious to him that her physical care needs far exceeded his ability to cope. After my mother had another operation for cancer, my father agreed that I should make immediate arrangements to have Mom placed in a nursing home. Unfortunately, this was all happening so quickly that I chose the first facility that would accept Mom. The plan was that I would view other facilities, and Dad and I would eventually decide what facility we wanted to become her "home."

Mom died only a month after we brought her back to the city. That month was one of the most difficult periods of my life. Thankfully, Mom and I had often talked about her wishes and she had made her feelings clear to me: when the quality of her life was bad and only going to get worse, she did not want any active treatment that would only prolong an existence that she would hate.

The night Mom died, I stayed late at the home. I worried that she might not survive the night. With the nurse's assurance that she would call if there was a change, I went home. To this day it bothers me that I was not there when Mom died. My mother was in a coma and, rationally, I know she wasn't aware of my presence, but in my heart, I wanted to be with her when she died.

The whole process of placing your loved one in a care facility is heartbreaking. If I can offer any advice, it would be try to get into the "system" as early as possible in your parent's illness. Call the local health department. Get a case worker and search out for yourself where you feel your parent would be most comfortable. Never be intimidated by the caregivers or the administration. Interview and inspect. Do remember that no matter how high the standard of care, it can never replace one's own home.

If your finances permit, it is wonderful to employ a "companion." Staff people are busy, and it is often the small, personal things they don't have time to do that make such a difference in the quality of life. I think this goes a long way to easing the guilt that all children feel. If a companion isn't possible, arrange with other members of the family to form a team, to visit and spend loving, quality time with your family member. Don't be afraid to call on them. In the end, they will be glad they helped and participated in caring for grandma or grandfather. It gives them a great foundation and enriches their lives. Sometimes they just need a good nudge—but do it.

The most difficult decision you might have to make is if you want to be present when your parent dies. This is a personal decision. Some children can't be there at the end and that is the only way they can handle it. If you can, for your own peace of mind after it is over, I would urge you to be there, physically touching your parent. I remember a daughter who lived in her mother's room for days. She used to lie in the bed, holding her mother close to her. Her mother died in her arms. The spiritual connection was so strong. It was an experience that I've never forgotten, and I often wish that I could have had this experience with my mother.

No matter what you do, you will feel guilt. Don't beat yourself up when it is over. Remember the love and good times. Know that you've handled one of the hardest situations you will ever face in the best way you could at the time. Take heart and courage knowing that parents' love is unconditional and if the circumstances had permitted, they would have supported your decisions with love and understanding.

CHAPTER 15

Out-of-Town Caregivers

If you are an out-of-town caregiver, you face some unique practical and emotional challenges. This can be true even when there is a family member living in the same town as your parent. Basically, the problem is that you can't see your parent's situation or their residence for yourself. The information you receive is secondhand. You have to put a lot of trust in the person or system giving you the information.

Developing trust is more difficult for long-distance caregivers. Generally, trust increases with information and experiences, and through relationships. It decreases in a void. Fear and mistrust, on the other hand, grow in a void because we fill in the gaps with our own thoughts and fears. What we make up is often much worse than the reality. You will be especially prone to fill in the voids with worry and worst-case scenarios because the process of care is so emotional and because of the frightening stories that we hear. (And maybe because of some of what you read in this book.)

It seems to me that degree of caregiver guilt increases with distance from the care receiver. (Doesn't that seem almost mathematical? Wow, I even impress myself sometimes. Anyway, to continue here . . .) Be prepared for this. It may show up in added worry because you can't drop by the home to find out what is going on. You may end up being overly critical of an in-town caregiver, of the home, and/or of the staff. You need to accept the fact that you live where you live; don't beat yourself up because of it.

You can make your situation easier, however. To begin with, be sure that you understand the long-term care system in the area where your brother lives. Try to know all the rules about nursing homes, placement, and funding. If something sounds funny or you are told that something can't be done, find out why and if there are any exceptions. It is harder for out-of-town caregivers to make decisions since they cannot be right in the area.

Long-distance caregivers do not have the opportunity to do a thorough preadmission process of visits and interviews or postadmission monitoring. This means you need to be especially diligent about checking out homes and selecting one or two that you feel you can trust. You can do this by looking at inspection reports or talking to local Alzheimer or caregivers organizations. For residences that you are considering, do a phone interview with a marketing person and then a care staff member, such as the director of nursing or social work. See if you can talk by phone to a family member of a resident at that home. You may want to hire a geriatric care manager to help with this process (see the section on care managers later in this chapter). There are also companies that claim to help people make decisions. Be wary about them. They sometimes receive payment from a residence for anyone they refer who is admitted. They also may not have a complete list of what is available in your area or may not suggest a place that does not provide them with an incentive.

After you have selected a residence, find someone who lives in the same vicinity as your brother who could be your representative while your brother is there. This may be a relative or a family friend. Just make sure it is someone who knows you both. The person should understand your values and be able to make decisions based on them. Let the residence know that this person is the primary contact and is authorized by you to make decisions, monitor care, and so on. Make clear, however, which decisions they are *not* authorized to make if there are some.

If you are able to spend a week or two visiting after admission, try to get to know some other family members and the family council. Ask them to keep an eye on your brother. Give them your phone number and take theirs. The more you feel you know the community of the home, the safer you will feel. If you have hired a geriatric care manager, you can keep them engaged.

Arrange to call the facility every week for an update, until you feel comfortable. You may have to search to find a staff member with whom you feel comfortable and whom you trust to be honest with you. It may be the music therapist, it may be a nurse, it may be a dietitian.

Long-distance caregivers need to be clear with the residence about their expectations. What information do you want, and how often do you want it? To what do you want the home to pay attention? You might want to make a list of things to ask about. Some would address your brother's specific care requirements and illnesses, but others would be about other concerns. For example, you could ask about

- changes in, and reactions to, medications
- whether he participates in recreation activities, and specifically which ones
- participation in bus outings
- how he is eating
- whether he has had visitors
- falls
- mood
- any newly identified concerns you or the staff may have
- changes and updates to care plans / individual service plans.

Try to put a phone in your brother's room. If that is not possible, see if the staff can arrange that he talk to you once a week. Try to visit at least once if not twice a year, and set up care conferences in advance. Make sure you have at least one conversation a year with your brother's doctor. If you are not able to attend a care conference, make sure the home is having one annually and ask for the results. Learn about his medications. I have had care conferences in which the out-of-town caregiver is linked in by telephone so he can listen in and participate to some extent. Maybe the home can do a video conference.

Use the Internet to stay in touch with your brother. If your brother has a computer, make sure he can take it with him. If he doesn't have one, most assisted living residences have them available. Set up your computer with a webcam and see if you your brother can have one in his room, so that you can see each other while you talk. Even if he cannot work it, someone else may be able to work it for him, even if you have to hire a companion or someone just for that. Find out how the residence handles residents' e-mail communications.

One practical reason for ongoing communication is that you may recognize a change in your brother's condition before the staff does. They are with your brother every day. From a distance it is sometimes easier to notice changes that occur so slowly that they are evident only at intervals.

Out-of-town caregivers especially might wish to employ a companion. This is further insurance that there is someone who reports directly to you and does not have any kind of obligation to the home. The person doesn't have to be a spy but can be your eyes and ears.

If there is a primary caregiver in the city where your brother lives, you need to have some trust in her and what she does. Clarify between you what your roles and responsibilities are, and the limits to those responsibilities, and in what areas you will make joint decisions. This may take some time to work out. Even if you had a working relationship before admission, it may help to review it. Circumstances have changed. It is not fair for the primary in-town caregiver to have the burden of the tasks but not the permission to make decisions that arise from them. Make sure you do not take out on her your guilt for being far away. While it is all right to discuss major decisions, if you are going to second guess her all the time, then you need to develop another decision-making process. This doesn't mean that you shouldn't keep informed; you should. But do it in a way that supports that person. When you talk about decisions she has made, ask if she is feeling that you disapprove or are critical. Even though that may be the farthest thing from your mind, remember that she is under stress. She may perceive what you say much differently from what you meant.

One of the best ways you can be supportive to your brother is to be supportive to his primary caregiver. This can be as simple as phoning her weekly to ask how things are going. Spend some time listening to her and what she is going through. This will help her feel she is not all alone. If you are willing to do more, ask her what you could do.

Maybe come stay with your brother for a week or two, or, if you can afford it, hire someone to come in to give the caregiver a break.

It is particularly helpful to the primary caregiver if you can be there when your brother has to move into the home. Stay for a week after the admission, to support her as she (and you) go through the initial phase of adjustment.

I spoke earlier in this book about family roles and conflicts. These can come into play in relationships you have with the residence and especially when you are a long-distance caregiver. You may not want the person who lives in town to be making decisions. You may not feel that her choices are in the best interest of your brother. Again, you need to be aware of what is going on for you. Is it jealousy? Old anger? Money? If you still do not feel that the person in town is making the best decisions and you have to intervene, you may have to have a conference with the facility to let them know what your concerns are and why. You may have to take some legal action, or at least have some mediation with the other caregiver.

It may or may not be a good idea to have your brother come stay with you as a vacation after he is admitted to a residence. If your brother has dementia, it could be confusing and upsetting to be in a strange place. It will take him a while to get used to being with you, and then when he returns to the home, he will have to become used to that routine again. If you do have him visit you, be prepared for what his caregiving needs are. You may be surprised at what it takes on a daily, round-the-clock basis.

If you are thinking about moving your brother to a residence near you, consider several points. A long-distance move is hard physically and emotionally on a frail, older person. He may miss old friends and the familiar climate, landscapes, or daily newspaper. Also, the change may lead to expectations from him that you had not anticipated. He may expect a daily visit; your idea may be different. A move can affect your work and family life. If your relationship with your brother was difficult, old conflicts can arise again. Before making the move, honestly look at all the repercussions: on you, your family, and your brother.

Professional Geriatric Care Managers

In many areas you can hire a private professional geriatric care manager. This is someone who specializes in working with elderly people and their families. (It is what I do.) A geriatric care manager has expertise in arranging and monitoring systems to help people stay at home rather than enter care. If you are out of town, we can act as your professional surrogate. If you are in town, we act as your partner. We know your brother's medical problems and his background. We usually know his finances. We know his values and yours.

We also are involved with people in nursing homes and assisted living. We can help your brother choose a residence, make the move, and follow him while he is there. We monitor the care he is receiving. We will read his chart, go to his care conferences, and make sure he has clean clothes, good food and proper social and recreational opportunities. We will help "interpret" him to the staff. We provide counseling to him if necessary (and to you if you need it). It is often easier for us to be the one working with the residence staff because we are also health care professionals and can relate on an equal footing. We are not intimidated by the jargon or the systems.

To find a geriatric care manager, you can contact the National Association of Professional Geriatric Care Managers at 520-881-8008 or www.caremanager.org. You can also try the phone book. As in hiring anyone, make sure you verify references and experience.

Lloyd

I am an only child. I am fifty years old and have a husband and two teenage sons. Two years ago, my dad, eighty-seven, and mom, eighty-four, were living in another city. I used to visit for two or three days a month. During my time with them, we would be busy doing errands and visiting—generally taking advantage of the fact that I had a car and could help them get around.

Dad started "failing" and having "bad days." We were unaware of the cause. We knew there had been "one or two small strokes," but his declining health was inconsistent and the reasons for his difficulties—what we now know is multi-infarct dementia—were never explained to us. I spoke to the physician several times, but I was never given a clear diagnosis or an indication of what to expect.

What I didn't know at the time was that Mom, the caregiver, was beginning to have some problems with dementia too. She was losing the ability to reason. She could not always be relied on to give me the facts. She couldn't cope with Dad's declining health and was always trying to make him be what he used to be.

Over the next year, my visits became more frequent and lasted longer. By telephone, I arranged for in-home help twice a week to give Mom a couple of hours home alone or time to go shopping. I also arranged for Dad to go to an adult day center. I wondered at the time if I was forcing something that my parents were not ready for, but I am fortunate that they have complete trust in me and did not oppose the steps I took.

I also put Dad's name on a waiting list for a facility. Nine months later, his name came up for a double room. By that time, Dad had lost most of his sight. The small strokes had made him almost totally confused, especially with regard to space. He shuffled slowly. But he could still reason. He was a sad, lost soul.

The facility was within walking distance of their apartment, so Mom could visit. She braced herself and coped well with his move. She enjoyed her walks to see him. Even with him in a home, she could look after herself but not after him. New batteries for his radio, new socks, his desire to have a phone in his room—all were insurmountable hurdles for her.

It didn't take me long to realize that I had to take charge. I remember that moment so clearly. The parents who had for so long been a strength for me now needed my strength. I was now the sole source of emotional support for Mom and Dad. At the same time, my teenage boys were learning to drive. Not good timing!

Against Mom's wishes, I bought a large-number telephone and had it installed in Dad's room. But being blind and confused, he could not always find the phone, let alone the memory button. He pressed other buttons and often erased my number from the phone's memory. Mom couldn't fix the phone. When I telephoned the nursing station, it was clearly explained to me that fixing telephones was not the responsibility of the nurse or the nurse's aides. When Dad's telephone did work, his calls to me tore me apart. He was so confused and knew that Mom was not able to help him.

Soon after that, I got a call from the social worker. She said that it wasn't working out in a double room. Dad was becoming agitated. She recommended a change to another facility.

So I had to shop around for another facility. This time we got one in the city where I live. After a short wait, he was admitted. We were happy with this facility and thought he would be able to stay there.

Then I had to deal with Mom, who was still seventy miles away. She became the major problem. She was unable to understand how the move had come about, even though she had been present for the discussions. She stayed in her apartment, afraid and overwhelmed at the thought of moving. I had Dad phone her every day, I brought her here for visits, and I showed her apartments in our area. But she always went away afraid and unable to make a decision. After a year, we had a call from a neighbor and then one from the physician. She was not coping.

I knew it was time to take over even more. We couldn't let Mom keep saying no to moving. We found her a small, assisted living complex where she was independent but had company and all her meals prepared. This filled the bill. I thought things were going smoothly.

Then, soon after Mom moved, we had a call from the facility where Dad was. He had been declining and needed more care. He was now confused, blind, and totally helpless. They were not licensed to provide additional care at that level. He had to move again. I had to start searching a third time. It did not help that many facilities offered tours only on Thursdays.

It has been just two years since my dad had his original assessment. He is now in his third facility. He still tries incredibly hard to keep the different staff members straight in his mind and to be socially correct. Three times now I have tried to help the staff understand who he was and what he has done in his life. I have tried to touch base with the nurses, the nurse's aides, the social workers, the recreation staff, the physical therapists, and the meal-time aides to tell them about this wonderful man who had such a rich past.

My parents are now, I believe, in situations that are suited to their needs. My sons have learned to drive. My husband continues to be a constant source of support and encouragement. Me, most days I keep my sanity!

CHAPTER 16

Making a
Home Better

Whether your brother is in a good home or one that is not so good, you can try to have an influence on what goes on there. It requires some time and effort. There are actions you can take by yourself or with other families.

Your efforts at change can be aimed at the system itself or at various groups or individuals in the home. Working with the system would mean, for example, targeting the philosophy, the communication patterns, and the policies and procedures. Ideally, work at this level filters down to affect individuals. Working with groups or individuals would mean working with nurse's aides on improving care skills or working with dietary personnel to change serving habits in the dining room. Working with individuals or groups may be extremely effective and, ideally, will filter up, but it may or may not have an impact on how the home functions as a larger system.

When I spoke earlier about good homes, I spoke about good caring, which at the most basic level comes through the quality of relationships that are available and fostered by the home. The groups involved in those relationships include residents, families (including children and pets), staff, administration, and community. When you are working with a family council or on your own, and whether you are working with the structure of the system or with individuals or groups, try to answer this question: What can I/we do to build relationships among all of these parties?

Include the Resident in the Change

I know this will sound silly, or like a given, but I want to remind you to involve the residents in making changes. It is their home. Their viewpoints should guide you. Cognitively aware residents, and especially younger residents, are valuable resources. Use their skills. Involvement in change helps give them a sense of ownership and of being needed and useful. It allows them to be leaders and in control of themselves. Encourage them to take control of seeking change. They are your allies, and, more important, you are their ally.

As I have tried to point out throughout this book, sometimes family members' needs are different from those of residents. What the residents see may differ from what you see; what they want may differ from what you want. If you don't know what they want or see, do a survey or help them do one. Think of yourself as supporting what they want in order to make their home better while working to meet the needs of families at the same time. Ask how to allow yourself to be used by residents.

Individual Actions

The easiest solution to making a difference is money, of course. Donations are always welcome. You can make a one-time donation and earmark it for something special or let the residence choose what is needed. They may wish to add it to other funds, such as an education or Christmas fund. If you wish to purchase something, look around and/or ask what kind of equipment is on the wish list of the residents' council, staff, or administration. You can also set up a fund and direct it toward a certain project or department. If you don't trust how the money will be spent, buy the gift yourself and donate it. You can also start a separate foundation or society that would act as a fundraising arm for the residence. These are effective when you wish to try to raise large sums or have large fundraising events.

Many nursing homes and some assisted living residences also usually need volunteers. If there is no volunteer coordinator, talk to the head of recreation. Maybe when you visit you can come in half an hour early or stay half an hour late and use that time to do something as a volunteer. Or maybe you can make one of your weekly visits a group visit in which you run an activity—it can be something as easy as reading or playing your guitar to two or three residents or playing cards with your mother and one other lady. If you take your mother out for ice cream, take another resident. This will also help your mother develop a friendship (although she may be jealous and not want to share you).

If the residents where your mother lives function at a high level, that may give you more opportunities for a wider range of activities, but you may have to organize many of them yourself. This may entail working with the administration to start setting things up. Depending on the activities you do, make sure that you would be covered by the residence's insurance if an accident happened.

You can act as a buddy to family members of new residents. Maybe you can answer phones or give tours. Look around and see what is missing or what you would have liked when your brother first came in. If you have an old computer, bring it in and teach some residents how to use it. Donate an Internet connection. Obtain e-mail addresses for different residents. Set up a webcam and computer so residents can see and talk with their families at home or out of town. Maybe you can bring in plants and make watering them part of the activity that you do with your mother. A warning: make sure what you are doing is not usually done by someone in a union position. If you start doing union work, that can lead to trouble. For instance, they can file a grievance, and you may have to stop. At any rate, it can create ill will between you and the staff.

If you have a pet or grandchildren, bring them in and share them with the residents. Children and pets provide some of the best stimulation possible. Warmth, caring, and love hold on and can be felt to the end, when everything else is gone. It is remarkable to witness the joy on a resident's face when she sees and holds a small baby. Seeing the same ones regularly will help residents develop a relationship with them. Just ten minutes can make a difference. Even cognitively impaired residents may be able to hold a child correctly and be able to talk to him.

Working with Other Families

Sometimes the most effective changes occur when you work with other families as a group. You can start with just one other family if you have to. This can also help you develop a sense of what is an individual problem that you have versus what is a systemic problem. If something is bothering you but no one else feels the way you do, this could indicate that it is your problem, not the residence's. If a number of other families have experienced the same difficulty, this is information that you can take to the administration and present as a problem to which the home needs to pay attention. If the administration resists making changes, you can offer to do a more systematic collection of the data. When you have information about when the problem occurs, who else is involved, and what else is occurring, this becomes a powerful and irrefutable tool for instigating change.

Many nursing homes have formalized family input through a family council. In the United States, a nursing home must provide meeting space for a family council. A family council is a group of family members and friends of residents whose focus is improving the quality of life at the home. They should be organized or at least run by family members and be legitimized by the administration. A family council is not a forum for a witch hunt, nor is it a forum to take revenge. When a family council is first formed, families often use it to "get" an individual staff member. If it is used that way, it will accomplish nothing and will cause increased friction and mistrust between staff and families. On the other hand, if the staff sees that the family council is working with them, they will come to view it as a valuable tool. Care can improve.

There is no mandate as of this writing for family councils in assisted living residences. You can start one, but you will have to negotiate with the administration for its existence. They are important in assisted living because these residences are often less regulated than nursing homes. Because of the sometimes higher functioning level of residents, you may find that other family members do not want to be so involved. You also have to be careful that the activities of your family council are consistent with the needs and wishes of the residents because often they are able to speak for themselves. You might want to consider holding occasional joint meetings with the residents' council, or even seeing if there is a way family members could be integrated into the residents' council, perhaps as nonvoting members.

Family councils can do incredible things—raise money, run activities, put on welcome teas for new residents and new families, problem solve, mediate between individuals and the home, set up libraries with books, films, and videos, start a day care or an after-school program for the staff's children, and bring in outside resources such as speakers. They can bring warmth and hope to families, staff, and residents.

In most nursing homes there is a huge need for education and upgrading. A family council can be instrumental in funding education and upgrading programs for the staff. Or they can fund a consultant who comes in and works with the staff on the floor to help them develop their skills. There is often either overt or covert illiteracy among the staff. A family council can fund literacy programs, or the members can help teach reading and writing.

The family council can be an effective forum for going to the state ombudsperson or state or provincial licensing agency for care facilities. If you are noticing neglect or abuse in the home, and it is not being addressed by the administration, use the family council's strength in numbers to begin to look for help outside the home. The council can do an informal (or formal) gathering of data on the problem to present to the state agencies.

A family council can help implement an ethics committee, or, conversely, an ethics committee could be a precursor to a family council. Ethics committees in health care started in hospitals to deal with issues such as the allocation of resources, which research to fund or allow, and when to allow a patient to die. However, in a nursing home they can be expanded to help decide a much broader range of issues. How do you decide whom to move if roommates are having difficulty? How do you decide when a home is no longer appropriate for a resident? When is a family member becoming unreasonable? When are the home's regulations becoming too onerous? When staff members and families sit down together to look at these questions from an ethical viewpoint, it helps shift them from a source of contention to a source for learning, so it takes away the power struggle. An ethics committee gives you the opportunity to develop some understanding of how other groups in the system think and what they view as important. It helps you see each other as people and work together.

The decisions made by ethics committees are complicated, and it may take some training time to get one off the ground. During the training time, you are building some trust among committee members—family and staff—and developing a common framework for viewing problems. This will help the committee to function effectively.

If the residence is a nonprofit organization, you may want to try to get a seat on the board of directors. Maybe the family council could be granted an official seat, or maybe the council or you and a group of families want to run a slate of candidates. I have seen families basically do a takeover of the running of a home by taking over the board of directors. Unfortunately, the two times I have seen this, the quality of the home deteriorated because the families were so destructive in the way they did things. One home has since been through fifteen top management people in ten years; this says something about the board that is running it.

Working with the System

ORGANIZATIONAL CHANGE

If you start working to change the system, you will be working with the administration, staff, and possibly unions. They all can be extremely wary of working with family groups and of where family-led initiatives will lead. They are often afraid that groups of family members will come together only to criticize the home, personnel, or care. This is especially true of the nursing staff, who usually end up receiving the brunt of complaints because they provide the primary care and because they are the largest department. Remember, the staff is one of the family council's client groups. If you do not have their support, they can sabotage what you are trying to do.

Staff members and groups will have to accept the changes you want. This may entail going to staff or department meetings. Explain what you are doing and ask them if they wish to have input. You can also let them know what is in it for them. If all they see is more work, they will not support what you are proposing.

Anyone working for change in an organization needs to be aware of the culture and history of the organization. This includes developing an understanding of the corporation or society that may own the home. When you understand this, you understand how the organization works and why. If you understand the organizational culture and history, it helps you understand the reasons for what people do. It will enable you to see the personnel as real people who often are as unhappy with the system as you may be. This understanding helps them feel validated and accepted. It sets up the conditions for positive change.

Another question you need to ask is, how will the changes affect the company's bottom line? This is just a reality that you have to accept—if you are involved in a for-profit system, then profits have to be a variable you consider. Sometimes the answer can be as simple as the change will increase staff satisfaction, which can lead to increased efficiency. If you can demonstrate that it will help or not add to costs significantly, the administration will be more receptive to change.

Start your efforts for change positively by finding what is right with a home. Building on the positive can help set the stage for working on the other parts. What do you see people doing that is positive? Under what circumstances are they doing it? How can you increase these circumstances so that the positive actions occur more often? For example, when is a nurse able to spend time with a resident to just listen to what is on his or her mind? Why at that time? What needs to shift so that those conditions can be replicated at other times? What can you and other families or resources do to help make that shift possible?

POLICY CHANGES

When something troubling has happened, you can look at it in two ways. One is that it is an individual issue between you and your mother and the residence. But you can also consider whether it indicates that something bigger is wrong and that what might be needed is change in policy.

An eighty-eight-year-old woman with advanced dementia I work with was recently taken to the hospital at ten at night. Her nursing home called me, but I was out, so they left a message. They did not call the second- or third-listed contacts, both of whom were family members, to let them know. So this poor woman went to the emergency room with no one who was familiar to her. I can be faulted for not having the proper system for backup, true. When I spoke about it with the director of care, she said it was their policy to call only one person on a call list, and that person is responsible for contacting others. I told her I thought that made sense sometimes, but not in an emergency or an unusual circumstance. I checked with the directors of care in other nursing homes for whom I have a high regard, and they all said that, more or less, this is a common policy. A nurse might call a second person, but it is not required. I told the director of care at the home where my client is that I thought they need to change their policy.

Sometimes you can work individually with someone in charge to effect policy change. It may mean sitting down with the person and talking it through. You may have to ask the person to talk to other family members. You may want to bring something up through the family council. Working for policy change might mean working with several departments or working your way up so that you are talking with an administrator or someone at a corporate level.

At some point, the need for policy change is more complicated. It signals the need for what we might call "structural change," change in how the organization functions as an entity. Then you are looking at vision.

VISION FOR CHANGE

It is helpful to have an overall vision of what you would like to see happen. Work with the staff and administration to develop a common vision. In some ways, the vision is like the enacting of the philosophy of care. It is like saying, "If all of our values were functioning, what would be happening here?" The vision needs to be able to be stated in a concrete and specific way. Perhaps the question you could ask is, "What can we do to make this a place where people would want to come to live?" You might not achieve your ideal, but it is a good starting point.

Be creative. What would you like to see happening? Children in day care? Pets and plants? After-school programs? What can you do with the rooms and the hallways?

What can be done to make the facility a home? What is life in our own home really like? What can be done to replicate that life in the residence? When people come into a nursing home, they give up many of their responsibilities and tasks. Everything is done for them. Sometimes people want to give them up—I can't tell you how many women have told me they are sick to death of cooking and have no desire to make another bed in their life. Sometimes, though, people don't want to give them up or find that they feel useless and have nothing to do. Having responsibilities and tasks gives structure, meaning, and normality to life. Figure out which tasks the residents can do. Can they help in the kitchen, the laundry, the office? The residence may have to make some shifts in job descriptions and insurance when residents start assisting the staff. For instance, a housekeeper may help a resident to wash his sink, rather than washing it herself. Changing job descriptions may involve unions and negotiating, so be realistic and be aware that it will take some time. This is why staff need to understand how it will benefit them, and you need their input and "buy-in." You may start in one section of the home or on one floor.

Think of the residence as what it could be beyond a nursing home or assisted living facility. The latter especially often have rooms and an atmosphere that outside groups would find attractive. Could it be a community center, a shelter, or an art gallery? Can the dining room become a small café for the community? Is there a yoga teacher who is looking for a space to teach a class? A night school looking for space? See if the American (or Canadian) Legion will hold a meeting or chapter there. Is there a church group looking for a meeting space? Bring the community to the residence, because so often the residents' access to the community is limited. They don't have to participate; often they like to watch activity. That in itself can be stimulating.

Essentially, vision and changes are about the model of care that an organization uses. I talked about this somewhat when I discussed good care and good caring. For more on inspirational models of what a residence can be, read *Life Worth Living: How Someone You Love Can Still Enjoy Life in a Nursing Home—The Eden Alternative in Action,* by William Thomas (www.edenalt.org. In Canada there is also www.edencan .com). There is also the Pioneer Network (www.pioneernetwork.net), whose Web site says: "We recognize the need to create ways of living and working together different from the traditional models. The Pioneer Network supports models where elders live in open, diverse, caring communities. Pioneers are working for deep system change by both evolutionary and revolutionary means, using Pioneer values and principles as the foundation for change."

Your vision for a nursing home might be to try to move it from a medical model to a social model, along the lines of assisted living. The difference between them sometimes is blurred, but it really is about a change of attitude and approach. One nursing home I know gave up the concept of therapeutic diets. They still made sure residents who had diabetes were taken care of, as were other residents with special needs, but they gave up the *concept* and just talked about nutritious, home-cooked food. (I can hear the dietitians screaming at me right now. This is not meant as disrespect or devaluation of your role or profession.) Remember that a model shift really is about history and culture, which is harder to change than rules and regulations.

HOW CHANGE HAPPENS, OR DOESN'T

Once there is a vision that is validated by all parts of the system, you are ready to create the methods to achieve it. Take a look at what it would take from you, the staff, and the administration to make it happen. Does it mean money? Does it mean a time commitment? Look around for other homes that have tried what you would like to do. How did they do it? You may want to consider hiring a consultant to help manage the change.

Remember that for most people and organizations, change doesn't happen overnight. It is a slow process. There are always some staff members in a home who will resist change and who will feel threatened by it. This can be for a number of reasons. They may have a vested interest in keeping things as they are, or they may be lazy. Sometimes they are afraid because they think they don't have the skills or capability to do something different. They may have tried to change things in the past and have been thwarted, threatened, or undermined; now they are so discouraged they don't have the energy to try again. Maybe they are so tired from their work they don't have the energy to try to do more. It will be easier if they see what is in it for them. A home may not want to be exposed. Sometimes the administration doesn't want to spend the money or is afraid of what the costs will be. If there is a union involved, the union can resist the change out of concern for loss of employment.

Sometimes people genuinely can't see how to make the changes or how they will benefit them. If you can find concrete examples, documented evidence, or other homes or residences in your area that are having success, and you can find ways to demonstrate how to make the changes, this may help.

I once proposed a new program for helping residents in a dining room. I worked with the administration and the head of food services, who loved the idea. Then I presented it to the kitchen and serving staff. One guy on the staff convinced all of the others that it would not work. Look for the key people in the organization. They may not be the ones identified by an organizational chart; they are the people of influence, for either good or bad. They are the ones who can galvanize and influence their coworkers, either to go ahead or to resist.

Don't allow yourself to be discouraged or put off! I was recently working in a good home, where the care and the caring were wonderful. It was a beautiful facility, small, homey, clean, and bright. But there were no pets. Well, trying to bring a cat into this place was like trying to buy New Zealand. We had to have a committee to examine how it would affect the staff, how it would affect the residents, who would feed it and clean it. We needed a policy about it, we needed family meetings. Discussion about this cat took months. I was ready to tear my hair out. But we just kept working, went as slowly as the system needed, and kept our eye on the goal. You can also hire an external person, someone who is experienced in organizational development and change. They can be expensive, and you may have to raise the money, but often an outsider is more easily accepted as impartial.

If you need a guide for managing change, explore these questions:

1. What is your vision?
2. What would it look like concretely if it were to happen?
3. What and where are the resources you need to make it happen?
4. Who are the people or groups, inside or out of the home, who need to be involved to make it possible?
5. What are the steps you need to take to make it happen?
6. Where are the potential problems, and who are the people or groups who could derail it from happening? How will you meet those challenges?
7. How will it affect the company's bottom line?
8. Could there be any unintended results because of the change?
9. What do you have to do to make sure the changes become part of the system and are functioning effectively?
10. What will the signs be that the change has occurred and been implemented? What kind of evaluation and follow-up will you do?
11. What will you do to make sure the change is working in the way that you planned it?

When you have answered all of these questions, make a flow chart to document the path you are choosing and the various issues that could take it in different directions—the "if this, then this" part of flow charts.

Good luck! When you feel that you are working positively, it will give you hope, energy, and enthusiasm. When people are working together, it will already start to make a difference.

Working with Government

Often the change people may want cannot be affected at an organizational or corporate level due to resistance or due to external regulations and laws. Or it may be that organizations are not willing to make the changes. Even if you advocate till you are blue in the face, you will get no results. Then something has to happen at a government level. It may be that the government or health authority or licensing policies will need to be tightened up or rewritten. Or it may be that new legislation is called for. This is happening with assisted living.

Most people figure they do not have the time or energy to "fight City Hall." Maybe on your own, it seems like a daunting task. But there are many advocacy groups and organizations, and that is what they are doing—fighting for better care. And they have been successful. On the national U.S. level, there is the NCCNHR (originally the National Citizens Coalition for Nursing Home Reform). There is the AARP and in Canada the CARP. There are state, provincial, and local groups. Contact your local ombudsperson or area agency on aging.

If there is no group around that you can join, you can start one. Once you have organized a group, you can often find some kind of supportive funding or grants from larger groups, churches/religious organizations, or businesses. What you will find is that instead of tiring you, or leading to more exhaustion, being part of an advocacy group can energize you. It helps you to feel that you are doing something and you are not helpless. It can be a legacy and a reason and give you a sense of pride in yourself and your community. It will also help you to develop a support network to aid you in your personal journey.

Groups are often necessary because they can gather statistics that prove that something needs to be changed at a system level. To that end, you might want to align yourself with a university department, such as social work, nursing, or public policy, that may have students or professors who can do some of the research with you.

Remember that advocacy groups don't exist just to harass seniors residences. They can support them by demanding better funding or different options for housing. You can ask for overbearing standards to be relaxed, as well as additional standards to be introduced.

If you don't want to involve yourself in a group, you can raise issues around election times at candidates' meetings. Meet with your state or federal congressional representative or senator. Talk to your provincial health critic or the opposition party health critic and keep them informed of issues. Write letters to newspapers about the care your sister has received. Newspapers love stories that can be centered on one person.

Ann

The move to the nursing home came at a time when Mom's condition precipitated a crisis. She had been forgetting to eat, and her food would be left in the microwave to spoil. My sister was going over there every day to check on her and make sure she was taking her medication. But one day Mom wandered away from her apartment. Only through a miracle was she able to tell the police that her son worked at Divine Providence Hospital and give his name.

The home was just opening, with a dementia wing that had access to a closed-in yard and was secured so the residents could not get out. It was a beautiful new home and tastefully decorated.

The first few months were painful not only for Mom but also for us as a family. It took many months for her to adjust to the home, to begin to make friends, and to join in some of the activities. The guilt, pain, and frustration of not knowing if we were doing the right thing caused differences of opinion and separation within the family. This was probably the hardest time for me, as Mom would ask to come home with me and I knew I could not take her. I dreaded having to say good-bye and explain why she could not come with me. I assured her that I would be back soon.

After almost a year, we finally felt that Mom was adjusting and seemed happy. My sister called and told me Mom went on an outing to Riverside Park and rode the carousel! The home took a picture of her; she was smiling and seemed to be enjoying herself. This was the first time in about four years that we had a feeling of contentment about Mom.

Our period of calm came to a halt when Mom started having falls for no apparent reason. One resulted in our taking her to the hospital for

X-rays. We took her to the doctor to see if there was a medical reason that she was falling. We purchased new shoes that were flat and easier on her feet. We ordered a walker to help steady her. We talked to the owner of the home about the falls and what could be done. She suggested putting a monitor on her at night. This monitor was to ring if she got up, and the staff would go in immediately to assist her.

Shortly thereafter, one of the employees said to us they were not treating Mom well there. We asked what she meant by that and she would not explain—just that they weren't treating the residents very well. We then had several talks with the owner. We explained what we heard and tried to get some answers as to why Mom was all of a sudden falling.

The owner was at first not receptive to our concerns and seemed to think that we were trying to make trouble. She intimidated us by telling us that she had asked a lady to leave the home because her daughters were making trouble. We learned later that other families had had the same threats. At the time, we did not understand that this was a tactic used by nursing homes to keep residents' families from asking too many questions.

When we brought to the owner's attention what the employee had told us, she was defensive and said she did have some employee problems but that she would never allow them to mistreat the residents. She reassured us that Mom was well taken care of. She wanted to know to whom we talked because she had some troublemakers.

Mom continued to fail both physically and mentally. She could not communicate with us, was lethargic, had difficulty eating, and was losing weight. We took her to the doctor again and again. He put her on a high-calorie drink to give her more energy and to supplement her diet. There were numerous visits to the doctor; at one point he thought she might have had a stroke. We talked to the owner again. She reassured us that Mom was doing okay. We did look into other homes at this time and put her on a waiting list for one, but it was a year long and we were concerned about having to move her again, as her dementia would have made the move frightening and devastating.

In November Mom took what we were told was a fall. They said a staff person tried to take her to the bathroom but she did not want to go and pulled away, falling face down to the floor. She was unconscious for five minutes and had severe bruising from the top of her head to her neck. My sister rushed her to the hospital.

We didn't find out what really happened until four months later, when we had a birthday party for Mom. She was like her old self again, smiling and laughing with the family. She was able to talk to us and seemed happy. She said, "Life is good," which was joy to our ears. When we were leaving the party, one of the Nurses made the remark, "Isn't it nice that your Mom is beginning to talk again?" We said that we thought it might be one of the new medicines. The nurse said, "No, that is not it. I would like to talk with you. Please call me at home." This was the beginning of a nightmare for us.

Later that night we called the nurse, who told us the reason Mom was talking was that she was no longer fearful because the two employees who had been abusing her and other residents were gone, and that Mom now felt safe. She went on to tell us that the fall Mom took in November was probably not a fall. She was the nurse on duty. When summoned, she found Mom on her back, knocked out. She also commented to us that the first thing Mom said when she regained consciousness was, "He hurt me," and pointed to the aide who was taking her to the bathroom. The bruising was on Mom's face; the nurse's concern was why she was on her back.

The nurse told us that she reported this incident to the management of the home and to the state department of health. Neither one did anything about it or said anything to the family. The employees, including the nurse herself, were threatened with their jobs if they talked to any of the families. We asked her if she herself had ever seen anyone abuse Mom or any of the other residents. She said she had not, but gave us a list of employees who had either turned the abuse in to the state agency or brought it to the management's attention. All this time we thought that Mom was falling. We thought we had done everything to help her.

After hearing from this nurse, we immediately took Mom out of the home and placed her in a nursing home, where she died three weeks later. We filed criminal charges with the city sheriff's office, which in turn sent it to the attorney general's office. The investigation revealed that records were hidden from the investigators. It turned out that there had been numerous complaints from employees who had witnessed abuse not only to our mother but also to other residents. They started to investigate only when we told them we were going to the media. After the investigation was completed, we initiated a lawsuit against the home and the department of health.

In hindsight, we found out that we trusted a precious life to those whom the investigation revealed were concerned only with making money. We see that we were too trusting and believed that they genuinely cared for elderly people. We learned that you have to trust your own feelings and question any action by caregivers that makes you suspicious. It is our right and obligation to do so. We were not of the mind-set to look for problems, nor did we go there to visit the staff; we went there only to spend time with our mother.

Looking back at this painful time in our lives, we have searched our souls, beat ourselves up, and read everything we could about nursing homes, trying to see what we could have done differently. We will spend the rest of our lives living with, and being haunted by, the guilt and memory of the pain and suffering that Mom went through.

Four years have passed. We are still involved in a lawsuit. Aunt May, my mother's sister, having suffered the knowledge of what happened to Mom, told us, "You have to fight for us old people because we can't." Those words give us the fortitude to keep fighting for justice. We have agreed to tell all, do all, and be all we can to see that elderly people are treated with the respect and love they deserve. We want to make positive use of our experience by advocating for continued improvement in care for elderly people.

CHAPTER 17

Difficult Decisions at the End of Life

Living and Dying

One of the differences between nursing homes and assisted living can result in how people see living in one of these residences as a stage in their life. As I mentioned earlier, assisted living is based on a social model as opposed to a medical model, and it often assumes more independence in ability and offers fewer services. It often provides a more homelike environment, more of an apartment feeling than a room in a hospital. It is easier for residents to see it as a shift in living.

On the other hand, many people feel that admission to a nursing home means they are going somewhere to wait until they die. They believe it is the last stop. Your husband may say, "The only way I am coming out of there is feet first." That may be where his resistance and sadness come from. A frank discussion of what he thinks is going to happen to him, how long he might live, and whether he is scared can be helpful to both of you. This may be an opportunity for you to talk about your feelings of living without each other.

At the same time, it is important to remind your husband and yourself that he is going into the nursing home to live, not to die (unless, in fact, he is in palliative care). While there is a process of loss and grief in the transition to living in a nursing home, the resolution of that grief is that life is going to go on. He needs to remember that, and you need to remember it, too. However painful the change may be at first, your life will go on. In the beginning you may not feel that way, and it may not help you to hear that from me, but we are remarkable beings, and people do adjust.

No matter the setting, be it your own home, a nursing home, assisted living, or other residence, there will come a point when your husband is truly dying and you will lose him in the near future. When a family member is dying, in some ways the death is a part of the relationship, and the relationship too will die. You are going through this together. There is no "right way" to "do death"; there is only what is right for you, for him, and for your relationship.

In our society we don't talk about death easily, or at least not about our own. Perhaps even less do we talk with someone we love about his or her death. We hush it up and close it off. The problem with that approach is that it robs us of the opportunity for a unique, intimate, and meaningful part of a relationship.

My mother died, after two years of fighting breast cancer, when I was twenty. One of the biggest regrets I had was that I had never said, "Thank you. I love you." I was able to forgive myself by letting myself think that she knew how I felt. What I learned from that and since then in my professional life is that the experience of saying good-bye to someone as she is dying is healing for both of you. It can be a moment of incredible love, sharing, and intimacy. It can be a time when you forgive what happened to you and in which you ask forgiveness for what you have done, even the small things. Allowing yourself this opportunity for forgiveness allows you to let go of whatever you are holding onto and what is eating at you. It can give you and the person dying some peace. It can set you free for the rest of your life.

Talking about Death

My experience has generally been that the person who is dying is willing to talk, at least to some extent. People who are dying have told me many things—sometimes they are ready, sometimes they are not; sometimes they are frightened, sometimes they just want to talk about their lives. Sometimes people talk about their sadness at leaving their family or the feeling of being cheated. Sometimes they talk about their worries about what will happen to their wife and children after they are gone. Sometimes they do not want to talk at all. But even when someone doesn't want to talk, sitting with them quietly can communicate an acknowledgment of what is happening and going to happen.

It can be easier for the person who is dying to talk about death than it is for those around him. Often, it is the relatives who are not ready to discuss it. By various means they let it be known to the person who is dying that they don't want to talk. Not mentioning it helps people avoid the pain. You may say that you don't want to upset your husband by talking to him about death, but it may be that you do not want to upset yourself.

So you need to think about, and maybe test out, whether it is you who needs to talk or doesn't want to. Is it your husband who wants to talk or doesn't want to? Are you ready to listen and/or is he ready to listen? Who is avoiding and who is willing?

It can be frightening to talk about death. That doesn't mean we shouldn't do it; it means that we need to face the fear. The fear may be harsher than the conversation itself; not talking about it may take more energy than talking about it. Ask yourself what you are afraid of, or what are you afraid will happen during the conversation. Once you can verbalize this, it may help you realize that you don't have to be frightened. You may want to write down what you want to say, maybe just in outline form, to help you face this.

The way to talk about death is to simply start. It can feel clumsy and awkward, but just start. I have started sometimes by asking people, "Do you know what is happening to you?" Sometimes I ask, "Do you know what your diagnosis is?" or "What have you been thinking about your condition?" Sometimes I ask directly, "Do you think you are dying?" You can also talk about your feelings. You can say, "I am afraid I am going to lose you," or "Can we talk about what is happening to you?" (For more on this, you may want to read *I Don't Know What to Say: How to Help and Support Someone Who Is Dying*, by Robert Buckman, or *What Dying People Want*, by David Kuhl.) You have to feel and grope your way through how to have this conversation.

If you cannot bring yourself to talk with your husband about his death or dying, try speaking with the home's social worker, nurse, or another professional first. They can tell you if they have already discussed it with him. Also, once you begin to talk about your fears and feelings, you may have the strength or courage to approach him.

If you feel that you simply cannot talk about it at all, do some reading about death and do some of your own writing. Keep a journal. Write a letter to yourself, to your husband, or to God. A first step in writing may be to write about what you still have instead of what you are going to lose. You don't even have to write directly about death; it may be easier for you to talk to yourself in metaphors. Write about endings, about how summer turns to fall, then winter, and how leaves fall off a tree. Write about yourself standing on a railway platform, watching the train move away down the tracks; about when you left your child at school on his first day; or about closing up the summer house for the last time. Read what you have written, maybe the next day or a few days later. The writing can be a first step and can prepare you to talk more directly.

When you talk with your husband, tell him about what *you* feel and think, about your fears and sadness. That is how you go through this together. Recently I had a friend who was dying, and I listened to her talk a lot about her illness. I kept having the feeling that something was missing or unbalanced in our conversations. Finally I realized that I wasn't participating. I was listening, but not giving of myself. I started to tell her of my sadness when I thought of not having her around and what a gap there would be in my life. I felt vulnerable and sad when I was telling her, but it put us on the same footing in a way. She was able to help me with my feelings. We felt much closer afterward.

When a loved one is dying is not necessarily the time to "be strong." Doing so may be robbing your husband of the opportunity to be strong for you. He may be able to comfort you, and that can be good for him.

Sometimes people are afraid that if they "break down" they won't recover. That is not true. The ability to let go can make you stronger. If you start to cry, you will stop.

Facing Feelings about Dying and Death

To be the relative of someone who is dying can bring up feelings of helplessness, failure, and guilt. When my mother was ill, it was like watching her slowly slip away and, no matter what I did, there was no way to stop it. You may find yourself asking again if you did all you could or reviewing what happened and thinking, "I should have taken him to the doctor," or "I should have had them give him that medication." You may find yourself angry with your husband for leaving you by yourself or with problems. You may be short-tempered with your children and at work. You may also find yourself angry with the nursing home and the staff, thinking, "They should have done more," or "If only they had sent him to the hospital earlier," or "The doctor should have paid more attention."

These are the same feelings and grief stages you went through when your husband moved into the home. They are all normal. If you ask other people who have lost a husband in a similar situation, many of them will tell you they felt the same thing. Use the strategies you learned about support and writing and sharing to help you through this time.

Unless your husband's condition is a result of abuse and neglect, you need to be aware that probably nothing anyone could have done would have changed things significantly. It is easy to look back and say "I should," with the knowledge that you have gained since that time. The truth is, people die. People are left behind. Underneath the helplessness you feel, you know that.

Decisions about Dying and Death

If your husband has not signed an end-of-life document, and sometimes even if he has, there may come a point when the residence will talk to you about his condition and ask you how you want to proceed with his care. They may tell you that if they take certain actions, his life will be prolonged; if they take another course, it will not be.

There are a number of fairly common circumstances in which these end-of-life decisions arise. Your husband may develop pneumonia, and the home will ask if you want them to treat it with antibiotics or by sending him to the hospital, or just allow nature to take its course. He may go into congestive heart failure. Do you want to let him go, or treat it? He may be diagnosed with some form of cancer for which an operation is possible. Do you want them to operate? He may have symptoms that tell the physician that something is wrong but no clear diagnosis. Do you want them to do some investigative procedures to find out what it is so that they can possibly treat it? If your husband has stopped eating or drinking, do you want a feeding tube inserted?

It is up to you how you handle this, unless the situation is clearly written in your husband's advance directives and those directives are legally binding. What the home and physician are asking you to think about is, "Do you think your husband's present quality of life is such that he would want to go on living?" They are also asking, "If we do this procedure, what quality of life will he have afterward, and is that something he would want or you want for him?"

These are life-and-death decisions, and they are immediate. With one choice, your husband will live longer; the other will allow him to die, probably shortly.

Having to make this kind of decision can be a painful experience. When my father became acutely ill after having a chronic condition for many years, he ended up in the hospital. The staff told us that if they took certain actions, his life might be prolonged for a while, but that he would ultimately die from the condition. One of the hardest things to do was to tell the staff to let him go, even though some of us in my family weren't ready to do so. They were hanging on, but for their sake, not his. My sister, crying, told me, "Peter, I'm not ready to let him go yet." This is another reason for having advance directives and conversations about death with your relative. They give you permission to do something that otherwise would be too painful.

I have known some families who insisted that their mother be taken to the hospital several times and given intensive care even though she was clearly not having any quality of life, was in pain, and did not wish to live any longer. They were not able to let her go. To me that seems a little cruel and selfish. I don't know about you, but I would want someone to act out of love for me, to do what was best for me, not what was best or easiest for them or what would make them feel good. We have to die of something. It was an incredible act of strength and love when my sister agreed to let my father go. Is it better to let your husband die of pneumonia in a few days or weeks, or is it better to let him continue for a year or more, becoming ever more disabled and confused from dementia? Would you want to continue if you were in his situation?

Think about what he would want. What kind of quality of life is he having now and will he have later on? What would he want for you and for the family? When you can answer some of these questions rationally, the decision may come more easily for you. This is a good time to talk to your pastor, priest, imam, or rabbi.

The decision to let your husband die can be one that will provide you and him with the relief that either one or both of you have wanted for a long time. This may be because he is in pain, because he has no quality of life, because he is completely unaware of his surroundings, or because you are exhausted from being a caregiver. Having made the decision can give you some serenity out of acceptance for the outcome, although it might not make his death easier on you.

Because you have wanted the relief, you may feel guilty about making the decision to let him go. Let me assure you that many relatives have a part of themselves that is "hoping" their loved one will die. Many people have seen a relative come close to the point of dying, get well, go downhill, then get better again. This can occur several times. The impact of having to prepare oneself several times is hard; it can lead people to think to themselves, "I wish he would just get it over with." Sometimes people hope a relative will die at a certain time because they have holiday plans and want to go away. I know of one family member who was by her dying mother's bedside for hours during the daytime. When she got home in the evening, she would stomp around her house yelling, "I wish you would die already." All of these are normal and common feelings.

You are not a bad or evil person for wanting an end to a difficult situation. Your feelings are your feelings. It is all right to have them. It just means that you have conflicting feelings—you can love someone and not want him to leave you and at the same time wish that he would die. What you want for your husband and the feelings you have for him can be different from what you want or need for yourself. This is another time when it is good to have a support group or just someone else with whom you feel comfortable enough to share these harder feelings. That person can support the part of you that knows it is okay to feel that way, so you don't get tripped up by the part of you that thinks it's not.

Hospice and Palliative Care

Decisions about feeding tubes, bringing someone to hospital, or instituting other interventions may mark the turning point at which someone will be allowed to start to die. At this point, if you decide to let your husband go, the home will begin to provide what is usually called *palliative care*. Palliative care is an approach to care in which the goal is symptom and pain management, making someone's dying and death as comfortable and pain free as possible. They often say, "from treatment to comfort." Aggressive or experimental treatments will not be used. The focus will be on pain control, comfort care, and quality of life for the dying person. Care will also include a great deal of emotional support for the person who is dying and the family. Sometimes a nursing home has a palliative/hospice care room. Many homes will keep someone while he is receiving palliative care until he dies, sometimes having special hospice workers come to the home. Otherwise, care may entail moving your loved one to a special hospice facility.

The term *hospice care* is sometimes used interchangeably with *palliative care*. Sometimes it is used to mean the setting (for example, a hospice unit). Sometimes hospice is used to mean the program, and palliative care the actual care that is provided through the program.

In many areas of Canada and the United States there are hospice programs or palliative care teams. They generally consist of a physician, nurse, social worker, and clergyperson and may include dietitians, physical therapists, and occupational therapists who are trained in caring for the dying. Their training includes an in-depth knowledge of pain control. Accessing hospice care may have to come via a referral by a physician who says that your husband is within six months of death. In the United States, this can be how you obtain Medicare-subsidized hospice care. If you access this care, you give up the right to choose other "curative" oriented treatments. In most parts of both Canada and the United States the subsidized care will include help with paying for equipment and for medications. They may provide or fund respite care, where someone will take over care-giving for you so you can do some of the other things you need to do in your life. You might also want to access volunteers through the hospice teams.

A nursing home may be licensed to provide Medicare-subsidized hospice/palliative care. If they are not, they still may keep your husband while he is dying, and provide excellent care, but they can't advertise themselves as having hospice programs. They may bring in the palliative care team or provider from outside, through a contract with a provider, or, as in some Canadian provinces, the team may be available through the local Health Authority. You should always ask about use of a palliative care team or program. Find out who provides it and when they can be called in.

Palliative care now is often advocated for people early in the disease process, before they are within six months of death, because of the approach to pain management. So even if your husband is not in his last six months, if he needs pain or symptom management, that is enough to consider palliative care experts, even if you have to pay for them yourself.

If your husband is in assisted living, they may not be able to keep him there while he is dying, depending on staffing levels and the services they are allowed to provide. Depending on the residence, the situation can be akin to someone dying at home; sometimes it can be arranged so that it is a comfortable experience, sometimes not. It may be that, like at home, you will have to hire private companions, a private nurse or other staff person, and rent equipment such as a hospital bed. The assisted living facility may call in the hospice service to provide the care necessary to allow him to die where he is. There may, however, still be an onus on you or your family to be more available than if he were in a nursing home, or to hire caregivers who can be, because assisted living facilities do not generally provide twenty-four-hour care.

Younger People and Death

In some ways, the younger your husband is, the harder the issue of death can be. It can be more difficult to talk about with him or to face it yourself. There are often much greater feelings of anger and much greater feelings about the unfairness of the situation. With an older person, at the very least there may be the comfort of knowing that he has had a long life; with a younger person, it is as though something is being stolen from him and from you. At the same time, your feeling of wanting relief from the strain can be greater because some of the practical issues—issues of payment or of juggling a growing family and career—can be greater, which in turn can give you an even stronger sense of guilt.

The younger a person is, the harder it is to make the decision that you are not going to ask for another operation or to decide to turn off life support (or not to start it). This is why it is especially important that you try to have a discussion with your husband about the possibility of this situation and what to do if it arises. It is also when the advance directives have greater value.

What Occurs during the Dying Process

Most of us know little about what happens when someone is dying. Essentially, dying is a process during which the body's systems shut down. This can happen quickly or more slowly. It can be upsetting to witness some of the processes that occur. Already feeling helpless, we may want to do something that is actually counterproductive and can interfere with a peaceful death.

When someone is dying, his need for food and liquid decreases. Feeding your husband or urging him to drink can interrupt what is a natural occurrence. You can wet his lips with a cloth or swab, or he may benefit from small amounts of water through a syringe. Consult with the staff about this because there may be a risk for choking.

During the dying process, metabolism slows and then stops. The excretory system starts to shut down, so there will be less output. Eventually, the extremities will start to feel cold as the circulatory system shuts down.

Toward the end, you may witness *Cheynes-Stokes breathing*. This is a change in the normal pattern of breathing, consisting of alternations between slow, shallow breaths and stopping breathing, and then repeating. It may look like your husband has died, but then he will start breathing again. The process has to do with changes in the part of the brain controlling respiration. It can appear to be uncomfortable for the dying person, so it can be difficult for you to watch. There may be gurgling sounds due to congestion that are fairly loud. Suctioning is contraindicated and may increase discomfort.

You may also witness what looks like anxiety—pulling at bed coverings, thrashing, or restlessness. This may be fear, or it may also be a result of less oxygen getting to the brain.

It may seem as though your husband begins to withdraw from you or others. He may come into and out of consciousness, or he may just seem distant. You may find that he is delusional or confused about where he is or who you are. At times the confusion is due to pain or medications, but sometimes it happens naturally as death approaches.

At an emotional level, your husband may experience fear, anxiety, or withdrawal. It may be helpful to hold his hand, to talk with him gently, to play some calming music, or to change his position. Ask the staff and/or the palliative care team what you might do to help.

After Death

After someone dies, the nurse on duty has to call a physician or official to have the person declared dead. If you were not present at the death, and you would like to view the body, you will usually have a chance to. Make sure the residence knows that you want to do so. If you want someone to be there with you, ask a friend or a pastor, one of the nurses, a social worker, or another staff member if there is someone to whom you feel close.

After you have stayed with your husband for a period, the home has to call someone to remove his body. You will have to know where you want the body to go. So you will have to know what kind of funeral to have or whether you will have one, where it will be, and all the other complicated and sometimes expensive decisions that have to be made about death. This is why it is a good idea to have made arrangements beforehand—it is upsetting to have to do it when you are in shock or in new grief. As I said earlier, when you are in an emotional state, it is hard to make decisions; it is easier to be influenced or let someone else make the decisions for you.

When your relative has died, if you are paying by the day, the residence may want the person's effects removed as soon as possible. They will want you to move your husband's things from his room that day or the next. In a period of grief, that may seem to you to be selfish and cold. In some ways, it is. However, no matter how much grief the staff may feel at the resident's death, the functioning of the home—the care they provide to residents—is usually based on beds being full close to 99 percent of the time. Without this income, staffing would be lower. If you pay by the month, then the accommodation is "yours" for the month.

One of the homes where I worked made it a habit to send a staff member to the funeral of residents when they died, but many places do not do that. Please do not think that this means that they do not care. It probably means that they do not have the luxury of sending a staff person.

Saying Good-bye to the Home

The death of a relative in a nursing home often means the loss of a number of relationships. As I have mentioned, during the time your husband is in the home, you will come to know the staff, the other family members, and many of the other residents. Even though he has died, these people are still there, and they may have come to mean a lot to you. If you have been in a support group or part of the family council, you have developed a role for yourself in the home. In some ways, these people and groups have become your family. The hallways of the home have become more than just hallways; they have become the pattern of your life.

With your husband gone, you may feel that you have no place in the home anymore. In a sense, that will be true. Just as you took on the role of "the family member," you are going to have let go of that identity. Once again, there will be a gap in your life. The adjustment that you will have to go through is similar to the one you went through when your husband first went into the home. It will be like finding a new life pattern for yourself.

It may take you some time to withdraw emotionally from the home. Partly this will be because it will be hard to let go of some of the relationships. Partly it will be because keeping involved in the home is a way of holding onto your husband. Partly it will be because it is hard to develop a new life pattern and role for yourself. This is why it is important for you to cultivate some activities, friends, and support outside the home even while your husband is there.

Some people do stay involved in the home for a while as a member of the family council or as a volunteer. If you have been a member of a support group, you can go a couple more times to say good-bye and talk about what you are going through now. This will be helpful for you and for the people who have not lost a relative. Some homes have memorial services or allow family members to have memorial services for their relatives in the home.

At some point you may want to do something that signals to you emotionally that you are leaving the home behind. Many people send flowers or a small gift to the staff to thank them for the care they provided. Some people set up a small fund or buy a piece of equipment as a memorial to their relatives. It does not mean that you are letting go of your husband's memory; it means you are allowing yourself to go on with your life.

Donald

My father was admitted to a nursing home in September. He had a diagnosis of Alzheimer disease and had developed something called sun-
downing syndrome. His confusion and agitation became worse at night,
and no one could care for him at home, because his schedule was different from everybody else's. We were afraid he was going to hurt himself
or wander off during the night.

My mother called and toured several facilities, but she finally decided
on the one facility that told her they had a "special Alzheimer unit." In
reality, this turned out to be nothing short of a jail, where mostly old people, but some younger people, were warehoused together in a locked
unit, with the barest of custodial care. At the time, it sounded good, and
we were naive enough to believe that this place did offer "special services" and was a "special" place for people with dementia.

I think that *naive* is the right word. When we look back on it, we ask
ourselves how we could have accepted this, but I guess in a small town
in rural Arkansas there wasn't much choice. We knew how it smelled in
there, we knew that there was only one orderly and one licensed nurse,
but they were the experts. My mother was eighty-one, my brother had
no idea about care for an elderly person, and I was living far away with
a young family.

Within a month after Dad went to the home, little things were happening: Dad would have a bruise on his arm; Dad was in bed because
he had had "a fall." Sometimes my mother would call me and tell me,
but sometimes she didn't want to worry me. When she visited, he would
ask her, "Why am I in jail?" and "Why won't you take me home?" My
mother would bring him food because he wasn't eating the food there.

319

She thought he just missed her cooking—he had been eating her food for fifty-five years.

The staff always had an answer for us. His skin is fragile, he hit his arm in the shower, and he was forgetting to eat or couldn't sit still long enough for them to get him some nutrition. They would say that people with Alzheimer disease often become confused about where they are and that it was common for them to think that they were in jail. To my family, all of those explanations made sense. We always had the feeling somewhere inside that things weren't the way the staff said, but we had no way to prove it. We are not a wealthy family; if we were, we would have hired private help to watch while we weren't there. That also meant that we couldn't move Dad easily—we couldn't pay $4,000 a month for another home.

If I were reading this, I would be wondering, "How could they not know?" The hard part is, like I said, we did know if we listened to ourselves. We were in crisis—about my mother and dad having to split up after fifty years, about how my mother was doing. It is like being in a nightmare and you don't know where to look first to try to make some sense of it all.

Finally in May we decided that we had had enough. My mother decided to try to sell some family property and use the money to move Dad to another home. But land wasn't selling well, and it didn't sell fast enough. If it had, Dad would still be alive. If it had, he would have been somewhere else on October 4. If, if, if, . . .

My journal starts from here. I omit some of the passages describing the horrible complications he suffered because of the injuries.

October 4

Dad either fell or was pushed down at the home, at 7:30 on the evening shift. He says he was pushed; the staff, of course, knows nothing. He wasn't seen at the emergency room until noon the next day. The ER doctor ordered X-rays, and discovered that Dad had a severe fracture of the left hip, a broken forearm, a puncture wound on the forearm, and a bone bruise on the knee. The home never had to explain these injuries because we couldn't see them. Dad was also dehydrated to the point of kidney failure. The surgery to repair his broken hip was delayed until the 7th. The orthopedic surgeon said Dad would never survive the surgery due to his weakened condition, so it had to be delayed until he stabilized medically.

October 16
Dad is having a feeding tube placed in his stomach, to keep him from starving. I object to that strongly, but the doctor wins. And everybody else is listening to him.

October 22
This morning Dad couldn't breathe, I called respiratory to come ASAP. X-rays show Dad to have pneumonia, doctor says bacterial, but I know better. Too much fluid, but who will listen? The doctor says Dad is hanging by a thread, won't make it through tonight, but again he is wrong. You will make it, Dad, you won't die in this stinking, god-forsaken place.

October 23
I heard you screaming from the chapel at the end of the hall, where I went when your nurses removed the fecal impaction. Oh, God, help me. Help Daddy make it out of here, he wants to go home. No one wants another feeding tube now for you, Dad, except that doctor of yours. I should have been stronger and demanded you not have one in the first place. You'd be home by now, eating. We've made another bad decision for you this time, Dad.

October 25
Your doctor, case manager, and social worker have all said how unrealistic it is for us to expect that we can manage you at home. The doctor suggested you go back to the nursing home. He wants to place another feeding tube in your stomach before he sends you, because once wasn't enough for him to learn. "How are we going to make sure he doesn't pull this one out, Doctor?" "We'll put him in restraints." Tied down, for how long? "Well, we'll have to keep him tied pretty much 24 hours a day." No thanks, doctor. He is not going to be in that nursing home again. We're taking you home, Daddy, which is where you always wanted to be, anyway. Did you have to do this to yourself to get there? No one should have to live, or die, tied down.

October 27

Well, you're home now. Do you know that you're home, Daddy? See the trees are all changing colors, Scorpio is in the yard, look at the pictures of the babies, Dad.

Now I know what happened to you at the nursing home. I got Mother to demand the chart. They didn't want to give it to me, they didn't even want to give it to her. At least we knew the law about that. Now I can see what really was happening there, how you got pulled out of bed by the staff. They pushed you around because in your confusion you were feisty with them and fought when they were trying to make you do something you didn't want to do. I can see how they lied to us. Where the bruise on your elbow was, one of the LPNs said that you got it in the bathtub but the nurse charted that you caught your elbow on the bedrail.

November 10

You have a UTI infection, as I suspected. We are at University Health Center now. I hate this feeding tube, and so do you. It won't work, will it? Is that why you asked today to have it cut out of you? Why won't you eat? Why do you tell me, "I don't do that no more"?

November 23

Daddy talked to me today. He was lying peacefully in bed, and said out of the blue, "I'm not afraid to die." "Do you want to die, Dad?" "No, but I'm not afraid to die. I'm at peace." Please, not yet, not yet, we have some things to do, Daddy. Not yet, please, please.

November 26

As I was rolling Dad over in bed today, he said, "Don't push me out of bed." Why, Dad? You're in bed, you can't fall. "I know I'm in bed. Please don't push me out of bed."

God, I'd never do anything to hurt you. Pain, Daddy, pain, how bad was it in that filthy nursing home? That's what they did to you there, isn't it? They pulled you out of bed.

December 13

I took Daddy out in the mid-December sunshine today. He actually laughed at Scorpio's dumb dog antics. I love you, Daddy. I'm so sorry,

I didn't know. Please forgive me. Please live for a while for me. I didn't know how bad it was for you there. What is killing you? Why do you say, "This is killing me." Let me help you, please.

December 25

Daddy's dying. There's no doubt that hospice is right. We have to come to terms with it. But I can't, not like this. He wants the feeding tube out.

January 3

Your blood pressure is bouncing around, you're not breathing right, I've called the hospice nurse. I sit here at 3 a.m. watching you and remembering what you have done for me. Remembering the last two months of this nightmare, watching you recapitulate your life. Listening to you talk of the babies, who will take care of the babies? The babies will be fine, Dad. Please don't worry about the babies, I'll take care of them. You did good with the babies anyway, and they love you very much. You can do whatever you need to do now.

January 4

Daddy broke down tonight at 9 p.m. and started crying. I pleaded with Michael to tell Daddy that it was okay for him to die, that he would be okay with it. Michael did. It won't be long now. He has released our father, whom we both loved and will always love.

January 5

Daddy died today at 4 p.m. He had been in a coma since 2 p.m. I know you heard the final words, didn't you, Dad? Peaceful death, no trauma. See you later, Daddy.

How will I fill this hole in my soul?

May 8

As I copied these paragraphs from my diary, I cried again. I thought that I had quit crying, but now I see that I never will. But, I have learned a lot since my father died from the abuse he received at the hands of an orderly. First, I learned that we gave my father a gift—if life is a gift, then a peaceful and tranquil release to death must also be a gift. My father left this awareness knowing that his children knew he was leaving and could cope with it. He wasn't afraid, and he was surrounded by all of us in the last hours, at home, where he wanted to be.

I don't think what I feel, and will always feel, is guilt. Guilt is something you feel when you've done wrong and know that you've done wrong. I feel regret, so much regret, for the horrible twelve months that my father spent locked up in conditions worse than what criminals in jail live in, regret for my and my family's naiveté and ignorance.

I am not ignorant now, and I devote a good part of my life to nursing home reform. Our system needs to be changed, in so many ways. My father's story is being played out all over the country every day, and I can't walk away from it, now that awareness has been dropped on me. If I had to offer one piece of advice to anyone looking to place a parent in a nursing home, I'd say this: Always, always, trust your heart. If something doesn't seem right, it isn't. Listen to your feelings, and not what the staff or administration, or even the state enforcement agency, tells you, but that tiny voice that somehow most always seems to be overridden.

Alvin (part 2)

Even though Alvin was at another facility, some of the staff at the House of Horrors was there for me during his last few days. One in particular told me she felt that she was part of our family.

In the end, Alvin made a beautiful exit. We were making a brain donation, and because none of his family lived in the area and his friends were from the staffs at both the House of Horrors and the new facility, we decided not to have a memorial, flowers, donations, etc.

For the next six weeks I worked on a memorial book for Alvin that would stay with his family and friends for a long time. I included pictures of our wedding seven years before and of our life together. Then came pictures of his life with his parents, children, and grandchildren. There was a letter I wrote to friends describing his last few days. The last section included photos of his "new life" in the new facility, showing him playing his harmonica, attending a St. Patrick's Day party, with his favorite nurse's aides, and next to me at the piano. In the last photos I took of him, shortly before his death, he looked wonderful and was smiling.

This memorial was absolutely beautiful. It was all I needed to do.

Accessing Care in Canada

Although the provinces and territories of Canada are struggling to make their systems accessible, it can still be frustrating to try to find information regarding residential care. The easiest way to begin to learn about your province's system is to call your local Health Authority or health department. You can also call your provincial Ministry of Health and ask about services for seniors. You might call or go to online directory assistance and ask for a number using terms like *long-term care, continuing care, home care,* or something similar. When you obtain a phone number and make a call, you may have to ask if you are speaking to an organization that deals with residential care and housing for seniors. If they do not, they will usually be able to give you the number of the agency that does. The local Alzheimer's Association chapter will also be able to tell you where to begin. You can access each province's Web site for care.

Most provinces have several types of residential care, including assisted living and group homes. In some provinces, as your care needs increase, you may have to move to another facility that can provide more services. This means that there can be several moves once you start in the residential-care system. Most of the provinces have funded residency in assisted living as well as nursing homes. Several provinces have small, group home types of facilities.

Each province and territory has a different system of providing residential care, but many aspects of care are common in different forms to all areas of the country. The names used to describe the various types of seniors housing may vary. Care systems are evolving continuously but tend to be headed in the same direction—a single-point entry system. A single-point entry system means that all services, whether in one's own home or in a residential facility, are coordinated and offered through the same or affiliated agencies. They all at least work closely together. If you need care, you call one agency and they follow you as long as you are in the system, from the early stages when you may need only homemaker services or adult day care through the time you may need placement in a nursing home. Ideally, you are assigned one case manager as you go through the system.

At the point of entry, an intake worker will take some basic information and pass it on to an assessor, who will do an in-depth assessment. This may start over the phone, but eventually someone will come to your home. The assessor examines a person's cognitive ability (for example, thinking, memory, judgment), physical functioning, and ability to manage at home. He or she will usually talk to family, physicians, and others who are involved. Most provinces have a standardized form that they use to help the assessor decide a level of care. The resulting assessments establish a level that corresponds to the type of care someone is eligible to receive and the amount of support he or she needs. For instance, level 1 might mean someone is eligible only for care in his or her own home, level 2 might mean someone qualifies for assisted living, and level 3 might qualify someone for a nursing home. The level system is different in each province, and the levels have different meanings.

Just because you want a certain type of help does not mean that you will be eligible to receive it. Your assessor/case manager ultimately decides eligibility, not the physician and not the family. If you believe that you are eligible for more or need more, you can appeal.

Governments prefer to help people stay in their own home for as long as possible with home support because it is less expensive than residential care. If you and the assessing agency feel you cannot manage at home any longer, they will put your name on the waiting list of at least one nursing home that you request, provided that the facility is able to provide the care you need. In some areas you may be able to put your name on more than one waiting list.

The criteria for eligibility for waiting lists vary from province to province. Whereas in one province you may qualify for nursing home care, in another you may not, even with the same conditions. You can appeal that decision by talking with the case manager or the agency administrator.

Policies regarding waiting lists and admission to a nursing home vary by province. In some provinces, admission priority is based more or less strictly on the date when your name was added to a list. In other provinces, priority for admission is based on comparing different candidates' needs and risk at home, as well as the date on the list.

Most provinces have exceptions to waiting-list admission policy. For instance, if someone living at home becomes at great and imminent risk, then he or she might be placed in a residence immediately, even if he or she is not on a waiting list. Or, if a husband is in care and his wife needs care, she may be placed immediately or at least added higher up on the waiting list, so that the two of them can be together. Also, it may happen that someone has been on a waiting list in one area of the province for a year and then decides that she wishes to live in another part of the province. She can "take" her waiting list date with her to another facility's list, and this would put her higher on the new list than some people who were added to it before she was.

Some provinces have moved to what is called a first-available-bed system. That means that you may request one or two places, but you *have* to accept the first bed that is offered. This is true also if they are moved there from a hospital. If you refuse to accept an offered bed, you are taken completely off the list of people who are awaiting places. You do not go to the bottom of the list and will have to request placement later. In some provinces, if your name comes up and you are not ready, you are allowed to be skipped or go back to the bottom of the list. In some provinces, you can turn down one or two offers of a bed, but you must accept the third offer or your name will go off the list or become inactive.

In most provinces, if you do not get into your preferred facility, you can ask to be placed on a transfer list. The wait for a transfer can be up to a couple of years. Ask the assessor how they figure out waiting-list dates. They may be figured from the day you requested to go to the place, or they may be figured from the day you went *somewhere* and then asked to wait for the place you prefer.

If you live in one part of a province but wish to receive care in another (for instance, if you wish to live closer to a son or daughter), call the agency in your area that is responsible for residential care. They will do the assessment and send it to the region where you wish to live. There may be some requirements before moving from one area or health region in your province to another in the same province, or they may give you a lower priority than people already in the area. In British Columbia, for example, if you wish to live in a nursing home in Vancouver but currently reside in Surrey, you may have to move to a care facility in Surrey and then go on a transfer list.

If you live in one province but wish to receive care in another, call the agency in the region where you wish to live. They will explain the process necessary. Some provinces allow you to apply for care from outside the province, so you are eligible to receive care as soon as you arrive. In others, there is a residency requirement, so you need to live in the province before you can apply for care. That can mean that you may have to live in the province for up to a year before you are even eligible to go on a waiting list. Residency requirement lengths vary among the provinces. Currently the provinces are trying to work out reciprocal agreements to make this system easier. Sometimes exceptions will be made to the policies.

Almost all provinces and territories have a system of for-profit facilities that coexist with the nonprofit and government-owned ones. Some of these are completely outside the public system and are not funded; others do have government-funded beds. The funded beds may be all or only a percentage of the total. The funded beds can only be accessed through an assessor/case manager, just as in the nonprofits.

The levels of care available privately vary from congregate living to assisted living up to nursing homes. Even when nursing homes are not subsidized, they are licensed by the governments and must meet certain standards. Assisted living may or may not be licensed or regulated. To find out for your province, go to the health region/authority. They can also tell you whom to contact to complain if a residence is not registered, such as in supportive housing. Even if there is no regulatory system for a facility, they may still fall under regulations for things like occupational health and safety and health department regulations for cleanliness and kitchen standards.

Remember that just because a facility is in the private sector, costs several thousand dollars more than a publicly funded one, and looks nice does not mean that the care or services provided will be better. Looks can be deceiving.

All provinces have adult day care centers. These are programs that someone can attend from one to five days per week, depending on the person's need and the space available. Adult day care centers can be helpful in giving caregivers a break and can allow someone to keep living in the community by providing social stimulation, good meals, and monitoring of health status. Some centers are open weekends and evenings.

All provinces have a respite bed system. This means that for up to four weeks a year someone may live in a facility to give their caregivers a rest. The provincially funded respite is an excellent way to begin to help your relative become accustomed to care and "try it out." If you would like to use the respite system, you may have to book the bed far in advance, especially in the summer. Many private residences also have some kind of respite available at a daily rate. This may be through a guest suite or room, or as a specifically designated respite care room or suite.

Costs for service in most provinces are based on income. The ability to pay is usually determined by a financial assessment. Some provinces include assets in estimated ability to pay; some take only income into account. They all have a minimum daily fee for someone who is on a fixed-income pension. This minimum fee is always less than a person's total monthly income, although there might not be much left over. This means that every Canadian has the funds to pay for residential care. There may, however, be an impact on a spouse remaining at home, for example, in terms of ability to pay rent on an apartment. Most provinces have a maximum top rate irrespective of income and assets. This means that even if you are worth $5 million or your yearly income is $100,000, the top ceiling rate is the same as for someone who makes one-tenth of that. A couple of provinces base costs on assets as well as income. They require that a majority of personal resources be exhausted before they will begin to subsidize. This means they will require you to "spend down" your resources until they are below a certain level. If they find that you have given away your resources to qualify for the subsidy, they will pursue payment from those to whom you distributed your wealth.

The way charges are figured for housing may vary according to the type of housing. For instance, charges or methods of figuring costs for a nursing home may be different from charges for assisted living.

The following is a list of questions you should ask the agency in your area:

1. Who handles the waiting list?
2. What are the eligibility requirements to be put on a waiting list for a nursing home?
3. What are the rules of waiting lists, and what are the exceptions to those rules?
4. How do the waiting lists function?
5. What happens if I turn down a bed that is offered to me?
6. Once I am in a home, under what conditions or circumstances would I have to move to another?
7. What services are available to me while I am waiting for a space in a nursing home?
8. Do you fund assisted living, group homes, or other alternatives to nursing homes?

9. What are the costs, and how are they determined?
10. To whom do I talk if I have a complaint about the home or the placement system?
11. What services are provided in nursing homes?

Make sure you understand the terminology that the system uses (for example, *nursing home, personal care home*) in your area, so that you obtain the care you need and you get what you think you are getting. If you do not understand what the differences are, make sure you ask; the people you will be speaking with may often use abbreviations and terminology that only someone in the system would know.

Questionnaires

1. GUIDE TO VIEWING NURSING HOMES AND ASSISTED LIVING FACILITIES

You may complete the table by using yes/no or a number system such as 1–5, or good, fair, poor.

STAFF	Facility A	Facility B	Facility C
Nurses *Number per resident*			
Training			
Nurses aides *Number per resident*			
Training			
Director of Care *Qualifications*			
Recreation workers *Number per resident*			
Training			
Recreation director *Training*			
Social worker *How often?*			
Training			

APPENDIX 2

STAFF (*cont.*)	Facility A	Facility B	Facility C
Physical therapist *On site?*			
Occupational therapist *On site?*			
Other rehabilitation staff			
Registered dietitian *On site?*			
House physician			
Access to geriatric physician			
Pastoral care			
Access to mental health / geriatric mental health			
Pharmacist available			
Complementary medical services *Allowed?*			
Present?			
PROGRAM	Facility A	Facility B	Facility C
Religious programs			
Art therapy			
Music therapy			
Other			
Recreation programs *Number*			
Variety			
Evenings?			
Weekends?			
For visually impaired			
For hearing impaired			
Exercise programs			

QUESTIONNAIRES

PROGRAM (*cont.*)	Facility A	Facility B	Facility C
Resident's council			
Family council			
Volunteers available			

POLICY	Facility A	Facility B	Facility C
Pets allowed/available			
Plants allowed/available			
Visiting hour restrictions			
Can take residents out as wish			
Care conferences—frequency			
Educational programs for staff			
Accredited			
Survey results			
Medicare accepted			
Medicaid accepted			
Policy on theft			
Policy on abuse			
Policy on restraints			
Policy on roommates			
Policy on room changes			
Policy on price increases			

FACILITY	Facility A	Facility B	Facility C
Cleanliness			
Lighting			
Smell			
Access to outdoor space			
Access to shops/shopping			
Equipped for wheelchairs			

FACILITY (*cont.*)	Facility A	Facility B	Facility C
Handrails			
Rails/bars in bathrooms			
Exercise equipment/room			
Cueing for visual impairment			
Cueing for hearing impairment			
Family visiting space			
ROOMS/ACCOMMODATIONS	Facility A	Facility B	Facility C
Single rooms			
Double rooms			
Appearance of rooms			
Size of rooms/room space			
Storage in rooms			
Lighting in rooms			
View from rooms			
Can bring in own furniture			
Can bring in TV			
Cable ready			
Can have telephone in room			
Call bells by bedside			
Call bells by toilet			
Distance of rooms *From dining/activity*			
From floors/elevators			
From staff/nursing station			
Noise level: high/low			
Equipped for wheelchairs			
Handrails			
Rails/bars in bathrooms			

ROOMS/ACCOMMODATIONS (cont.)	Facility A	Facility B	Facility C
Cooking facilities in room/suite			
Fridge in room			
Balcony			
ATMOSPHERE	Facility A	Facility B	Facility C
Residents appear well dressed			
Residents appear clean			
Residents appear happy/content			
Staff appear helpful, interested			
Staff appear to have good relations			
Staff turnover rate			
Management is open to family input			
Residents' council			
Family council			
Ethnic sensitivity			
Gay/lesbian/transgendered friendly			
CARE/HOUSING OPTIONS	Facility A	Facility B	Facility C
Independent living			
Assisted living			
Nursing home			
Acute care			
Rehabilitation			
Palliative/hospice care			
Dementia unit			
Campus-of-care/continuing-care retirement			
Limitations on care/services			

DINING ROOM / MEALS	Facility A	Facility B	Facility C
Dining room cleanliness			
Dining room atmosphere			
Dining hours appropriateness			
Appearance of food			
Variety of menu			
Portions appropriate			
Choices/alternatives available			
Meals served in rooms			
Family can join residents			
Private family dining area			
LAUNDRY	Facility A	Facility B	Facility C
Laundry done on premises			
Laundry frequency			
Family can do laundry			
Dry cleaning services			
PAPERWORK	Facility A	Facility B	Facility C
Copy of admission agreement			
Copy of recreation schedule sample			
Copy of menu			
Survey/deficiencies/corrections			

HOW DOES IT FEEL TO YOU? NOTES:
Facility A

QUESTIONNAIRES

Facility B
Facility C

2. DAILY SCHEDULE

What time do you wake up?
_____

What time do you have breakfast?
_____

What do you have for breakfast?
_____

_____

_____

What is your morning hygiene routine?
_____

_____

_____

What do you do in the morning?
_____

_____

_____

_____

What time do you have lunch?
_____

What do you have for lunch?
_____

_____

_____

What do you do in the afternoon?
_____

_____

_____

_____

What time do you have dinner?
_____

What do you have for dinner?
_____

_____

_____

QUESTIONNAIRES

What do you do after dinner?

_____

_____

What is your evening hygiene routine?

_____

_____

What time do you go to bed?

_____

How often do you get up at night?

_____

Weekly activities (such as bridge club, dinner with your family, meetings, church)?

_____

_____

_____

_____

_____

_____

_____

_____

_____

Special needs/equipment, etc.?

_____

_____

_____

_____

_____

_____

3. SOCIAL HISTORY

Below is an outline of a social history. It is detailed, so you might not be able to answer all the questions. I want you to see what kinds of things can be included. Social histories are done more often for a nursing home than for assisted living. However, when someone is impaired and is receiving a high level of services, the distinction is not important. A social history helps people know who you are and, it is to be hoped, give you the kind of service you need in the way that you can use it.

1. Where were you born?

2. Describe your family. What was your father like? Your mother? How many brothers and sisters did you have?

3. What were relationships like in your family? Between your parents? Between you and your parents? Between you and your siblings?

4. What was your childhood like? What kind of child were you?

5. Describe your schooling.

6. Describe your young adulthood. What were your friendship and dating circles like? Your activities and interests?

7. Describe your work life and history.

8. Describe your marriage. What was your wife/husband like? What kinds of things did you do together? Describe some of the ups and downs in your marriage.

9. Did you have children? What was your family life like? What were you like as a parent?

10. Have you had any particular life crises? How did you handle them?

11. What were your retirement years like?

12. Describe your use of alcohol and other substances.

13. Have you ever had any psychiatric treatment, or was there any psychiatric illness in your family?

14. Do you have any chronic illnesses in your family?

15. What brought you to the point where you need to go into a nursing home?

16. What did your parents and any siblings die of? How old were they when they died?

17. Describe your personality. What are you like? How do other people see you? What are some of your strengths and weaknesses?

18. What are you like socially? Are you a joiner or more of a one-on-one person?

19. How do you react to stress and anxiety? Are you easily angered or frustrated? What kinds of things bother you?

20. When are you happy or content?

21. What do you want people to know about you?

22. What is important to you that will mean that you are getting good care?

23. What things are important to you in your day-to-day life? Little things you do or habits you have that help to "make your day"?

4. EVENT AND ACTION LOG

Use this chart (or a similar one) to help you keep a record of your caregiving. Because it is a caregiving record based on your loved one's needs, it is objective. Over a long period, it will show the progression and escalation of his or her needs, and it will help to show others, and convince you if you need convincing about, what you do and what you have given over time.

Event/ appointment/ behavior	Date	Care receiver's reaction	Your actions/follow-up

Some Common Medical Abbreviations

For Medications

BID	twice a day
HS	at night
NPO	nothing by mouth
OD	daily
PO	by mouth
PRN	when or as needed
Q (as in, Q 4 hrs)	every (every four hours)
QID	four times a day
STAT	immediately
TID	three times a day

Illness

ASHD	atherosclerotic heart disease
BP	blood pressure
CA	cancer
CAD	coronary artery disease
CHF	congestive heart failure
COPD (COLD)	chronic obstructive pulmonary disorder (— lung disorder)
CVA	cerebrovascular accident (stroke)
GERD	gastroesophagal reflux disease
GI	gastrointestinal
HTN	hypertension
MI	myocardial infarction (heart attack)
NIDDIM (IDDIM)	non-insulin-dependent diabetes mellitus (insulin-dependent diabetes mellitus)

NYD	not yet diagnosed
RBC	red blood cells
SOB (SOBOE)	short of breath (short of breath on exertion)
TIA	transient ischemic attacks (small strokes)
TSH	thyroid-stimulating hormone
TUPR	transurethral prostatic resection
URTI	upper respiratory tract infection
UTI	urinary tract infection
WBC	white blood cells

Dementia and Care

AD	Alzheimer disease
ADL	activities of daily living
Ax	assessment
DAT	diet as tolerated
DNR	do not resuscitate
DOI	degree of intervention
Dx	diagnosis
ETOH	alcohol
Hx	history
IADL	instrumental activities of daily living
LTM	long-term memory
MCI	mild cognitive impairment
MMSE	Mini-Mental State Examination
MOCA	Montreal Cognitive Assessment
SDAT	senile dementia of the Alzheimer type
STM	short-term memory
Sx	symptoms

Professions

OT	occupational therapy
PT	physical therapy, physiotherapy
RD	registered dietitian
SLP	speech-language pathologist
SW	social work (MSW = master, BSW = bachelor)

Last but Not Least

OMG	oh my God (as in, oh my God, how will I ever remember all these abbreviations?)

Resources

Books and Pamphlets

These are just some of the books I have found useful. I recommend that you also go to amazon.com or a similar online bookstore and see what they carry on grief and loss, nursing homes and seniors housing, pain, and caregiving. There are many excellent books on these subjects.

Abrahm, Janet L. *A Physician's Guide to Pain and Symptom Management in Cancer Patients*, 2nd ed. Baltimore: Johns Hopkins University Press, 2005. A thorough and compassionate manual with a separate bibliography for patients and their families.

Blaivas, Jerry G. *Conquering Bladder and Prostate Problems: The Authoritative Guide for Men and Women*. New York: Plenum Books, 1998.

Boss, Pauline. *Ambiguous Loss: Learning to Live with Unresolved Grief*. Cambridge, MA: Harvard University Press, 1999.

Bradshaw, John. *Healing the Shame That Binds You*. Deerfield Park, FL: Health Communications, 1988. An in-depth look at the issues of shame that run our lives.

Bridges, Barbara J. *Therapeutic Caregiving: A Practical Guide for Caregivers of Persons with Alzheimer's and Other Dementia-Causing Diseases*. Mill Creek, WA: BJB Publishing, 1995. An excellent guide with practical advice for the caregiver who is caring for someone at home.

Burger, Sarah Greene. "Avoiding Drugs Used as Chemical Restraints." Washington, DC: National Citizens' Coalition for Nursing Home Reform, 1994.

———. "Avoiding Physical Restraint Use: New Standards in Care." Washington, DC: National Citizens' Coalition for Nursing Home Reform, 1993.

————. *Nursing Homes: Getting Good Care There*. San Luis Obispo, CA: American Source Books, 1996. This is an excellent in-depth guide to care planning in nursing homes.

Callone, Patricia R., ed. *A Caregiver's Guide to Alzheimer's Disease: 300 Tips for Making Life Easier*. New York: Demos Medical Publishing, 2006.

Caplan, Louis R., Mark L. Dyker, and J. Donald Easton. *American Heart Association Family Guide to Stroke, Treatment, Recovery, and Prevention*. New York: Times Books, 1996.

Carlson, Eric M., and Katharine Bau Hsai. *Baby Boomer's Guide to Nursing Home Care*. New York: Taylor Trade Publishing, 2006. Explains much about what nursing homes can and cannot do legally, and what you are entitled to.

Colgrove, Melba, Harold H. Bloomfield, and Peter A. McWilliams. *How to Survive the Loss of a Love: 58 Things to Do When There Is Nothing to Be Done*. Los Angeles: Prelude Press, 1991.

Gas, Thomas Edward. *Nobody's Home: Candid Reflections of a Nursing Home Aide*. Ithaca, NY: Cornell University Press, 2005. A much-needed book that tells it like it is, from the point of view of a nursing home aide.

Kübler-Ross, Elisabeth. *On Death and Dying*. New York: Scribner Classics, 1997.

Kuhl, David. *What Dying People Want: Practical Wisdom for the End of Life*. New York: Public Affairs, 2002.

Kushner, Harold S. *When Bad Things Happen to Good People*. New York: Schocken Books, 2001. How to cope with the senselessness of tragedy in life.

LeBow, Grace. *Coping with Your Difficult Older Parent: A Guide for Stressed Out Children*. New York: Avon Books, 1999.

Loverde, Joy. *The Complete Eldercare Planner: Where to Start, Questions to Ask, and How to Find Help*, rev. and updated ed. New York: Hyperion Books, 2009.

Mace, Nancy L., and Peter V. Rabins. *The 36-Hour Day: A Family Guide to Caring for People with Alzheimer Disease, Related Dementias, and Memory Loss in Later Life*, 4th ed. Baltimore: Johns Hopkins University Press, 2006. The classic book in the field for caring for someone with dementia. It has a section on nursing homes.

Marcell, Jacqueline. *Elder Rage, or Take My Father . . . Please! How to Survive Caring for Aging Parents*, 2nd ed. Irvine, CA: Impressive Press, 2001. A humorous and helpful book for when your parents are driving you crazy.

Morris, Virginia. *How to Care for Aging Parents*. New York: Workman Publishing, 2004. A good guide for caregivers.

National Senior Citizens Law Center. "Twenty Common Nursing Home Problems and How to Resolve Them." National Seniors Citizen's Law Center (www.nsclc.org). Practical advice regarding legal issues in nursing homes.

O'Donnell, Jill et al. *The Canadian Retirement Guide: A Comprehensive Handbook on Aging, Retirement, Caregiving, and Health and How to Plan and Pay for It*. London, ON: Insomniac Press, 2004.

Quinn, Mary Joy, and Susan K. Tomita. *Elder Abuse and Neglect: Causes, Diagnoses, and Intervention Strategies*. New York: Springer Publishing, 1997.

Sankar, Andrea. *Dying at Home: A Family Guide for Caregiving*, rev. and updated ed. Baltimore: Johns Hopkins University Press, 2000.

Tapp-McDougall, Caroline. *The Complete Canadian Eldercare Guide: Expert Solutions to Help You Make the Best Decisions for Your Loved Ones*. Toronto: Wiley, 2004.

Thomas, William H. *Life Worth Living: How Someone You Love Can Still Enjoy Life in a Nursing Home—The Eden Alternative in Action*. Acton, MA: Vander Wyk and Burnham, 1996. An inspiring guide to what a nursing home can be.

Organizations and Web Sites

There are numerous organizations and Web sites for caregivers, including an organization for almost every disability and disease. Most have both U.S. and Canadian counterparts. If you wish to call a U.S. resource from Canada, and the 800 number is valid only for the United States, try dialing 880.

It is essential for you to have an understanding of the disease that you are facing. Because people at these organizations are specialists in their areas, they have the most up-to-date information on treatments, research, medications, and so on. They know more than many professionals because they are able to focus on their areas of interest. They can be excellent resources to help you choose a nursing home. If there is not a local chapter of a particular organization near where you live, you can call the national office. In addition, most of them have Web sites.

It is well worth your time to go online and look at the Web sites below or go to search engines and search for "nursing homes," "eldercare," "seniors," "long-term care," "long-term care insurance," "death and dying," etc. No matter where you live, there are people on the Web who can be there for you. This is one of the best examples of the positive power of the Internet.

AARP, 601 E Street, N.W., Washington, DC 20049. 800-424-3410. www .aarp.org; email: member@aarp.org. Advice and information on a range of topics affecting seniors, including long-term care insurance.

Administration on Aging, Department of Health and Human Services, 330 Independence Avenue, S.W., Washington, DC 20201. 202-401-4541. www.aoa.dhhs.gov. They have a complete listing of resources on aging. Their directory is well worth a look.

Agenet Information Referral Network, www.agenet.com. A comprehensive Web site of resources and information on geriatrics and aging. Among other services, they provide a medication assessment, a resource directory, and a housing directory.

Aging with Dignity, P.O. Box 1661, Tallahassee, FL 32302-1661. 850-681-2010. www.agingwithdignity.org; email: fivewishes@aol.com. You can download Aging with Dignity's Five Wishes, a guide for health care proxy decision making. It is legally recognized in thirty-four states. Aging with Dignity is also an advocacy group for elderly persons and their caregivers.

Alzheimer's Association, 225 N. Michigan Avenue, Floor 17, Chicago, IL 60601-7633. 800-272-3900. www.alz.org; email: info@alz.org.

Alzheimer Society of Canada, 20 Eglinton Avenue W., Suite 600, Toronto, ON M4R 1K8. 800-616-8816. www.alzheimer.ca; email: info@ alzheimer.ca.

American Association of Homes and Services for the Aging, 901 E Street, N.W., Suite 500, Washington, DC 20004-2037. 202-783-2242; fax 202-783-2245. www.aahsa.com.

American Diabetes Association, 1701 North Beauregard Street, Alexandria, VA 22311. 800-342-2383. www.diabetes.org; email: customerservice@ diabetes.org.

American Heart Association, 7272 Greenville Avenue, Dallas, TX 75231. 800-AHA-USA1. www.americanheart.org.

American Parkinson Disease Association, 1250 Hyland Boulevard, Suite 4B, Staten Island, NY 10305. 800-223-2732. www.apdaparkinson.org.

Arthritis Foundation, 1330 West Peachtree Street, Atlanta, GA 30309. 404-872-4100, 800-283-7800. www.arthritis.org.

Arthritis Society of Canada, 393 University Avenue, Toronto, ON M5G

1E6. 800-321-1433, 800-323-1400. www.arthritis.ca; email: info@arthritis.ca.

Assisted Living Federation of America, 1650 King Street, Suite 602, Alexandria, VA 22314-2747. 703-894-1805; fax: 703-894-1831. www.alfa.org; email: info@alfa.org. This is the industry association for assisted living facilities.

Canadian Diabetes Association, 15 Toronto Street, Suite 800, Toronto, ON M5C 2E3. 800-BANTING or 416-363-3373. www.diabetes.ca; email: info@diabetes.ca.

Caregiver Network, 561 Avenue Road, Suite 206, Toronto, ON M4V 2J8. 416-323-1090. www.caregiver.on.ca; email: Karen@caregiver.on.ca. A Canadian Web site for caregivers.

Caregivers.com. A general site for caregivers, associated with Agenet. They have a number of resources, including a directory of geriatricians and geriatric care managers in your area and links to other information sites.

CareGuide, Inc., 739 Bryant Street, San Francisco, CA 94107. 415-474-1278. www.careguide.com. A private company that provides care management services. Their Web site is especially helpful.

Caring Connections, c/o National Hospice and Palliative Care Organization, 1731 King Street, Suite 100 Alexandria, VA 22314. 800-658-8898. www.caringinfo.org; email: caringinfo@nhpco.org. Caring Connections is a program of the National Hospice and Palliative Care Organization (NHPCO). They have numerous brochures on palliative care and end-of-life issues and state-specific advance directives.

CARP, 27 Queen Street East, Suite 1304, Toronto, ON M5C 2M6. 800-363-9736; fax 416-363-8747. www.carp.ca; email: carp@carp.ca. Similar to AARP, for Canadians—help, information, and advocacy.

Centers for Medicare and Medicaid Services (formerly Health Care Financing Administration, HCFA). 800-MEDICARE (800-633-4227). www.cms.hhs.gov. This government site is helpful on everything about Medicare and Medicaid. See also the listing for Medicare, below.

Children of Aging Parents, 1609 Woodbourne Road, Levittown, PA 19057. 215-945-6900. www.caps4caregivers.org. An organization dedicated to caregivers. They have lots of great pamphlets on issues pertinent to caregiving.

Consumer Consortium on Assisted Living, Oak Street, Falls Church, VA 22046. 703-533-8121. www.ccal.org; email: info@ccal.org. A coalition of groups interested in assisted living.

Diamond Geriatrics, Inc., 25 West 11th Avenue, Vancouver, BC V5Y 1S6.

604-874-7764. www.diamondgeriatrics.com. The author's care management and consulting company.

Eldercare Locator. www.eldercare.gov/eldercare.net/public/home/aspx. The Department of Health and Human Services site for finding state ombudspeople and other resources.

Eldercare Online. www.ec-online.net. A comprehensive Web site that offers information of interest to caregivers. Also has information about issues related to nursing homes and finding a good one.

Elderpost. www.elderpost.com. A free online listings and ads service for seniors, caregivers, and providers of products and services. Find anyone and anything you need on Elderpost.

Family Caregiver Alliance, 180 Montgomery Street, Suite 1100, San Francisco, CA 94104. 415-434-3388 or 800-445-8106; fax: 415-434-3508. www.caregiver.org. An excellent site for information and resources. Their "Family Care Navigator" lists resources state by state.

Gilbert Guide. www.gilbertguide.com. An excellent site for information on caregiving, aging, and seniors housing. They have an excellent newsletter.

Government of Canada. www.seniors.gc.ca/home.jsp. Complete information for Canadians. Guides you to provincial services also.

Government of Canada Services for Seniors. www.servicecanada.gc.ca/en/audiences/seniors/. Information for Canadians.

Heart and Stroke Foundation of Canada, 222 Queen Street, Suite 1402, Ottawa, ON K1P 5V9. 613-241-4361.

Life Care Planning Law Firms Association. 10320 N. Bald Head Place, Oro Valley, AZ 85737. 520-270-1541. www.lcplfa.org. This is an association of law firms practicing holistic, elder-centered law, with a broader approach to helping clients.

Medicare. 800-MEDICARE. www.medicare.gov. The Medicare website has a number of tools to help you compare nursing homes, Medigap and other funding possibilities, drug plans, etc. The site is similar to that of the Centers for Medicare and Medicaid Services, above.

Medicare Rights Center. www.medicarerights.org. Independent organization for health care information and assistance for recipients of Medicare.

Multiple Sclerosis Society of Canada, 250 Bloor Street East, Suite 1000, Toronto, ON M4W 3P9. 800-361-2985. www.mssoc.ca; email: info@mssoc.ca.

Myziva. www.myziva.net. Comprehensive guide to searching for nursing homes.

National Academy of Elder Law Attorneys, 1577 Spring Hill Road, Suite 220, Vienna, VA, 22182. www.naela.org; email: info@naela.org.

National Association of Professional Geriatric Care Managers, 1604 North Country Club Road, Tucson, AZ 85716-3102. 520-881-8008; fax 520-325-7925. www.caremanager.org.

National Association of Professional Organizers. www.napo.net. The U.S. association of people who assist in moves and downsizing. (In Canada, www.organizersincanada.org.)

National Association of Senior Move Managers. 1-877-606-2766, www .nasmm.com, email: Jennifer@nasmm.org. A national association of companies and individuals who focus on helping seniors move.

National Center for Home Equity Conversion, 360 Robert Street N, Suite 403, St. Paul, MN 55101. 651-222-6775. www.reverse.org. The Web site explains all you want to know about reverse mortgages.

National Center on Elder Abuse. www.ncea.aoa.gov. This is the Administration on Aging's site on elder abuse. Information and guidance to local and government resources.

National Clearinghouse for Long-Term Care Information. www.long termcare.gov. Some excellent information on planning and paying for long-term care, especially about long-term care insurance.

National Family Caregivers Association, 10604 Concorde Street, Suite 501, Kensington, MD 20895-2504. 800-896-3650. www.nfcacares.org; email: info@nfcacares.org.

National Hospice and Palliative Care Organization. *See* Caring Connections.

National Long Term Care Ombudsmen Resource Center, 1828 L Street N.W., Suite 801, Washington, DC 20036. 202-332-2275. www.ltc ombudsman.org; email: ombud@nccnhr.org. A site for ombudsmen and help for people seeking the services that the ombudsmen can provide.

National Multiple Sclerosis Society, 733 Third Avenue, New York, NY 10017. 800-FIGHT-MS. www.nmss.org; email: info@nmss.org.

National Pace Association, 801 N. Fairfax Street, Suite 309, Alexandria, VA 22314. 703-535-1565; fax: 703-535-1566. www.npaonline.org; email: info@npaonline.org. "The National PACE Association (NPA) exists to advance the efforts of Programs of All-inclusive Care for the Elderly (PACE). PACE programs coordinate and provide all needed preventive, primary, acute and long term care services so that older individuals can continue living in the community."

National Parkinson Foundation, Bob Hope Parkinson Research Center, 1501 N.W. 9th Avenue, Bob Hope Road, Miami, FL 33136-1494. 305-243-6666 or 800-327-4545; fax 305-243-5595. www.parkinson.org; email: contact@parkinson.org.

National Senior Citizens Law Center. www.nsclc.org. Excellent site for advice and information on legal issues relating to older people.

NCCNHR (formerly National Citizens' Coalition for Nursing Home Reform), 1424 16th Street, N.W., #202, Washington, DC 20036. 202-332-2275. www.nccnhr.org; email: nccnhr@nccnhr.org. The NCCNHR is an advocacy group. They put out a number of excellent booklets, including "Avoiding Drugs Used as Chemical Restraints" and "Avoiding Physical Restraint Use."

Parkinson Foundation of Canada, 4211 Yonge Street, Suite 316, Toronto, ON M2P 2A9. 800-565-3000. www.parkinson.ca; email: alicia.pace@parkinson.ca.

Pioneer Network, P.O. Box 18648, Rochester, NY 14618. 585-271-7570. www.pioneernetwork.net. A national organization dedicated to transforming nursing homes and care facilities.

Professional Organizers in Canada. www.organizersincanada.org. The Canadian association of professionals who help with downsizing and organizing and packing for moves.

Public Health Agency of Canada. www.phac-aspc.gc.ca/sh-sa-eng.php. See their section, in either English or French, on seniors.

Senior Housing Net. www.seniorhousing.net. This site explains senior housing and has a comprehensive guide by state to all kinds of housing for seniors.

Senior Sites. www.seniorsites.com. Use this site to search by county and state for nonprofit nursing homes and other residential care alternatives.

Web of Care. www.webofcare.com. A comprehensive site for caregivers that deals with many different issues and diseases.

Information about Payment

AARP, 601 E Street, N.W., Washington, DC 20049. 800-424-3410. www.aarp.org. They have several excellent booklets describing Medicare and Medicare options such as Medigap (supplemental insurance) and Medicare HMOs. The booklets are clearly written, with comparative information.

Centers for Medicare and Medicaid Services, Room 314G, Humphrey Building, 200 Independence Avenue, S.W., Washington, DC 20201. 800-MEDICARE. www.cms.hhs.gov. CMS is the U.S. government agency responsible for overseeing Medicare and Medicaid. Each state also has an Information Counseling and Assistance office to help beneficiaries with questions about CMS, Medicare, and Medicaid.

Health Insurance Association of America, 555 13th Street, N.W., Suite 600 East, Washington, DC 20004. 202-824-1600. www.hiaa.org. This is a lobbying group for insurance companies. They can provide you with information on long-term care and other types of insurance.

Medicaid. For Medicaid eligibility and benefits, you need to contact your state office. For general information, you can contact CMS (see above).

Medicare. 800-MEDICARE. www.medicare.gov. Various sections on the site have information about billing, payment, and appeals.

National Center for Home Equity Conversion, 360 Robert Street N, Suite 403, Saint Paul, MN 55101. 651-222-6775; fax: 651-222-6797. www .reverse.org. Information on reverse mortgages.

National Senior Citizens Law Center, 1101 14th Street, N.W., Suite 400, Washington, DC 20005. 202-289-6976; fax: 202-289-7224. www .nsclc.org. Legal information, articles, and advocacy on issues affecting lower-income senior citizens.

Social Security Administration. 800-772-1213. Handles enrollment.

Index

AARP, 114, 301, 350, 354
abandonment, 21–22, 76, 137
abbreviations, medical, 345–46
abuse. *See* elder abuse
acceptance
  process of, 22, 23, 202, 243
  stories of, 83, 163, 215–16
  working at, 212–13
accessing care, 95–96, 327–32
accreditation, 132
activities, 209–10. *See also*
  recreation
activities of daily living (ADL),
  147, 159, 222–23, 244
addictions, 80, 238–41
adjustment. *See* caregiver adjustment; resident adjustment
administration, 105–6, 140–41,
  259. *See also* policies
Administration on Aging, 117,
  350
admission. *See also* assessments;
  hospital discharge; moving
  behavior and, 95–96, 193–96
  documents, 119–20, 130, 186
  monitoring care after, 193, 249
  of person with dementia,
  183–84, 195
  preadmission meetings and,
  247–48

stories of, 162–63, 216
subsidies and, 11
waiting lists and, 328–29
adult day care, 17, 55, 82, 83, 88,
  244, 293, 297, 328, 330
advance directives, 35–39, 187,
  222, 311, 315
advocacy. *See also* problem
  solving
  individual actions, 290–91
  residents and, 197–98, 290, 292
  stories of, 136–37, 190–91,
  304–5, 324
  types of, 289, 294–96, 300–301
  vision and, 296–300
aggression, 91, 96, 109, 195, 201
aging, 87–88, 200
Aging with Dignity, 35, 39, 350
agitation, 195–96, 197, 198, 269
alcohol, 28, 96, 156, 201, 238–41
alternative health practices, 151
Alzheimer disease
  about, 200–201, 202. *See also*
  dementia
  stories of, 53–57, 133–38, 161,
  188–91, 245–46
Alzheimer's Association, 8, 202,
  327, 350
Alzheimer Society of Canada, 54,
  56, 350

anger, 21, 23, 27, 79, 168, 194, 195

anxiety, 3, 6, 30, 31, 79, 90, 107, 160, 167, 171, 176, 193, 269, 316

application process, 95–96, 327–39

assessments
  behavior, 95–96
  care, 7, 143, 147, 231, 328
  income, 331
  instruments for, 223–24
  questionnaires for making, 333–39

assisted living facilities
  about, 8, 9–11, 26, 157, 241
  adjustment to, 58, 213, 306
  advocacy and, 260, 292–93
  assessing, 125, 127, 132, 333–39
  care model for, 9, 155, 222
  complaints about, 11, 129
  costs of, 10, 119, 331
  discharge from, 14–15, 129
  end of life and, 314
  expectations and, 150, 157, 171
  finding, 92–93, 94, 327–28
  regulations and, 92–93, 130
  service plans for, 222–23, 224, 225
  services, 9, 160, 173–74, 175, 206

Assisted Living Federation of America, 7, 11, 351

bedsores, 27, 92, 100, 126, 237–38, 266

behavior. See resident behavior

benefits. See subsidies

blindness, 126, 161, 202, 264, 287–88

board-and-care homes, 13

brain function, 176–77, 179, 205, 207. See also memory loss

bruises, 102, 106, 237–38, 253

building maintenance, 131, 148–49

burnout, 29, 30, 254, 268, 269

campus-of-care facilities, 13–14, 96. See also continuing-care retirement communities

Canada
  care system of, 95, 105, 327–32
  costs of care in, 111, 115, 331
  regulations in, 8, 93, 130, 257
  subsidies in, 88, 115, 118, 148, 314

care. See also care system; quality of care; standards of care
  about, 7–14
  and caring, 96–98, 100
  organization of, 222–24
  working to improve, 289–94

care aides, 11–12, 103, 141–42

care conferences, 189, 190–91, 224–27, 248, 251, 282

caregiver adjustment
  after admission, 210–14
  after death of relative, 270, 317–18
  emotions and, 196, 207–8, 210, 255
  filling the gap, 208–10
  stories of, 17, 134, 163
  support and, 200, 212
  visiting and, 268

caregiver course, 54, 56

caregivers, family
  burden of care and, 27–30, 68
  burnout and, 29, 254, 268, 269
  caregiving at home and, 88–91
  process of becoming, 3–4
  record keeping and, 45, 57, 91, 344
  respite care and, 83, 89, 314, 330–31
  self-care and, 30, 80
  setting limits and, 31–32, 51, 61, 72, 268
  stories of, 16–18, 40–41, 53–57, 71, 82–83, 244–45
  support for, 67, 72–73, 89

care planning, individual. See also preadmission planning
  care conferences, 189, 190–91, 224–27, 248, 251, 282
  care/service plans, 222–24

families and, 248, 250–51, 280–81
involving the elderly, 225
out-of-town caregivers and, 282,
  283, 284
paid companions and, 274
care standards. *See* standards of care
care system
  about, 6–14, 88, 97–98, 104
  in Canada, 95, 105, 327–32
  client-centered model for, 98–99
  medical vs. social model, 9, 155,
    222, 306
  problems with, 105, 106, 137
  understanding, 94, 331–32
  working to improve, 289, 294–300
Caring Connections, 35, 351
Centers for Medicare and Medicaid
    Services (CMS), 111, 114,
    351, 354
certified nursing assistants (CNAs).
    See nurse's aides
charts, resident, 160, 223, 227–28,
    250, 254, 322
clothing, 174–76
coercion, 100, 184
cognitive impairment. *See* brain
    function
comfort account, 173–74
committee of person, 34, 36
communication
  about care, 19–26, 45
  about death, 307–9
  in facilities, 108, 157, 158, 171,
    224
  with staff, 191, 247–51, 261–62,
    282–83
  techniques, 47–48, 49, 135
communication book, 248, 250
community. *See* social interaction
companions, paid, 273, 274–76,
    278, 283
competency, 32–34, 54
complaints. *See also* advocacy;

inspection reports; problem
  solving; surveys
administration and, 105–6
assisted living and, 11, 129
procedure for, 132, 254–60, 258–60
residents and, 145, 153, 197–98
computers, 241, 282–83, 291.
  See also Internet
conflict(s)
  family, 34–35, 42–43, 44, 48, 49,
    284
  psychological, 60–61
confusion, 189, 247
congregate care, 8. *See also* independent living
continuing-care retirement communities (CCRCs), 13–14,
  146–47, 148
contracts, 14, 119–20, 129, 130
control, 6, 32, 155–56, 196, 290
cost/benefit analysis, 71
cost cutting, 104, 130
costs. *See also* payment; subsidies
  about, 10, 111, 118–19
  of buying or renting, 14
  in Canada, 115, 331
  understanding, 130, 131
counseling, 80, 196
couples, 10, 13, 19–26, 61–62, 329.
  See also marriage
crisis theory, 176

day care, adult, 17, 55, 82, 83, 88,
  244, 293, 297, 328, 330
deafness, 161, 202, 248
death and dying
  about, 315–16
  decisions about, 35–39, 310–13
  discussions about, 307–9
  emotions and, 267, 309–10, 312,
    315, 316
  events after, 316–17
  hospice/palliative care and, 313–14

death and dying (*cont.*)
  policies, assessing, 130
  saying good-bye and, 307,
    317–18
  stories of, 278–79, 322–24, 325
  support and, 312–13, 318
  younger people and, 314–15
decision making
  competency and, 32–33
  dementia and, 183, 184
  emotions and, 162, 176, 316
decisions, care. *See* care planning
degree of intervention orders, 37–38
dehydration, 205–6
delirium, 201, 202
dementia. *See also* Alzheimer disease
  about, 52, 200–202
  admission and, 183–84, 195
  care decisions and, 19–20, 168
  caregiver guilt and, 68–69
  going out and, 272, 284
  malnutrition and, 205
  pain control and, 230, 231
  resident relationships and, 204–5
  story of, 16–18
  visiting person with, 270–71
dementia care units, 110–11, 190,
    272, 302, 319
denial, 28, 202, 226
depression
  adjustment and, 194, 196–97
  behavior and, 109, 201–2
  caregivers and, 27
  residents and, 238, 239, 241
  stories of, 161, 263
design, physical, 126, 131
deterioration, 11, 90, 101, 161, 184,
    189, 202, 237
dietitian, 144
dignity, 25, 156, 235, 236
dining. *See* food services
director of care, 143–44, 255

disabilities, 20, 36–37, 51, 161, 202,
    248, 276
discharge, 14–15, 129–30. *See also*
    hospital discharge
disorientation, 189
DNR orders, 37, 39
doctors, 149–50, 200
documents, 46, 50–51, 119–20,
    130, 172. *See also* legal issues;
    social history
donations, 290, 291, 325
do not resuscitate (DNR) orders,
    37, 39
downsizing, 169
driving, 40, 53–54
drug abuse, 28, 238–41

Eden Alternative, 99, 238, 298
education, 54, 56. *See also* staff
    training
elder abuse. *See also* neglect
  about, 100–105
  addressing, 119, 260, 293
  assessing facilities for, 129
  complaints and, 105–6, 198
  falls and, 236, 237
  financial, 50, 101, 240
  preventing, 106–8, 109, 242,
    258
  resident-on-resident, 109
  stories of, 302–5, 319–23
Eldercare Locator, 7, 92, 260, 352
Elderpost.com, 352
emotions. *See also specific emotions*
  adjustment and, 196, 207–9,
    210, 255
  death and, 267, 309–10, 312,
    315, 316
  decision making and, 162, 176,
    316
  family journey and, 5–6
  visiting and, 267, 273

end-of-life decisions, 35–39, 310–13, 315
equipment, 147, 153, 172–73, 290
ethics committees, 293–94
evaluations. *See* assessments
eviction, 14–15, 129–30
exercise(s), 128, 205, 206, 235. *See also* physical therapy
expectations
    for assisted living, 150, 157, 171
    about care, 5, 90, 150, 181, 284
    communicating, 247–48, 282
    cultural/familial, 46, 64

falls, 106, 232, 236–37, 302–4
families. *See also* family relations; staff relations
    advocacy and, 292–94
    becoming a "family member," 4–6
    caregiving by (*see* caregivers, family)
    care planning and, 24, 38, 39–40, 44–52, 248, 250–51
    conflict and, 42–43, 44, 48, 49, 284
    dynamics in, 31–32, 43, 50, 291
    expectations and, 46, 282
    letting go by, 74–77, 79
    moving on by, 209–10, 317–18
    and role of family member, 6–7, 211, 252–54, 317–18
    roles in, 43–44, 45, 47
    rules in, 47, 63
family caregivers. *See* caregivers, family
family councils, 108, 128, 260, 292–94
family relations, 30–31, 66–68, 80–81, 246, 284
fear, 21–22, 76, 100, 101, 176, 211, 308, 316
finances, 33–34, 49–50, 173–74,

290, 293. *See also* costs; payment; subsidies
finding a residence, 91–94, 281. *See also* viewing facilities
Five Wishes, 39
food services, 130–31, 136, 144–45, 153, 162. *See also* kitchen facilities
foot care, 127, 150
forgiveness, 68–69, 74, 307
fraud, 105, 241
fulfillment, 87–88, 150. *See also* quality of life
funding. *See* Medicare
fundraising, 290, 293

gays and lesbians, 203–4
geriatric care managers, 48, 49, 88, 93, 171, 259, 285
government. *See* regulations, government
grief and loss
    at end of life, 306, 310
    experiencing, 77–79, 83, 99–100, 168, 207–8
    handling, 79–81, 209–10
    stages of, 79
group homes, 13, 327
guest rooms, 168, 331
guilt
    about, 58–60, 280
    dementia and, 68–69
    experiencing, 53, 57, 315, 324
    handling, 69–74, 259, 279
    monitoring, 51
    psychology of, 60–61, 65–66

hallucinations, 40
Healing the Shame That Binds You (Bradshaw), 73
health, 156, 203, 205–7
health care proxy, 34, 36

hearing problems, 161, 202, 248
helplessness, 103, 238
home, breaking up of, 168–69
home care, 82, 118, 216, 328.
    See also living at home
hospice care, 313–14
hospital discharge, 41, 126, 135,
    170, 196, 251, 272
housekeeping, 148–49

identity, 252, 272
I Don't Know What to Say
    (Buckman), 308
incontinence, 101, 205, 234–36
independence, 51, 128, 142,
    155–57, 236
independent living, 8–9, 10
individual service plan (ISP), 222
individuality, 155, 156–57
information. *See also* communica-
    tion; social history
    complaints and, 256, 260
    residents' rights to, 186–87
    for staff, 137, 170–71, 247–51
    transfer of, 251
inheritance, 39, 46, 50
injuries. *See* elder abuse; falls
inspection reports, 105, 121, 126,
    132, 237
insurance, 39, 46, 50, 116–18
Internet
    addictions involving, 239, 241
    to monitor care, 258
    organizations found on, 349–54
    sites for caregiving journals, 45
    use of, for staying in touch, 282
    using support groups on, 259
intimacy, 203–5, 213–14, 242,
    276, 307
intimidation, 256, 303
involuntary separation, 118
isolation, 239, 241. *See also*
    withdrawal

journal keeping, 45, 57, 71, 77,
    213, 309

Kabat-Zinn, Jon, 70
kitchen facilities, 9, 156, 242, 271.
    See also food services
Kübler-Ross, Elizabeth, 79

laundry, 174–76
legal issues, 14, 33–39, 119–20, 149,
    151, 240. *See also* residents' rights
legislation. *See* regulations,
    government
lesbians, 203–4
letters, 213, 271, 301, 309
letting go, 74–77, 79–80, 83, 212,
    217, 226
life support, 34, 310–12
Life Worth Living (Thomas), 99,
    298, 349
living at home, 88–91, 117
living at risk, 28, 30–32, 234
living wills, 35
long-distance caregivers, 44, 45–46,
    270, 280–85
loneliness, 76, 238, 239
losing things, 106, 173, 251–52
loss. *See* grief and loss
love, 81, 138, 270, 291, 307

maintenance, building, 131, 148–49
malnutrition, 205–6, 265
management. *See* administration
marriage, 75, 204–5, 270. *See also*
    couples
massage therapy, 150, 151
meals. *See* food services; nutrition
Medicaid
    about, 112–13
    applying for care and, 95
    assisted living and, 11, 94
    coverage, 115, 127, 129
    resources, 114, 354, 355

medical abbreviations, 345–46
medical director, 150
Medicare
  about, 111–12, 113–15
  coverage, 12–13, 122, 147
  resources, 92, 121, 123, 124, 132,
    352, 355
Medicare Rights Center, 114, 352
medications
  addiction to, 238–41
  adjustment and, 153, 196–97
  administration of, 141, 149
  elder abuse and, 101
  effects of, 230, 232, 238
  food and, 205
  monitoring of, 228–30
  naturopathic, 149
  pain control and, 229, 230–32
  as a restraint, 232, 233
  subsidies and, 114–15
meditation, 69–70
memorials, 318, 325
memory loss, 16–17, 20, 40–41,
    244. *See also* brain function;
    dementia
mental stimulation, 205, 207, 274
Michigan Consumer's Guide to
    Nursing Homes, 123
mindfulness, 69–70
*Mindful Way Through Depression,
    The* (Williams et al.), 70
mobility, 147, 172–73, 206, 237.
    See also transfer
money. *See* finances
monitoring of care. *See also* com-
    plaints; video monitoring;
    visiting
  after admission, 193, 249
  assisted living and, 10–11,
    206, 249
  and body checks, 238, 265, 266
  deficiencies and, 92, 253–54
  elder abuse and, 106

nutrition and, 205–6
  by out-of-town caregivers, 45,
    281–82
  paid companions and, 274
  personal needs account, 174
  roommates and, 242
  story of, 265–66
moving
  action plan for, 176–79
  arrival procedures when, 185–86
  from hospital. *See* hospital
    discharge
  more than once, 154, 327
  from out of town, 284
  personal items, 173–76
  policies for, 129, 329–30
  preparing for, 167–79, 182, 188
  residents' perspective on, 184–85
  resistance and, 169–70, 183–84
  stories of, 16, 83, 180–81, 189,
    287–88
  support for, 178–79
moving on, 209–10, 317–18.
    See also letting go
multi-infarct dementia, 17, 201,
    244, 286–87
music, 18, 134, 138, 271

National Academy of Elder Law
    Attorneys, 14, 352
National Association of Professional
    Geriatric Care Managers, 93,
    285, 353
National Association of Professional
    Organizers, 169, 353
National Center for Home Equity
    Conversion, 116, 353, 355
National Citizens' Coalition for
    Nursing Home Reform
    (NCCNHR), 224, 234, 301, 354
National Clearinghouse for Long-
    Term Care Information,
    117, 353

National Hospice and Palliative
Care Organization (NHPCO),
35, 351
National Senior Citizens Law Center, 256–57, 354, 355
NCCNHR, 224, 234, 301, 354
neglect. *See also* elder abuse
about, 101–2, 104, 105
addressing, 119, 293
incontinence and, 234
preventing, 242, 258
story of, 264–65
noise, 242, 272
nurses, 103, 143–44
nurse's aides, 11–12, 103, 141–42
Nursing Home Compare Web site,
121, 123, 124, 132
Nursing Home Reform Law, 12, 15,
130, 197, 222, 226, 256
nursing homes
about, 11–13, 155–56
compared to assisted living, 9,
155, 222, 306
for-profit vs. non-profit, 124, 294,
295, 330
as places to live, 306
nursing home system
about, 6–14, 157–58
advocating for change in, 294–99
and good caring, 97–98
problem solving in, 247
problems with, 224, 229, 251
nutrition, 144, 205

occupational health, 156, 330
occupational therapy, 147
Older Americans Act, 92, 94
ombudsperson, state, 7–8, 11, 92,
260, 293
On Death and Dying (Kübler-Ross), 79
online addictions, 239, 241
only children, 64, 75–76, 277,
286–88

out-of-town caregivers, 44, 45–46,
270, 280–85
ownership, 124, 141

PACE, 88, 353
packing. *See* home, breaking up of
pain control, 229, 230–31, 240,
313, 314
palliative care, 130, 313–14
Parkinson disease, 201, 202, 263
Parkinson Foundation(s), 353, 354
pastoral care, 17, 72, 134, 137, 150
payment, 111–18, 354–55. *See also*
subsidies
personal boundaries. *See* setting
limits
personal care, 8, 10, 34–35, 45, 91,
141–42, 150. *See also* activities
of daily living (ADL)
personal items, 162, 168–69,
173–74, 251–52
personal needs account, 173–74
pets, 289, 291
pharmacists, 97, 149, 230
philosophy of care, 99, 100, 296.
See also care system
physical activity, 128, 205, 206,
235. *See also* mobility; physical
therapy
physical plant, 131
physical therapy, 147, 148, 237,
274, 276
physicians, 149–50, 200
Pioneer Network, 298, 354
placement. *See* admission
podiatry, 127, 150
policies, 129–30, 256, 274–75,
295–96, 328–30. *See also*
administration
possessions. *See* personal items
power of attorney, 34, 35, 36, 53, 54
preadmission planning. *See also*
viewing facilities

couples and, 19–26, 61–62
dementia and, 19–20, 168
elderly and, 20–21, 51–52, 126,
    156–57
families and, 24, 44–46
family meetings and, 38, 39–40,
    46–52
legal issues and, 31, 33–39
preadmission meetings for, 247–48
pressure sores, 27, 92, 100, 126,
    237–38, 266
primary nurse model, 143
privacy, 45, 228, 242–43, 258,
    270, 276
private-care agreements, 46, 50–51
problem solving. *See also* advocacy;
    complaints
and behavior issues, 193, 232–33
emotions and, 255–56
finding missing items, 251–52
other families and, 292
resident charts and, 227–28
role of family member in, 193,
    252–54, 257, 258–60
Professional Organizers in Canada,
    169, 354
programming. *See* recreation

quality of care, 96–97, 98, 125, 126,
    193, 212, 253–54. *See also* elder
    abuse; standards of care
quality of life, 87–88, 99–100, 139,
    146, 150, 311–12
questionnaires, 333–44

recreation
about, 146, 147
assessing facilities for, 127–28
paid companions and, 276
social interaction and, 206–7
staff for, 137, 145–47, 160
stories of, 162
visiting and, 271, 273, 290–91

reform. *See* advocacy
regret, 267, 324
regulations, government. *See also*
    Nursing Home Reform Law;
    residents' rights; subsidies
and advance directives, 35, 36
assisted living and, 10, 92–93, 130
costs and, 119
discharge and, 15, 129–30
finding out about, 7–8
group homes and, 13
nursing homes and, 12, 91–93,
    159–60
and privacy laws, 228
social worker and, 145
standards and, 257, 330
regulations, nursing home. *See*
    policies
rehabilitation, 23, 147–48, 226–27,
    263, 274
rehabilitation centers, 12–13
relationships, 203–5, 213–14.
    See also family relations; resi-
    dent relations; staff relations
religion, 73
resident adjustment
assisted living and, 58, 213, 306
and behavioral changes, 193–96
compared to caregiver adjust-
    ment, 208
complaints and, 197–98
keeping track of, 199
medication and, 153, 196–97
memory loss and, 192–93
new relationships and, 204–5
paid companion and, 276
resistance and, 183–84
signs of, 273
stories of, 41, 55, 134–35,
    153–54, 302
vacations and, 274, 284
visiting and, 198–99, 268–69
resident abuse. *See* elder abuse

resident behavior
  addictions, 238–41
  admission and, 95–96, 193–96
  aggression, 96, 109, 201
  agitation, 195–96, 197, 198, 269
  dementia symptoms and,
    200–202
  pain control and, 231
  and problem solving, 193, 232–33
resident charts, 160, 223, 227–28,
  250, 254, 322
residential care, 13, 327
resident relations, 109, 203–5, 206,
  207. *See also* roommates
residents' councils, 128, 293
residents' rights. *See also* regula-
    tions, government
  to be free from restraints, 233
  to information, 186–87, 254
  to live at risk, 31, 234
  to make care decisions, 149, 184
  overview of, 221–22
  to quality of life, 139
  to rehabilitation, 147–48
resistance
  to care, 24, 51, 169–70, 183–84
  to change, 294–95, 298–99
resources
  books, 347–49. *See also specific*
    titles
  organization Web sites, 349–54
  on payment, 354–55
respite care, 83, 89, 314, 330–31
restraints, 232–34, 321
reverse mortgages, 115–16
rights. *See* residents' rights
role reversal, 62–63, 287
roommates, 241–43, 276
routines, 158–60, 171, 212, 235
  questionnaire about, 340–41

sadness. *See* grief and loss
safety, 27, 129, 156, 330

schedules. *See* routines
security. *See* special care units
    (SCUs)
selecting a residence, 91–94, 281.
    See also viewing facilities
self-care, 30, 80
separation, 118. *See also* couples
services, therapeutic. *See* therapy
settling in. *See* resident adjustment
sex, 203–5, 213–14, 242, 276
sexual disinhibition, 96, 109
shame, 59–60, 73, 234, 241
skin, 237–38. *See also* bruises; pres-
    sure sores
social history (document), 137,
    172, 224
  questionnaire about, 342–43
social interaction, 26, 206–7, 272.
    See also withdrawal
social workers, 145, 255
special care units (SCUs), 110–11,
    190, 272, 302, 319
staff. *See also* care conferences;
    unions; wages
  assisted living, 38, 104, 127
  communication with, 147–51,
    255
  elder abuse and, 106–8
  family councils and, 292
  information for, 137, 170–71
  levels of, 104, 106–7, 110,
    126–27, 261
  monitoring of, 136
  organizational change and,
    294–95, 298–99
  roles of. *See* staff roles
  routines, 157, 158–60, 250
  stories of, 134, 136–37, 246,
    263–64
  training. *See* staff training
  workload, 103, 137, 142, 261
staff relations, 108, 137, 211,
    261–62, 250–51, 289

staff roles
    dietitian and food services,
      144–45
    director of care, 143–44, 255
    housekeepers/maintenance,
      148–49
    marketing director, 124
    medical director, 150
    nurses, 103, 143–44
    nurse's aides, 11–12, 103, 141–42
    other, 150–51
    pharmacists, 97, 149, 230
    physicians, 149–50, 200
    receptionist, 139–40
    recreation therapists, 137,
      145–47, 160
    rehabilitation, 147–48
    social worker, 145, 255
staff training
    good care and, 96–97
    of hospice staff, 313
    of nursing staff, 141, 143
    resident abuse and, 107–8
    standards and, 104, 105
    upgrading of, 293
standards of care, 11, 91, 104–5,
    221–22, 257, 301
state licensing agencies, 260, 293
state ombudsperson, 7–8, 11, 92,
    260, 293
statistics, 98, 101, 122, 149, 200,
    201, 231, 238
stimulation, mental, 205, 207, 274
stress, 28–29, 40, 67, 77, 83, 123,
    192, 274
strokes, 17, 134, 135, 201, 244
subsidies. *See also* Medicaid;
    Medicare
    about, 111–15
    for assisted living, 11
    in Canada, 115, 148, 327–31
    coverage by, 88–89, 147–48,
      313–14

    insurance and, 177
    understanding of, 118–19
support. *See also* resources
    care decisions and, 22, 25
    for family caregivers, 67, 72–73,
      89
    for family members, 80, 200, 212
    organizations for, 349–54
    for residents, 137
    at time of death, 312–13, 318
support groups, 72, 246, 318
support services, 148–49
surveys, 92, 132

terminology, 7, 332, 345–46
theft, 149, 252
therapy, 71, 147–48, 150, 151, 213,
    309. *See also* counseling; physi-
    cal therapy
threats, 265, 303
toileting, 101, 104, 234–36
tours. *See* viewing facilities
transfer, 156. *See also* hospital dis-
    charge; mobility
transition to care. *See* admission;
    moving
transient ischemic attacks (TIAs),
    17, 201

unions, 106, 291, 297, 299

vacations, 273, 284
valuables, 173–74, 251
values, cultural, 64
video monitoring, 45, 258. *See also*
    webcams
viewing facilities
    asking questions when, 100,
      124–32, 147
    comparison chart for, 126,
      333–39
    out-of-town caregivers and, 281
    stories of, 121–23, 152–53

vision problems, 161, 202
visiting. *See also* monitoring of care
    about, 125, 267–70
    activities for, 271, 291
    ending a visit, 198–99, 273–74
    going out or going home, 272–73
    paid companions and, 274–76
    person with dementia, 270–71,
        273
    policies, assessing, 129
    preadmission, 167–68, 169–70
    privacy and, 242, 270
    stories of, 55–56, 266
volunteering, 290–91

wages, 104, 105
waiting lists, 328–29
wandering, 27, 153

webcams, 45, 283, 291
Web sites. *See* resources
What Dying People Want (Kuhl), 308
wills, 35, 46
withdrawal, 194–95, 198, 202, 234,
    271–72, 316. *See also* social in-
    teraction
women, 62, 65, 122
writing, as therapy, 71, 213, 309.
    See also journal keeping; letters

younger people
    admission and, 195–96
    advocacy and, 290
    care decisions and, 22–23, 157
    life in care for, 241, 272, 276
    placement of spouse, 62, 76

About the Author

Peter S. Silin is originally from Newton, Massachusetts, and has lived in Canada since 1973. He has worked in the field of aging and elder care since 1980. He currently is the owner of Diamond Geriatrics (www .diamondgeriatrics.com), a geriatric care management and consulting company. He is the founder of the Web site Elderpost (www.elderpost .com). He lectures frequently in Canada and the United States and writes for journals and magazines.